Cardiological Society of India
Yearbook of Cardiology 2023
CVD in Women

Cardiological Society of India
Yearbook of Cardiology 2023
CVD in Women

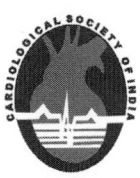

Editor-in-Chief

Shibba Takkar Chhabra MD DM FACC FCSI
Professor
Department of Cardiology
Hero DMC Heart Institute
Dayanand Medical College and Hospital
Ludhiana, Punjab, India

Co-Editor

Ankur Goyal

Section Editors

Asha Mahilmaran
Sujatha Vipperla
Kunal Mahajan
J Cecily Mary Majella
Hetan C Shah
Sarita Rao
Bhupinder Singh
Ankur Goyal

Foreword

Vijay Bang

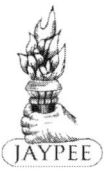

JAYPEE BROTHERS MEDICAL PUBLISHERS
The Health Sciences Publisher
New Delhi | London

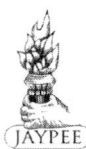 **Jaypee Brothers Medical Publishers (P) Ltd**

Headquarters
EMCA House
23/23-B, Ansari Road, Daryaganj
New Delhi 110 002, India
Landline: +91-11-23272143, +91-11-23272703
+91-11-23282021, +91-11-23245672
E-mail: jaypee@jaypeebrothers.com

Corporate Office
Jaypee Brothers Medical Publishers (P) Ltd.
4838/24, Ansari Road, Daryaganj
New Delhi 110 002, India
Phone: +91-11-43574357
Fax: +91-11-43574314
E-mail: jaypee@jaypeebrothers.com

Overseas Office
JP Medical Ltd.
83, Victoria Street, London
SW1H 0HW (UK)
Phone: +44-20 3170 8910
Fax: +44(0)20 3008 6180
E-mail: info@jpmedpub.com

Website: www.jaypeebrothers.com
Website: www.jaypeedigital.com

© 2024, Jaypee Brothers Medical Publishers and Cardiological Society of India

The views and opinions expressed in this book are solely those of the original contributor(s)/author(s) and do not necessarily represent those of editor(s) or publisher of the book.

All rights reserved. No part of this publication may be reproduced, stored or transmitted in any form or by any means, electronic, mechanical, photocopying, recording or otherwise, without the prior permission in writing of the publishers.

All brand names and product names used in this book are trade names, service marks, trademarks or registered trademarks of their respective owners. The publisher is not associated with any product or vendor mentioned in this book.

Medical knowledge and practice change constantly. This book is designed to provide accurate, authoritative information about the subject matter in question. However, readers are advised to check the most current information available on procedures included and check information from the manufacturer of each product to be administered, to verify the recommended dose, formula, method and duration of administration, adverse effects and contraindications. It is the responsibility of the practitioner to take all appropriate safety precautions. Neither the publisher nor the author(s)/editor(s) assume any liability for any injury and/or damage to persons or property arising from or related to use of material in this book.

This book is sold on the understanding that the publisher is not engaged in providing professional medical services. If such advice or services are required, the services of a competent medical professional should be sought.

Every effort has been made where necessary to contact holders of copyright to obtain permission to reproduce copyright material. If any have been inadvertently overlooked, the publisher will be pleased to make the necessary arrangements at the first opportunity.

Inquiries for bulk sales may be solicited at: jaypee@jaypeebrothers.com

CSI Yearbook of Cardiology 2023: CVD in Women / Shibba Takkar Chhabra

First Edition: 2024

ISBN: 978-93-5696-685-7

Printed at Replika Press Pvt. Ltd.

Dedication

From a daughter to her Father
"Who raised her, enabled her, and gave her the vision"

From a daughter to her Mother
"Who gave her birth, inspired her and nurtured with strength"

From a wife to her Husband
*"Who was her armor, her strength, her confidence,
her belief and shield through everything"*

From a disciple to her Mentor
"Who trained, carved and polished her into a physician"

From a mother to her Child
"Who is her angel and her world"

Shibba Takkar Chhabra

Contributors

Editor-in-Chief

Shibba Takkar Chhabra MD DM FACC FCSI
Professor
Department of Cardiology
Hero DMC Heart Institute
Dayanand Medical College and Hospital
Ludhiana, Punjab, India

Co-Editor

Ankur Goyal MD (Medicine)
Senior Resident
Dayanand Medical College and Hospital
Ludhiana, Punjab, India

Section Editors

Asha Mahilmaran MD DNB DM FCSI FACC FESC FSCAI
Senior Interventional Consultant Cardiologist
Apollo Hospitals
Chennai, Tamil Nadu, India

J Cecily Mary Majella MD DM (Cardiology) FESC FSCAI
Professor and Senior Interventional Cardiologist
Department of Cardiology
Tamil Nadu Government Multi Super Speciality Hospital
Chennai, Tamil Nadu, India

Bhupinder Singh MD DM (Cardiology)
Additional Professor and Head
All India Institute of Medical Sciences
Bathinda, Punjab, India

Sujatha Vipperla MD DM FIC FSCAI
Consultant Cardiologist
Indus Hospitals
Visakhapatnam, Andhra Pradesh, India

Hetan C Shah MD DNB (Cardiology) FACC FESC FSCAI
Professor of Cardiology
Seth GS Medical College and KEM Hospital
Mumbai, Maharashtra, India

Ankur Goyal MD (Medicine)
Senior Resident
Dayanand Medical College and Hospital
Ludhiana, Punjab, India

Kunal Mahajan DM (Cardiology) FACC FESC FSCAI FAPSC FAPSIC FISH FISC
Chief Interventional Cardiologist
Himachal Heart Institute
Mandi, Himachal Pradesh, India

Sarita Rao MD DNB DM FACC FSCAI
Senior Interventional Cardiologist
Director, Cath lab
Apollo Hospitals
Indore, Madhya Pradesh, India

Associate Editors

Rukmani Prabha MD DrNB
(Cardiology)
Consultant Cardiologist
Thaibala Medical Centre
Valliyur, Tamil Nadu, India

S Anne Princy MD DM
Assistant Professor
Department of Cardiology
Tamil Nadu Government Multi
Super Speciality Hospital
Chennai, Tamil Nadu, India

Rajeshwari Nayak DNB
(Medicine) DNB (Cardiology)
Fellowship Heartfailure and Echo
FRCP (Glasgow)
Senior Consultant
Interventional Cardiologist
Apollo Hospitals
Chennai, Tamil Nadu, India

Vatchala Sree Varadharajan
MD MRCP MPhil
Consultant Cardiologist and
Director
Muhil Heart Centre
Vellore, Tamil Nadu, India

K Meenakshi MD (General
Medicine) DM (Cardiology)
Professor and Head
Department of Cardiology
Saveetha Medical College
Chennai, Tamil Nadu, India

S Jayalakshmi MD DM
(Cardiology)
Associate Consultant
Apollo Hospitals
Chennai, Tamil Nadu, India

Radha Priya Yalamanchi
DNB (General Medicine) DrNB
(Cardiology)
Associate Consultant
Cardiologist
Apollo Main Hospital
Chennai, Tamil Nadu, India

Aruna D DrNB (Cardiology) FSCAI
Senior Consultant Cardiologist
Apollo Main Hospital
Chennai, Tamil Nadu, India

Narra Lavanya MD DNB
(Cardiology)
Associate Cardiologist
Apollo Main Hospital
Chennai, Tamil Nadu, India

Prabhakar Dorairaj MD DM
FACC
Preventive Interventional
Cardiologist
Ashwin Clinic, Apollo Group of
Hospitals
Chennai, Tamil Nadu, India

G Justin Paul MD DNB (Medicine)
DM DNB (Cardiology) FACC FESC
Director and Head (I/C)
Department of Cardiology
Madras Medical College
Chennai, Tamil Nadu, India

Anil Kumar Mahapatro MD
DM FSCAI
Consultant Cardiologist
Indus Hospitals
Visakhapatnam, Andhra
Pradesh, India

Achukatla Kumar Pharma D
Consultant Scientific
Regional Medical Research
Centre (ICMR)
Port Blair, Andaman and
Nicobar Islands, India

Tanuj Bhatia DM (Cardiology)
Associate Professor Cardiology
SGRR Medical College and
SMI Hospital
Dehradun, Uttarakhand, India

Jaikrit Bhutani DM (Cardiology)
Senior Resident Cardiology
SMS Medical College
Jaipur, Rajasthan, India

Sai Devvrat MD
2nd Year (DM)
SGRR Medical College and
SMI Hospital
Dehradun, Uttarakhand, India

Abhishek Rastogi MBBS MD
2nd Year (DM)
SGRR Medical College and
SMI Hospital
Dehradun, Uttarakhand, India

Prashant Patel PGDCC
Associate Consultant
Cardiology
Himachal Heart Institute
Mandi, Himachal Pradesh, India

Contributors

Lokesh Verma MD (Medicine)
Assistant Professor
Department of Medicine
SLBS Government Medical College
Mandi, Himachal Pradesh, India

Rohith Velusamy DNB
Postgraduate of Internal Medicine
Sundaram Arulrhaj Hosiptals
Thoothukudi, Tamil Nadu, India

S Arulrhaj MD PhD FRCP
(Glasgow and London) MBA
Chief Physician and Intensivist
Sundaram Arulrhaj Hospitals
Thoothukudi, Tamil Nadu, India

Arun Ranganathan MD DM
(Cardiology)
Assistant Professor of Cardiology
Stanley Medical College
Chennai, Tamil Nadu, India

Bhavik Shah MD
Senior Registrar Cardiology
Seth GS Medical College and
KEM Hospital Mumbai
Mumbai, Maharashtra, India

Roshan Rao MD DM FESC FACC
Head and Senior Interventional Cardiologist
Apollo Hospitals
Indore, Madhya Pradesh, India

Pankaj Manoria MD DM FACC
FESC FSCAI FAPSIC
Director Cath Lab
Manoria Heart Hospital
Bhopal, Madhya Pradesh, India

T Neelambujan MD DNB
(Cardiology) FESC FCSI FIAE FSCAI
Consultant Cardiologist and Interventionalist
Sundaram Arulrhaj Hospitals
Thoothukudi, Tamil Nadu, India

J Nandhini MD DNB (Cardiology)
Senior Consultant
Interventional Cardiologist
Mumme Hospital
Vellore, Tamil Nadu, India

Manikandan DNB (General Medicine)
Post Graduate
Sundaram Arulrhaj Hospitals
Thoothukudi, Tamil Nadu, India

P Deepa MD (Biochemistry)
Assistant Professor of Biochemistry
Stanley Medical College
Chennai, Tamil Nadu, India

Chandrakant Chavan MD
DM (Cardiology)
Electrophysiologist
Bharati Vidyapeeth Hospital
Pune, Maharashtra, India

Roopali Khanna MD DM
Professor
Sanjay Gandhi Postgraduate Institute of Medical Sciences
Lucknow, Uttar Pradesh, India

Prerna Goyal MD (Medicine)
FIACM
Consultant Physician and Deputy Medical Superintendent
RG stone and Superspeciality Hospital
Ludhiana, Punjab, India

Aarathy Kannan MD Dip Diab MBA
Consultant Physician and Diabetologist
Sundaram Arulrhaj Hospitals
Thoothukudi, Tamil Nadu, India

Sundar C MD DNB DM FNB
Senior Consultant
Interventional Cardiologist
Kauvery Hospital
Chennai, Tamil Nadu, India

Nikhil Govind DNB
Post Graduate
Sundaram Arulrhaj Hospitals
Thoothukudi, Tamil Nadu, India

Tamagna Ghosh MD DM
(Cardiology)
Assistant Professor of Cardiology
Seth GS Medical College
KEM Hospital
Mumbai, Maharashtra, India

Malav Jhala MD DM (Cardiology)
Electrophysiologist
Criticare Hospital
Mumbai, Maharashtra, India

Hema S MD DM (Cardiology)
Associate Professor in Cardiology
Sri Jayadeva Institute of Cardiovascular Sciences and Research
Mysuru, Karnataka, India

Priya Palimkar MD (Medicine)
DNB (Cardiology) FACC
Director Cath Lab
Sahyadri Hospital
Pune, Maharashtra, India

Contributors

Amjad Ali MD DM (Cardiology)
Consultant Interventional Cardiologist
Sagar Multispeciality Hospital
Bhopal, Madhya Pradesh, India

Abha Pandit DNB (Medicine)
Professor
Department of Internal Medicine
Index Medical College and Research Centre
Indore, Madhya Pradesh, India

Mahpaekar Mashhadi MBBS MD DM
Senior Interventional Cardiologist
Apollo CVHF Heart Institute and Apollo Hospital International Limited
Ahmedabad, Gujarat, India

Harsh A Chaudhary MD
Final Year DrNB Cardiology Fellow
Apollo Hospitals International Limited
Ahmedabad, Gujarat, India

Suraj Kumar MD DM (Cardiology)
Assistant Professor
All India Institute of Medical Sciences
Bathinda, Punjab, India

Surender Deora MD DM (Cardiology)
Additional Professor and Head
All India Institute of Medical Sciences
Jodhpur, Rajasthan, India

Jai Bharat Sharma DM (Cardiology)
Assistant Professor of Cardiology
Geetanjali Medical College and Hospital
Udaipur, Rajasthan, India

Rahul Yadav DM (Cardiology)
Consultant Cardiologist
Himachal Heart Institute
Mandi, Himachal Pradesh, India

Surender Kumar DM (Cardiology)
Consultant Cardiologist
Himachal Heart Institute
Mandi, Himachal Pradesh, India

Suresh Kumar P MD DM (Cardiology)
Assistant Professor of Cardiology
Chengalpattu Medical College
Chengalpattu, Tamil Nadu, India

Raghothaman Sethumadhavan MD DM (Cardiology)
Assistant Professor of Cardiology
Chengalpattu Medical College
Chengalpattu, Tamil Nadu, India

Raagini Gupta MBBS
Student
Dayanand Medical College and Hospital
Ludhiana, Punjab, India

Nikita Sharma MBBS
Student
Dayanand Medical College and Hospital
Ludhiana, Punjab, India

Zoofi Shan MBBS
Student
Dayanand Medical College and Hospital
Ludhiana, Punjab, India

Muzammil Farooqi MBBS
Student
Dayanand Medical College and Hospital
Ludhiana, Punjab, India

Rabia Aggarwal MBBS
Student
Dayanand Medical College and Hospital
Ludhiana, Punjab, India

Khushi Goyal MBBS
Student
Dayanand Medical College and Hospital
Ludhiana, Punjab, India

Anshdeep Saluja MBBS
Student
Dayanand Medical College and Hospital
Ludhiana, Punjab, India

Harsh Kishore M Pharma (Pharmacology)
Senior Researcher
Dayanand Medical College and Hospital
Ludhiana, Punjab, India

Samman Verma DM (Cardiology)
Senior Resident
Department of Cardiology
Postgraduate Institute of Medical Education and Research
Chandigarh, India

Akash Batta DM (Cardiology)
Assistant Professor
Dayanand Medical College and Hospital
Ludhiana, Punjab, India

Foreword

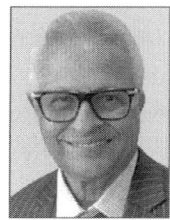

Vijay Bang MD DM FCSI FESC FSCAI FACC
Senior Interventional Cardiologist
Lilavati Hospital and Research Center, Mumbai, Maharashtra, India
President, CSI 2023 (Platinum Jubilee)
President-Elect and Chairman, Scientific Committee
CSI Annual Conference 2022 at Chennai
Honorary Professor and Head, Grant Government Medical College and
Sir JJ Group of Hospitals, Mumbai (Former)
- Founding President, Cardiovascular Academic Research Foundation
- Founding Course Director, India Act Conference
- Founding Director and Moderator, International Cardiology CME
- Founding Course Director, National Cardiology PG Course

I am happy to write foreword for "*CSI Yearbook of Cardiology: CVD in Women, 2023*" which is being published by a group of experts in the field of cardiovascular disease (CVD) in women. The authors have picked up landmark articles with good clinical relevance from high-impact medical journals with special emphasis on the articles from the Indian subcontinent. This comprehensive collection of articles will enable our cardiology fellows and practicing cardiologists and gynecologists to get an overview of the new developments in the field of CVD in women. The abstracts of the article tell us the science and evidence on the topic. The commentaries give you an expert's opinion on interpreting these trials published.

Cardiovascular disease in women remains a global health challenge, affecting millions of individuals and burdening healthcare systems around the world. In today's era of advancement in technology, a physician needs to be aware of the latest developments in various fields. This helps in taking better care of the patient and improving the outcomes. In this collection of articles, authors delve into the most recent advancements in our understanding of CVD in women, the innovative approaches to diagnosis, and the evolving landscape of CVD management in women in India, defining the impact and the exploration of women CVD care in India. The insights and strategies to address disparities in different population are also discussed. Precision medicine and patient-centered care in CVD management are the paths of the future and will be a reality in the coming years in the management of CVD in women.

The quest for knowledge is a perpetual one, and this book is a remarkable testament to our collective commitment to improving the care and outcomes of women CVD patients. As we read these articles and commentaries, we are presented with a tapestry of discoveries in diagnosis and treatment.

I hope this exercise will continue in the coming years by CSI Pink Council and we wish good luck to the editors for this CSI Yearbook on women CVD.

Message

I applaud the team for bringing out this important, much timely, publication. Many of us have believed in the past that heart disease mostly affects men. Most of the medical literature, till recently, has also focused on studies conducted mainly in men and the results have been extrapolated to women. But as we know, there are several physiological differences related to the cardiovascular system between men and women and hence a need for dedicated information on cardiovascular disease in women.

I am glad that physicians and cardiologists across the country have collaborated and attempted to address the issue by compiling the literature specifically pertaining to women's cardiovascular medical ailments in the form of this book. Besides accumulating the relevant women-oriented scientific literature for the reader from the latest articles published in leading journals, this book sensitizes the medical fraternity to manage their female patients with the evidence-based, state-of-the-art medical care that they deserve. I congratulate Dr Shibba Takkar Chhabra and her entire team for coming out with this unique and innovative project to deliver up-to-date key messages pertaining to cardiovascular disease in women, amalgamated and simplified by cardiologists across the country. I believe this book will become essential reading for all those caring for women's heart health.

I also congratulate the Cardiological Society of India (CSI) and entire executive board for coming up with CSI Pink Council and embarking steps toward woman cardiac care in the country. It also strengthens the woman cardiologists across country to work in unison with CSI for the cause.

Anita Saxena MD DM FACC
Vice Chancellor
Pandit Bhagwat Dayal Sharma University of Health Sciences
Rohtak, Haryana, India

Message

In my 46 years of long journey through the medical profession, I have seen unfathomable tremendous progress in the way women have excelled not only academically but have also proven their skills as astute physicians and surgeons. However, women still have to face discrimination in our society as well as in the hospital premises as both doctors and patients. Also, there persists a lag regarding gender representation in major trials and other aspects of medical literature which is the sad reality we have to face while practicing the medical profession in the largest vibrant democracy of the world. It gives me immense pleasure to know that this book compiled by physicians and superspecialists attempts to address this issue of gender bias. The effort to highlight various aspects of cardiovascular diseases in every aspect appears to be innovative and one of its kind. I congratulate Dr Shibba Takkar Chhabra and her talented team for the endeavor and hope that this unique book changes the perception of medical practice with respect to women.

I congratulate the Cardiological Society of India (CSI) President and entire executive board for coming forward with CSI Pink Council and embarking on steps toward woman cardiac care in the country. It also strengthens the woman cardiologists across country to work in unison with CSI for the cause and prove their mettle in encouraging youngsters to provide better treatment and care for mankind by excellent and most efficient women cardiologists. **This book will enrich the knowledge of the clinicians in future**. I wish all the best for all their endeavors.

IB Vijayalakshmi
MD DM DSc FICC FIAE FICP FCSI FIAMS FAMS FISH FRCP (London)
Professor Emeritus
Former Professor and Head
Department of Pediatric Cardiology
Sri Jayadeva Institute of Cardiovascular Sciences and Research
Bengaluru, Karnataka, India

Message

Acknowledging the existing gender imbalances in healthcare provision for women and the limited representation of their health concerns in medical literature, particularly in the realm of cardiovascular research, is essential. Hence, the creation of a textbook dedicated to addressing the intricacies of female cardiovascular health is a commendable initiative. I take great pleasure in learning that medical professionals and cardiologists from diverse regions are collaboratively gathering and reinforcing data on cardiovascular issues specific to women.

Women exhibit physiological, hormonal, and anatomical distinctions that necessitate a unique consideration of their health concerns. Given this, a distinct and tailored approach to healthcare for women is imperative. I am optimistic that this collaborative effort will inspire healthcare practitioners to revolutionize their approach in managing female patients. The insightful recommendations compiled in this textbook have the potential to reshape physicians' perspectives on women's health, fostering improved care.

My sincere congratulations extend to the entire team involved in this nationwide endeavor. I am confident that the ignited spark will illuminate and invigorate our collective commitment to advancing the cause. Special commendation is due to the Cardiological Society of India (CSI) and the entire executive board for the establishment of the CSI Pink Council, a significant step toward enhancing cardiac care for women in the country. This initiative not only fortifies the resolve of woman cardiologists nationwide but also encourages their collaborative efforts with CSI for this important cause.

Dipti Itchhaporia MD MACC FAHA FESC FRCP
Eric & Sheila Samson Endowed Chair in Cardiovascular Health
Director of Disease Management
Hoag Memorial Hospital Presbyterian
Clinical Professor, University of California, Irvine
California, United States
Past President, American College of Cardiology
Board Member, World Heart Federation

Preface

Cardiovascular disease (CVD) in women is now globally well recognized as the leading cause of mortality attributing to 35% of deaths in women, more than all the cancers combined together. However, it continues to be under-recognized, underdiagnosed, and undertreated globally as well as in our country. As India witnesses an obstetric transition with more and more maternal mortality attributed to CVD, it becomes all the more imperative for the physician to acquaint himself or herself with variant presentation of CVD in women across all the reproductive phases of life. Women have women-specific risk factors [e.g., pregnancy-induced hypertension (PIH), preeclampsia, eclampsia, gestational diabetes, stillbirth, maternoplacental syndrome, intrauterine growth restriction (IUGR), polycystic ovarian syndrome (PCOS)] and women-predominant risk factors [autoimmune diseases, systemic lupus erythematosus (SLE), Takayasu arteritis, etc.] contributing to ever-rising burden of CVD in women. Moreover, the women of the present-day society stand at par with men as regards multitasking and professional stresses. Rising maternal age, assisted reproductive techniques, infertility treatments, and increased number of postoperative mothers with congenital and valvular heart disease represent the changing scenario of women subject to cardiovascular ailment not just during the phase of pregnancy but in their future life as well. With variant anatomy, smaller stiffer hearts, diffuse atherosclerosis, plaque erosions, and outward remodeling defining a woman's heart, it becomes imperative that a physician become aware of challenges while dealing with CVD in women.

The Cardiology Society of India (CSI) in the Platinum Jubilee year has initiated the CSI Pink Council to work in this direction of increasing the awareness and improving diagnosis, management, and access to cardiovascular care for women in our country. The *Yearbook of CVD in Women* is an effort in this direction with an amalgam of latest articles published in leading journals in the years 2022–2023. The cardiologists across the country have amalgamated, analyzed, and simplified the delivery of the latest key messages pertaining to CVD in women. This shall update the physicians with the latest in the field and uplift the approach and management of CVD in women.

"No beauty shines brighter than a healthy heart! *Especially when it is a woman's heart*"

"The Foundation of a Healthy Society"

Shibba Takkar Chhabra

Preface

Acknowledgments

I thank my parents Rita and Ved Parkash Takkar and Rama and Ramesh Chabbra and my heartbeats Ritesh and Vidyut. They are my world. Their love and support make this endeavor possible.

I am indebted to my mentors Professor GS Wander, Professor Jyotsna Maddury and Dr Debabrata Roy. Professor GS Wander has been a guide with vision and belief, always encouraging academic ventures with his wisdom, inputs and unrelenting support at every juncture. I am grateful to Professor Jyotsna Maddury for her person, being a role model with grit and passion, for the inspiration she ignites through her tremendous, focused work on cardiovascular diseases in women. I am grateful to Dr Debabrata Roy, Honorary General Secretary, CSI for vesting his faith and confidence, for enabling, encouraging, guiding and showing the path to tread. I acknowledge and wholeheartedly thank Dr MK Das, Dr PS Banerjee, Dr Vijay Bang and Dr PC Rath; the presidential chairs of CSI who have embarked the cause of CSI Pink Council with great zeal and vision.

I also acknowledge untiring efforts of my co-editor Dr Ankur Goyal who made the yearbook of CVD possible. I extend my abundant thanks to Mr Harsh Kishore who worked day and night assimilating and organizing the script with great enthusiasm. I am extremely grateful to Dr Nitika Sharma, Dr Rabia Aggarwal, Dr Zufi Shan, and Dr Khushi Goyal for extensive research and data collection.

I express my thanks to the entire team of Jaypee Brothers Medical Publishers (P) Ltd, including Shri Jitendar Pal Vij (Group Chairman), Mr Ankit Vij (Managing Director), Mr MS Mani (Group President), Ms Chetna Malhotra (Senior Director—Professional Publishing, Marketing and Business Development), Ms Pooja Bhandari (Director—Production), Ms Sunita Katla (Executive Assistant to Group Chairman and Publishing Manager), Ms Tamali Deb (Manager—Copyediting), Mr Ajay Kumar Sharma (DGM—Production), Mr Keshav Kumar (Assistant Manager—Production), Mr Manoj Kumar (Team Leader—Production), Mr Sumit Kumar (Cover Visualizer), and Gopal Singh Kirola (Senior Graphic Designer). Special thanks to Ms Nedup Bhutia Pillai (Team Leader—Print Publishing) for being so prompt and efficient in drafting the entire script with an amazing commitment and coordination.

Above all, I thank Almighty, The Supreme Power, who has guided us throughout.

Contents

Section 1: Pregnancy and CVD in Women
Section Editor: Asha Mahilmaran

Associate Editors: Rukmani Prabha, S Anne Princy, Rajeshwari Nayak, Vatchala Sree Varadharajan, K Meenakshi, S Jayalakshmi, Radha Priya Yalamanchi, Aruna D, Narra Lavanya, Prabhakar Dorairaj, G Justin Paul

1. Prenatal Factors Associated with Maternal Cardiometabolic Risk Markers during Pregnancy: The ECLIPSES Study — 1
2. Peripartum Screening for Postpartum Hypertension in Women with Hypertensive Disorders of Pregnancy — 3
3. Adverse Pregnancy Outcomes and the Development of Short-term Maternal Cardiovascular Disease Risk Factors — 6
4. Risk of Future Cardiovascular Diseases in Different Years Postpartum after Hypertensive Disorders of Pregnancy — 7
5. Meta-analysis of Cardiovascular Risk Factors in Offspring of Preeclampsia Pregnancies — 9
6. Early Pregnancy Cardiometabolic Risk Factors and the Prevalence of Metabolic Syndrome 10 Years after First Pregnancy — 11
7. Association of Gestational Diabetes Mellitus with Overall and Type Specific Cardiovascular and Cerebrovascular Diseases: Systematic Review and Meta-analysis — 12
8. Coronary Artery Bypass Graft Surgery for Spontaneous Coronary Artery Dissection in Early Pregnancy: Medical and Ethical Decision-making Issues — 14
9. Contemporary Rates of Pre-pregnancy Hypertension and Diabetes Among a Multi-ethnic Sample of Pregnant Individuals in a Diverse US State — 16
10. Pregnancy Loss and Risk of Incident CVD Within 5 Years: Findings from the Women's Health Initiative — 18
11. Management of Hypertension in Pregnancy — 20

Section 2: Hypertension and CVD in Women
Section Editor: Sujatha Vipperla
Associate Editors: Anil Kumar Mahapatro, Achukatla Kumar

1. Sex Differences in Arterial Hypertension: A Scientific Statement from the ESC Council on Hypertension, the European Association of Preventive Cardiology, Association of Cardiovascular Nursing and Allied Professions, the ESC Council for Cardiology Practice, and the ESC Working Group on Cardiovascular Pharmacotherapy — 25
2. Sex and Gender in Hypertension Guidelines — 28
3. Evaluating Sex Differences in the Effect of Increased Systolic Blood Pressure on the Risk of Cardiovascular Disease in Asian Populations: A Systematic Review and Meta-analysis — 30
4. Effect of Sacubitril/Valsartan or Valsartan on Ventricular Remodeling and Myocardial Fibrosis in Perimenopausal Women with Hypertension — 32
5. Salt Sensitivity of Blood Pressure in Women — 33
6. Placental Syndromes and Long-term Risk of Hypertension — 35
7. Hypertension: Sex-related Differences in Drug Treatment, Prevalence, and Blood Pressure Control in Primary Care — 37
8. The Effect of Calcium and Vitamin D Supplements on Blood Pressure in Postmenopausal Women: Myth or Reality? — 38
9. The Impact of Antihypertensive Treatment of Mild-to-moderate Hypertension during Pregnancy on Maternal and Neonatal Outcomes: An Updated Meta-analysis of Randomized Controlled Trials — 40
10. Medications for Preventing Hypertensive Disorders in High-risk Pregnant Women: A Systematic Review and Network Meta-analysis — 42
11. Effects of Yoga on Cardiometabolic Risks and Fetomaternal Outcomes are Associated with Serum Nitric Oxide in Gestational Hypertension: A Randomized Control Trial — 44
12. The Association between Hypertensive Disorders in Pregnancy and the Risk of Developing Chronic Hypertension — 46
13. Is Blood Pressure 120–139/80–89 mm Hg before 20 Weeks a Risk Factor for Hypertensive Disorders of Pregnancy? A Meta-analysis — 49
14. Low-dose Aspirin for the Prevention of Superimposed Preeclampsia in Women with Chronic Hypertension: A Systematic Review and Meta-analysis — 51
15. Differential Sex-specific Effects of Angiotensin-converting Enzyme Inhibition and Angiotensin Receptor Blocker Therapy on Arterial Function in Hypertension: CALIBREX Trial — 53
16. Comparing the Effects of Different Exercises on Blood Pressure and Arterial Stiffness in Postmenopausal Women: A Systematic Review and Meta-analysis — 55

17. Effectiveness of a Community-based Education and Peer Support Led by Women's Self-help Groups in Improving the Control of Hypertension in Urban Slums of Kerala, India: A Cluster Randomized Controlled Pragmatic Trial ... 56
18. Focus on Today's Evidence While Keeping an Eye on the Future: Lessons derived from Hypertension in Women ... 58

Section 3: Dyslipidemia and CVD in Women
Section Editor: Kunal Mahajan
Associate Editors: Tanuj Bhatia, Jaikrit Bhutani, Sai Devvrat, Abhishek Rastogi, Prashant Patel, Lokesh Verma

1. Sex Differences in Lipid-lowering Therapy of Familial Hypercholesterolemia ... 67
2. Gender Disparity in the Relationship between Lipid Profile and the Incidence of Cardiovascular Disease in Young Adults ... 68
3. Correlation between the Nutrition and Lipid Profile among Adult Women ... 70
4. Calorie Restriction to Improve Metabolic Health among Overweight or Obese Females ... 72
5. Effect of Regular Exercise on Lipids and Apolipoprotein Profiles in Middle-aged Women ... 74
6. Significance of Levothyroxine Treatment on Serum Lipid in Pregnant Women with Subclinical Hypothyroidism ... 75
7. Association of Lipid Levels with the Prevalence of Hypertension in Chinese Women ... 76
8. Effect of Optimized Food-based Recommendation Promotion on Lipid Profiles among Minangkabau Women with Dyslipidemia ... 78
9. Association between Serum Lipid Profile and Osteoporosis in Postmenopausal Women ... 79
10. Temporal Sequence of Blood Lipids and Insulin Resistance in Perimenopausal Women ... 81
11. Usefulness of Lipid Screening during First Trimester of Pregnancy ... 82
12. Sex-specific Differences in Premature ASCVD and its Risk Factors among Patients with Familial Hypercholesterolemia ... 84
13. Effect of Food-away-from-home on Lipid Profile ... 85
14. Association between Serum Lipids and Hemostatic Factors ... 87
15. Impact of Insulin Resistance on Serum Lipoprotein Profile in Women with Gestational Diabetes Mellitus ... 88
16. Correlation of Trends in Lipid Profiles from First to Second Trimester with Trends in Insulin Indices and Gestational Diabetes Mellitus ... 90
17. Impact of Early Midlife Cardiovascular Health on Future HDL Metrics in Women ... 91

Section 4: Diabetes Mellitus and CVD in Women
Section Editor: J Cecily Mary Majella

Associate Editors: Vatchala Sree Varadharajan, K Meenakshi, T Neelambujan, Aarathy Kannan, Rohith Velusamy, J Nandhini, Sundar C, S Arulrhaj, Manikandan, Nikhil Govind, Arun Ranganathan, P Deepa

1. Cardiovascular Risk and Lifetime Benefit from Preventive Treatment in Type 2 Diabetes Mellitus: A Post Hoc Analysis of the CAPTURE Study — 95
2. Association of Gestational Diabetes Mellitus with Overall and Type Specific Cardiovascular and Cerebrovascular Diseases: Systematic Review and Meta-analysis — 98
3. Cardiovascular Outcomes in Type 1 and Type 2 Diabetes Mellitus — 100
4. Cardiovascular Risk Factors in Diabetic Patients with Metabolic Syndrome — 105
5. 14 Sex-specific Predictors of Coronary Microvascular Function in a Multiethnic Cohort of 455 Asymptomatic People with Type 2 Diabetes Mellitus — 107
6. Pregestational Diabetes Mellitus and Congenital Heart Defects — 109
7. Rising Prediabetes, Undiagnosed Diabetes, and Risk Factors in Young Women — 112
8. Can Artificial Intelligence Predict Heart Disease in Diabetic and Prediabetic Women: Hype or Hope? — 114

Section 5: Metabolic Syndrome and CVD in Women
Section Editor: Hetan C Shah

Associate Editors: Tamagna Ghosh, Bhavik Shah, Chandrakant Chavan, Malav Jhala

1. Assessment of Cardiovascular Risk in Women: Progress So Far and Progress to Come — 123
2. Cardiometabolic Biomarkers in Women with Polycystic Ovary Syndrome — 124
3. Cardiovascular Health in the Menopause Transition: A Longitudinal Study of up to 3,892 Women with up to Four Repeated Measures of Risk Factors — 126
4. Cumulative Burden of Metabolic Syndrome and Its Components on the Risk of Atrial Fibrillation: A Nationwide Population-based Study — 128
5. Fitness Attenuates Long-term Cardiovascular Outcomes in Women with Ischemic Heart Disease and Metabolic Syndrome — 130
6. Gender Differences and Cardiometabolic Risk: The Importance of the Risk Factors — 131
7. Menstrual Cycle Regularity and Length Across the Reproductive Lifespan and Risk of Cardiovascular Disease — 133
8. Metabolic Disorders in Menopause — 134
9. Cardiovascular Disease in Women: Clinical Perspectives — 135

10.	Metabolic, Behavioral, and Psychosocial Risk Factors and Cardiovascular Disease in Women Compared with Men in 21 High-income, Middle-income, and Low-income Countries: An Analysis of the PURE Study	137
11.	Modifiable Cardiovascular Risk Factors in Adults Less than 40 Years of Age	139
12.	Scoring Systems of Metabolic Syndrome and Prediction of Cardiovascular Events: A Population-based Cohort Study	140
13.	Sex Differences in Adiposity and Cardiovascular Diseases	142
14.	Subclinical Cardiovascular Disease and Polycystic Ovary Syndrome	143
15.	Women's Reproductive Milestones and Cardiovascular Disease Risk: A Review of Reports and Opportunities from the CARDIA Study	144

Section 6: CVD in Women: Acute Coronary Syndrome
Section Editor: Sarita Rao

Associate Editors: Roshan Rao, Roopali Khanna, Hema S, Pankaj Manoria, Prerna Goyal, Priya Palimkar, Amjad Ali, Abha Pandit, Mahpaekar Mashhadi, Harsh A Chaudhary, Achukatla Kumar

1.	Gender Disparities in Prevalence by Diagnostic Criteria, Treatment and Mortality of Newly Diagnosed Acute Myocardial Infarction in Korean Adults	149
2.	Sex-specific and Hormone-related Differences in Vascular Remodeling in Atherosclerosis	151
3.	Incidence and Outcomes of Cardiogenic Shock Among Women with Spontaneous Coronary Artery Dissection	152
4.	Sex-related Differences in Thrombus Burden in STEMI Patients Undergoing Primary Percutaneous Coronary Intervention	153
5.	Ischemia with No Obstructive Coronary Arteries (INOCA): A Review of the Prevalence, Diagnosis and Management	155
6.	Less Revascularization in Young Women but Impaired Long-term Outcomes in Young Men after Myocardial Infarction	157
7.	Updates on MINOCA and INOCA through the 2022 Publications in the International Journal of Cardiology	159
8.	Updates on Pharmacologic Management of Microvascular Angina	160
9.	Association between Hormone Therapy and Short-term Cardiovascular Events in Women with Spontaneous Coronary Artery Dissection	162
10.	Sex Differences in 10-year Outcomes Following STEMI: A Subanalysis from the EXAMINATION-EXTEND Trial	164

Section 7: Coronary Artery Disease and CVD in Women
Section Editor: Bhupinder Singh
Associate Editors: Suraj Kumar, Surender Deora

1.	Sex Differences in the Clinical Presentation of Acute Coronary Syndromes	168
2.	Sex-related Differences in Plaque Characteristics and Endothelial Shear Stress-related Plaque-progression in Human Coronary Arteries	169
3.	Sex-specific Associations of Myocardial Perfusion Imaging with Outcomes in Patients with Suspected Chronic Coronary Syndrome	170
4.	The Prevalence of Risk Factors and Pattern of Obstructive Coronary Artery Disease in Young Indians (<45 Years) Undergoing Percutaneous Coronary Intervention: A Gender-based Multicenter Study	172
5.	Sex Difference in the Association of the Triglyceride Glucose Index with Obstructive Coronary Artery Disease	173
6.	Relationship between Breast Arterial Calcification and Coronary Artery Disease by Invasive Coronary Angiography in Postmenopausal Women	174
7.	Early Coronary Atherosclerosis in Women with Previous Preeclampsia	176
8.	Comparative Effectiveness of Initial Computed Tomography and Invasive Coronary Angiography in Women and Men with Stable Chest Pain and Suspected Coronary Artery Disease: Multicenter Randomized Trial	177
9.	Sex Difference in Coronary Artery Spasm Tested by Intracoronary Acetylcholine Provocation Test in Patients with Nonobstructive Coronary Artery Disease	179
10.	Psychosocial Well-being and Progression of Coronary Artery Calcification in Midlife Women	180

Section 8: Miscellaneous
Section Editors: Kunal Mahajan, J Cecily Mary Majella, Ankur Goyal
Associate Editors: Jai Bharat Sharma, Rahul Yadav, Surender Kumar, Suresh Kumar P, Raghothaman Sethumadhavan, Raagini Gupta, Nikita Sharma, Zoofi Shan, Muzammil Farooqi, Rabia Aggarwal, Khushi Goyal, Anshdeep Saluja, Harsh Kishore, Samman Verma, Akash Batta

1.	Gender Differences in Benefits of Empagliflozin in Patients with HFpEF	184
2.	Sex Differences in Bleeding Events in Patients Receiving Aspirin and P2Y12 Inhibitor after Percutaneous Coronary Intervention for Acute Coronary Syndrome	186
3.	Gender Differences in Mortality Rate after Surgical Aortic Valve Replacement	188
4.	Sex Differences in Outcomes after Single Antiplatelet Maintenance Therapy after Percutaneous Coronary Intervention	189
5.	Sex Differences in Quality of Life of Heart Failure Patients	191

6.	Gender Differences in Heart Failure Trends in China from 1990 to 2019	193
7.	Gender Disparities after Transcatheter Aortic Valve Replacement with Newer-generation Transcatheter Heart Valves: A Systematic Review and Meta-analysis	194
8.	Gender Differences in Atrial Fibrillation: From the Thromboembolic Risk to the Anticoagulant Treatment Response	196
9.	Sex Differences in Characteristics, Outcomes, and Treatment Response with Dapagliflozin Across the Range of Ejection Fraction in Patients with Heart Failure: Insights from DAPA-HF and DELIVER	197
10.	Gender Differences in Acute Aortic Dissection	199
11.	Sex and Gender Differences in the use of Oral Anticoagulants for Non-valvular Atrial Fibrillation: A Population-based Cohort Study in Primary Health Care in Catalonia	201
12.	Maternal and Fetal Outcomes in Pregnant Patients with Mechanical and Bioprosthetic Heart Valves	207
13.	Validation of Risk Stratification for Cardiac Events in Pregnant Women with Valvular Heart Disease	208
14.	Pregnancy Outcomes in Women with Heart Disease: The Madras Medical College Pregnancy and Cardiac (M-PAC) Registry from India	209
15.	2023 HRS Expert Consensus Statement on the Management of Arrhythmias During Pregnancy	210
16.	2023 ESH Guidelines for the Management of Arterial Hypertension the Task Force for the Management of Arterial Hypertension of the European Society of Hypertension Endorsed by the International Society of Hypertension (ISH) and the European Renal Association (ERA)	212
17.	Sex-based Differences in Risk Factors for Incident Myocardial Infarction and Stroke in the UK Biobank	213

Index   221

SECTION 1

Pregnancy and CVD in Women

Section Editor: Asha Mahilmaran

Associate Editors: Rukmani Prabha, S Anne Princy, Rajeshwari Nayak, Vatchala Sree Varadharajan, K Meenakshi, S Jayalakshmi, Radha Priya Yalamanchi, Aruna D, Narra Lavanya, Prabhakar Dorairaj, G Justin Paul

ARTICLE 1

Prenatal Factors Associated with Maternal Cardiometabolic Risk Markers during Pregnancy: The ECLIPSES Study

Motevalizadeh E, Díaz-López A, Martín-Luján F, Basora J, Arija V. Prenatal Factors Associated with Maternal Cardiometabolic Risk Markers during Pregnancy: The ECLIPSES Study.
Nutrients. 2023;15(5):1135.

Abstract

Background and objective: Pregnancy is associated with significant changes in the physiological, vascular, and metabolic milieu of the mother like increased insulin resistance, raised adiposity, reduced vascular resistance, hypercoagulability, and cardiovascular remodeling.[1] These changes are essential to promote fetal development; however, an inadequate adaptation to these changes leads to adverse health outcomes. This study aims at analyzing the impact of maternal factors, both modifiable [e.g., prepregnancy weight, gestational weight gain (GWG), smoking, alcohol consumption, diet, lifestyle, and physical activity] and nonmodifiable (age, socioeconomic status), on maternal cardiometabolic risk.

Materials and methods: Designed as a prospective cohort study, the population comprised of 265 healthy pregnant women who participated in the ECLIPSES study.[2] Medical, obstetric history, and data on socioeconomic status, lifestyle habits (smoking, alcohol consumption, diet, physical activity) along with BP and anthropometric measurements were obtained in the first and third trimesters. Cardiometabolic biomarkers including fasting values of blood sugar, lipid profile, and insulin were obtained at 12 and 36 weeks of gestation. Insulin resistance was then calculated based on the homeostasis model assessment of insulin resistance (HOMA-IR). A clustered cardiometabolic risk (CCR) score was then calculated by the summation of z-scores of seven biomarkers obtained, namely body mass index (BMI), systolic blood pressure (SBP), fasting glucose, HOMA-IR index (log), triglyceride (log), low-density lipoprotein cholesterol (LDL-C), and high-density lipoprotein cholesterol (HDL-C). A continuous CCR score was then calculated for both first and third trimesters.

Results: All cardiometabolic biomarkers except for fasting blood sugar increased between first and third trimesters ($p < 0.05$). Higher educational qualification was associated with lower BMI and SBP and age above 30 years was associated with higher HDL-C levels. Obesity/overweight early in pregnancy revealed independent and positive correlation with SBP, DBP, insulin, HOMA-IR, and LDL-C ($p < 0.05$). The positive association between obesity and lower HDL-C persisted into the third trimester. Similarly, subjects with excessive GWG had higher levels of SBP and HDL-C. Blood pressure measurements, both systolic and diastolic, BMI, and fasting blood sugar were inversely related to insufficient GWG. Higher social class was associated with lower fasting glucose, lower insulin, and HOMA-IR levels. Further analysis revealed a statistically significant positive correlation between CCR score and obesity/overweight; likewise, a significant negative correlation was observed between CCR score with university education and higher levels of physical activity during early stages of pregnancy. This positive association between CCR and obesity/overweight persisted into the third trimester as well. The first-trimester CCR score showed a statistically significant correlation with the third-trimester CCR score [β 0.31; 95% confidence interval (CI) 0.19, 0.43; $p < 0.001$].

Discussion and conclusion: The results reveal that among the prenatal factors, the modifiable factors such as ideal BMI, appropriate GWG, and increased physical activity along with other factors like higher educational qualification and good socioeconomic status were significantly and independently associated with lower cardiometabolic risk. Smoking and alcohol, though having a nonsignificant correlation, showed a trend toward a higher CCR score in the third trimester. The positive correlation between the CCR scores at 12 and 36 weeks highlights the fact that cardiometabolic risk progresses through pregnancy.

Body mass index at baseline was found to be the strongest predictor of high cardiometabolic risk in both first and third trimesters. Obesity was associated with an unfavorable cardiometabolic profile like elevated systolic and diastolic BP, elevated insulin levels, increased insulin resistance, and a proatherogenic lipid profile. High levels of HDL-C observed in women with excessive GWG are considered a high risk factor for small size for gestational age in the child. Smoking was associated with high levels of triglycerides and LDL-C in the third trimester; similarly, alcohol consumption in pregnancy leads to elevated BP and LDL-C levels.

The main factor that sets this study apart is the cluster approach in the assessment of cardiometabolic health, which provides a holistic idea rather than about individual factors on their own. The use of both clinical and biochemical parameters, which can easily be obtained during clinical practice, in calculating the CCR score makes it an important tool. Furthermore, the continuous CCR score calculation at first and third trimesters makes it more sensitive and less error prone than other categorical forms.

COMMENT

Healthcare systems are often segmented, making pregnancy and maternal health primarily a concern of obstetricians. However, this study has proved the vital role of modifiable factors on the cardiometabolic health of women in the prepregnant state as well as in early pregnancy which then translates into long-term cardiovascular health.[3] The most protective modifiable prenatal factors of cardiometabolic risk are maintaining a normal weight, higher educational qualification, engaging in greater physical activity, and avoiding smoking and drinking alcohol. The continuous cardiometabolic risk (CCR) score assessment at 12 and 36 weeks enables us to monitor the progression of risk as pregnancy advances. Thus, this cluster approach to the assessment of cardiometabolic risk has demonstrated the importance of patient education before and/or during early pregnancy to ensure optimal outcomes to both mother and child.

ARTICLE 2

Peripartum Screening for Postpartum Hypertension in Women with Hypertensive Disorders of Pregnancy

Giorgione V, Khalil A, O'Driscoll J, Thilaganathan B. Peripartum screening for postpartum hypertension in women with hypertensive disorders of pregnancy.
J Am Coll Cardiol. 2022;80(15):1465-76.

Abstract

Background: In women with hypertensive disorders of pregnancy (HDP), chronic hypertension (CHT) is the main cardiovascular risk factor.

Objective: The objective of the study was to assess the effectiveness of peripartum screening to prognosticate the incidence of CHT, the cardiovascular risk, after HDP.

Methods: This observational longitudinal cohort study was conducted at St George's University Hospitals NHS Foundation Trust. The study period was between February 2019 and August 2021. Women with a pregnancy complicated by HDP who had undergone a peripartum and postpartum cardiovascular assessment were included in the study and recruited consecutively. Exclusion criteria include patients with a diagnosis of CHT and on antihypertensive medications before the pregnancy, patients with known cardiac conditions, and pregnancies complicated by genetic syndromes and fetal abnormalities. Pregnancy data and outcomes were ascertained from the maternity databases, discharge letters, and direct patient enquiry. All study data were collected and managed using electronic data-capture tools.

Cardiovascular assessments were done at both peripartum and postpartum visits according to a predetermined protocol, which included anthropometric measurements, BP profile, and maternal transthoracic echocardiogram (TTE). BP profile was obtained using an upper arm automatic BP monitor in a resting state and sitting position with at least three measurements with 1 minute. Mean arterial pressure (MAP) was calculated, and an average of the last two measurements was used to diagnose hypertension. TTE was performed in all participants, and parameters assessed included two-dimensional Doppler TTE, speckle tracking, and strain imaging [global longitudinal strain, left ventricular (LV) radial and circumferential strain, LV twist]. Univariable and multivariable analyses were done to assess the association between the observed clinical and transthoracic echocardiographic data and a postpartum diagnosis of CHT.

Result: Total 211 (81.8%) of 258 patients were included in the final analysis. Out of the 211 patients, 70 patients (33.2%) were found to remain hypertensive or were on antihypertensive medications at postpartum follow-up. Baseline characteristics of the HDP cohort ($n = 70$) were compared with normotensive patients ($n = 141$). The postpartum evaluation was performed at a median of

123.5 days [interquartile range (IQR) 98–147 days] in hypertensive women ($p = 0.192$) and 126 days (IQR 108–155 days) in normotensive women. It was noted that compared to normotensive women, women with CHT were older (35.5 ± 5.0 vs. 32.9 ± 5.6 years; $p = 0.001$), more likely to be Afro-Caribbean (27.1% vs. 7.8%; $p < 0.0001$), had higher body mass index (33.4 ± 5.9 vs. 31.2 ± 5.4 kg/m^2; $p = 0.006$), higher mean arterial pressure (106.5 ± 8.4 vs. 103.3 ± 7.0 mm Hg; $p = 0.004$), higher LV mass index (84.0 ± 17.9 vs. 76.3 ± 14.8 g/m^2; $p = 0.001$), higher relative wall thickness (0.46 ± 0.10 vs. 0.40 ± 0.10; $p < 0.0001$), and lower global longitudinal strain (–15.6% ± 2.7% vs. –16.6% ± 2.2%; $p = 0.006$).

On postpartum TTE, it was noted that a total of 134 (63.5%) women had hypertension or persistent LV myocardial dysfunction and those with postpartum LV myocardial dysfunction [$n = 103$ of 211 (48.8%)] had worse cardiac indices in comparison to those with normal myocardial function. Various prediction models were proposed and multiple predictors were evaluated. However, the prediction model combining clinical features (first-trimester MAP and maternal age) and echocardiographic features (E/é ratio > 7, LV mass index > 75 g/m^2, and relative wall thickness > 0.42) showed excellent accuracy for the identification of women with persistent hypertension after HDP [area under the curve 0.85; 95% confidence interval (CI) 0.79–0.90].

Conclusion: This peripartum screening approach may be useful to identify the women at risk of CHT following an HDP. Intensive monitoring of BP along with appropriate medical therapy beginning from the early postpartum period can prevent the future risk of cardiovascular disease in these women.

COMMENT

The overall prevalence of hypertensive disorders of pregnancy (HDP) is up to 10% of all pregnancies, with prevalence of chronic hypertension (CHT) constituting 14%, preeclampsia 2–8%, and gestational hypertension 2–5% of all pregnancies.[4] Many studies have well established the association with cardiovascular risks. It has further been noted that there is a two-fold to eight-fold increased future risk of CHT in women with HDP than normotensive pregnancies. One of the important cardiovascular risk factors in women with HDP was CHT and up to 32% of women with HDP developed CHT in the first 10 years after pregnancy and 10% of women aged 20–29 years with a previous HDP developed CHT in 8 years postpartum. A meta-analysis by Heida et al. demonstrated that women with preeclampsia have a relative risk (RR) 2.76 (95% CI 1.63–4.69) increased risk of having CHT after pregnancy in comparison to normotensive pregnant women with a normotensive pregnancy.[5]

In the background of an increased risk of classical cardiovascular risk factors, especially CHT, the time of screening these mothers becomes critical. Although it is evident that a postpartum screening for cardiovascular risk assessment is essential, there is a wide variation in the existing recommendations, thus making cardiovascular follow-up of women with a previous HDP noncoherent and confusing. Some recommend CV follow-up at 6–12 months after pregnancy. Concurrent with BP monitoring, other CV risk factors such as lipid and glucose assessment should be done. This is done annually to every 5 years until the age of 50 years after whence the women qualify the CV risk assessment according to prevention guidelines.

Although majority of studies focus on the association between HDP and long-term CVD risk, there are only limited data available addressing the early risk, and the present study assesses the early risk. This study delineates that earlier screening in women with HDP should be initiated much earlier, initiating in the peripartum period itself. This can be substantiated by the outcome of the study which shows that one-third of patients had persistent postpartum hypertension after HDP.

The cardiovascular assessment which includes various clinical and echocardiographic parameters increases the accuracy of the prediction. A prediction model based on demographic, clinical, and echocardiographic indices has been found to show good or excellent discrimination.

Although MAP is not included in the definition of HDP, studies have shown that first-trimester MAP is a strong predictor of gestational hypertension and preeclampsia in nulliparous women. A prospective cohort study[6] of 4,749 nulliparous women showed that first-trimester MAP was associated with gestational hypertension, term PE, preterm PE, and early onset preeclampsia. The present study has evaluated both first-trimester MAP and peripartum MAP and the former has been found to be statistically significant.

The risk of CHT after HDP also depends on the number of pregnancies. However, data on the recurrence of preeclampsia which has a higher risk of CHT is not brought out in the study.

The echocardiographic parameters evaluated include LV geometry, LV diastolic and systolic function, and LV mechanics. Of these, increased relative wall thickness and LV mass and impaired global longitudinal strain had been found to be statistically significant. However, the associations between peripartum echocardiographic findings and persistent short-term CV impairment may not be accurate for long-term CVD in these HDP cohorts, which is a limitation.

The presence of HDP serves as an early indicator of a future cardiovascular risk in a woman and offers an opportunity to timely initiate risk-reduction strategies. As the study states, screening of the women affected by HDP for CV risks during the peripartum period instead of the postpartum period would benefit the patient more and keep the patient under surveillance, because loss of follow-up becomes more common during the postpartum period, especially in low- and middle-income countries (LMICs). Hence, peripartum screening provides an effective universal screening tool for women with HDP and allows the early initiation of lifestyle modifications and tailored antihypertensive therapy. Early and appropriate antihypertensive treatment controls diastolic BP and improves LV geometry, which are diastolic indices, and helps regression of LV hypertrophy, which is a good prognostic index.

Hence, peripartum cardiovascular screening, both clinical and TTE, can be used to effectively identify women affected by HDP who are at an increased risk of persistent postpartum hypertension or asymptomatic LV myocardial dysfunction. However, further study is necessary to validate the predictive models and evaluate the short- and long-term effectiveness of early cardiovascular interventions after HDP.

ARTICLE 3

Adverse Pregnancy Outcomes and the Development of Short-term Maternal Cardiovascular Disease Risk Factors

Quist-Nelson J, Meng ML, Stuart JL, Fuller M, Rogers U, Pencina M, et al. Adverse pregnancy outcomes and the development of short-term maternal cardiovascular disease risk factors.
Am J Obstet Gynecol. 2023;S497.

Abstract

Objective: There is evidence that adverse pregnancy outcomes (APOs), such as pregnancy-induced hypertension, preeclampsia, gestational diabetes, preterm delivery, small for gestational age delivery, and pregnancy loss, increase the risk of future development of cardiovascular disease (CVD) risk factors and CVDs such as coronary artery disease, stroke, and peripheral vascular disease. The aim of this study was to evaluate the association between APOs and development of CVD risk factors.

Materials and methods: A retrospective cohort study of pregnant women who delivered from January 2016 till December 2020 and who were free of CVD risk factors during pregnancy was conducted. APOs were defined using International Classification of Diseases 10th Revision (ICD-10) codes for gestational hypertension, preeclampsia, gestational diabetes, preterm delivery, and delivery of a small for age infant. Patients were followed-up till December 2021 for development of CVD risk factors. The cumulative hazard for CVD risk factors was estimated at 3 and 5 years after delivery.

Results: Median length of follow-up was 1.9 years. Patients with APOs had a significantly higher risk of developing CVD risk factors compared to the control group without APOs (18.1% vs. 6.7%). 25.7% of the patients had more than one APO. 7.7% of the patients developed APO within 1 year. The estimated cumulative hazard of developing a CVD risk factor after APO was 21.7% after 3 years and 54.3% after 5 years of delivery. Women with an APO were more likely to develop hypertension (11.4%) in the follow-up period and women with gestational diabetes were more likely to develop type 2 diabetes mellitus (3.5%).

Conclusion: In this retrospective follow-up study, patients with an APO had a significantly higher risk of developing CVD risk factors within 1 year of delivery and the risk increased exponentially with the increasing years of follow-up.

COMMENT

The main aim in obstetric care is to reduce maternal and fetal risk to very minute. The development in the therapeutic armamentarium is reflected as better perinatal outcome in the last few decades. However, adverse pregnancy outcome (APO) continues to pause a major challenge to the treating obstetrician and physician. In the growing realm of cardiovascular disease (CVD), APO is the newest of the risk factors. This study highlights the importance of recognizing APO while evaluating CVD risk factors in women. Women with history of APO call forth more vigorous primary prevention methods for CVD.

ARTICLE 4

Risk of Future Cardiovascular Diseases in Different Years Postpartum after Hypertensive Disorders of Pregnancy

Sukmanee J, Liabsuetrakul T. Risk of future cardiovascular diseases in different years postpartum after hypertensive disorders of pregnancy.
Medicine (Baltimore). 2022;101(30):e29646.

Abstract

Background: Pregnancy-induced hypertension (PIH) or hypertensive disorders of pregnancy (HDP) is a common clinical condition and complicates nearly 6–10% of pregnancies. HDP can be classified into four types, namely: (1) preexisting hypertension, (2) gestational hypertension and preeclampsia (PE), (3) preexisting hypertension plus superimposed gestational hypertension with proteinuria, and (4) unclassifiable hypertension.[7] Gestational hypertension is defined as a new-onset blood pressure (BP) after 20 weeks of pregnancy with a systolic BP ≥ 140 mm Hg and a diastolic BP ≥ 90 mm Hg, with no proteinuria and a normal BP recording before 20 weeks of gestation. PE is gestational hypertension with proteinuria. New-onset seizure and coma in a preeclamptic pregnant women is called eclampsia.[8] Cardiovascular disease (CVD) includes disease of the heart and blood vessels comprising ischemic heart disease (IHD), venous thromboembolism (VTE), peripheral artery disease (PAD), and stroke. HDP in general and eclampsia and PE in particular are major contributors of maternal and neonatal morbidity and mortality. There is paucity in the data regarding the progression of HDP to future CVD and there is no consensus on the follow-up schedule of women with HDP to prevent CVD and hypertension (HT).[8] The meta-analysis aims to assess the occurrence of CVD-related mortality and morbidity and onset of HT in later life in women with prior HDP, particularly in various years of postpartum as compared with normotensive pregnant women.

Methods: Studies published in Medline, Cochrane Library, Web of Science, and Scopus of any language were included for review. Standardized international guidelines pertaining to selection and removing duplicate articles were applied. Both prospective and retrospective studies were included. The studies that looked at mortality 6 weeks postpartum and morbidity such as HT, heart failure (HF), VTE, PAD, stroke, and dementia in women with prior HDP (1,262,726) were compared with controls (14,711,054). A total of 3,754 studies were screened of which a qualitative review was done in 59 studies. 56 of them were quantitatively reviewed in the meta-analysis. Statistical analysis was carried with R version 4.0.4 (2020 The R Foundation for Statistical Computing).

Results: 37/56 studies assessed the risk of HT in later life in pregnant women with HDP against pregnant women who were normotensive. Of the 37 studies, 16 included women with gestational hypertension alone whereas 21 included both gestational hypertension and PE. There was a significantly higher risk of HT within the first 5 years of postpartum in pregnant women with HDP compared to normotensive pregnant women [relative risk (RR) 5.34; 95% confidence interval (CI) 2.74–10.39]. There was a trend toward increased risk of HT at 6–10 years and 11–15 and ≥15 years postpartum period in pregnant women with prior HDP against normotensive pregnant women; however, they were not significant. Similarly, the incidence of late-onset HT was higher in pregnant women with varying severity of PE (mild-to-severe,) compared to pregnant women with normal BP; however, the values had low certainty of evidence with a wide range of CI (RR 6.67; 95% CI 1.51–29.40). 10, 7, 4, and 3 studies evaluated the risk of development of IHD, HF, VTE, and PAD, respectively, in pregnant women with HDP in later life compared with normotensive pregnant women. There was a two-fold increased risk of development of IHD (RR 2.06; 95% CI 1.38–3.08), a significantly higher incidence of HF in later life (RR 2.53; 95% CI 1.28–5.00) in pregnant women with HDP compared to normotensive pregnant women. On the other hand, there was no significant difference in the occurrence of VTE and PAD in pregnant women with HDP compared to pregnant women with normal BP. Data from two studies show that there was no significant difference in the incidence of IHD and VTE in pregnant women with varying severity of PE against pregnant women with normal BP. A significantly higher incidence of stroke was found in pregnant women with prior HDP (RR 1.59; 95% CI 1.08–2.33) in 12 studies that compared normotensive pregnant women. A review of three studies showed that the incidence of dementia in later life was higher in pregnant women with prior HDP compared to pregnant women with normal BP (RR 1.37; 95% CI 0.70–2.71) with very low certainty of evidence. The cardiovascular mortality and all-cause mortality in pregnant women with HDP compared with normotensive pregnant women were RR 2.82; 95% CI 2.55–3.09 and RR 1.32; 95% CI 1.27–1.36, respectively. The study numbers included for analysis are small involving only three studies regarding cardiovascular mortality and two involving all-cause mortality.

Interpretation: Studies that looked at the occurrence of HT in later life in pregnant women with prior HDP compared to normotensive pregnant women were higher in numbers (37). Rest of the analysis was performed in studies involving smaller numbers ranging between 2 and 12. With the available data regardless of the sample size, there was a significantly higher incidence of IHD, HF, stroke, and onset of HT in later life, particularly in the first 5 years of postpartum, in pregnant women with prior HDP compared with pregnant women with normal BP. There was a trend toward increased incidence of VTE and dementia in later life in pregnant women with HDP compared to normotensive pregnant women; however, the sample size was small, there was no significant difference with wide range of CI and very low certainty of evidence. There was no difference in the occurrence of PAD between pregnant women with HDP and normotensives. The cardiovascular mortality and all-cause mortality were higher in pregnant women with HDP compared with normotensive pregnant women although the sample size was small.

COMMENT

There are no precise data regarding the impact of hypertensive disorders of pregnancy (HDP) on future occurrence of hypertension (HT) and cardiovascular disease (CVD)-related mortality and morbidity in pregnant women with prior HDP. Better understanding regarding this commonly occurring clinical entity will have a positive impact on a woman's health by providing insight related to optimal strategies for prevention, early detection, and treatment of cardiovascular ailments in women. This study that has included more than 50 studies and 10 million pregnant women with or without HDP throws some background information. However, the study is limited by the heterogenicity of the data and most of the parameters not reaching statistical significance and being of low certainty of evidence. Nevertheless, the study has demonstrated in accordance with other previous studies that the incidence of ischemic heart disease (IHD), heart failure (HF), stroke, and onset of HT, particularly in the first 5 years of postpartum, and cardiovascular mortality is increased in pregnant women with HDP compared to normotensive pregnant women. Further prospective collection of data mitigating the heterogenicity of the population may a better option to glean statistically significant data in the future than can be applied in clinical practice with much confidence.

ARTICLE 5

Meta-analysis of Cardiovascular Risk Factors in Offspring of Preeclampsia Pregnancies

Wang W, Lin R, Yang L, Wang Y, Mao B, Xu X, et al. Meta-analysis of cardiovascular risk factors in offspring of preeclampsia pregnancies.
Diagnostics (Basel). 2023;13(4):812.

Abstract

Introduction: Preeclampsia (PE) is a constellation of clinical abnormalities occurring after 20 weeks of pregnancy, characterized by new-onset hypertension and/or end-organ dysfunction with or without proteinuria, which can have lifelong adverse effects on the mother and child.

Methodology: The data for the meta-analysis were collected from PubMed, Web of Science, Ovid, other foreign language databases, SinoMed, China National Knowledge Infrastructure, Wanfang, and China Science and Technology Journal Databases, from January 1, 2010 to December 31, 2019 and aimed to assess the prevalence of cardiovascular risk in offspring of pregnancies complicated by PE. A random-effects model or a fixed-effects model was used, and RevMan 5.3 software was used for meta-analysis to determine the odds ratio (OR) value and 95% confidence interval (CI) of each cardiovascular risk factor. The English retrieval terms were "cardiovascular," "risk factor," "influence factor,", and "preeclampsia pregnancy." For a more complete analysis, the references of the included literature were also manually searched after the databases were searched.

Results: The meta-analysis included a total of 16 case–control studies involving a total of 4,046 cases in the experimental group and 31,505 in the control group.

This meta-analysis demonstrated the following differences in the offspring of PE and non-PE pregnancy. The PE pregnancy had offspring with higher body mass index (BMI) ($p < 0.00001$), higher systolic BP ($p < 0.00001$), and higher diastolic BP ($p < 0.00001$) when compared to the non-PE group. Higher total cholesterol ($p < 0.00001$), non-high-density lipoprotein (non-HDL) cholesterol ($p < 0.00001$), and HDL cholesterol ($p = 0.0002$) occurred in PE offspring than in non-PE offspring. The low-density cholesterol levels were comparable to those in children of non-PE pregnancy ($p = 0.48$). The triglyceride levels in PE offspring group were lower ($p < 0.00001$) as were the glucose levels ($p < 0.00001$) and insulin values ($p = 0.0004$) when compared to the non-PE group.

Conclusion: The safety of the mother and child are jeopardized in PE. Early diagnosis and early intervention and its prevention by recognizing high-risk factors and screening high-risk groups would go a long way in preventing the lifelong risk.

COMMENT

Preeclampsia (PE) is not just a derangement that occurs only at the time of pregnancy and delivery but an entity which imparts a lifelong risk of metabolic abnormalities and cardiovascular risk to the mother and child. The American Heart Association (AHA) guidelines in 2011, for the first time, listed PE as a risk factor for cardiovascular disease in women.[3] Women who had PE should be educated on the higher prevalence of the risk of lifelong elevated high blood pressure (BP) and cardiac complications, both in them and the child. The meta-analysis had shown mainly metabolic abnormalities in the offspring, in addition to elevation in systolic and diastolic BP and a higher body mass index (BMI). Postpartum pressures were more abnormal in recurrent PE. Studies have also shown that infants born to PE mothers show ventricular hypertrophy at birth, reduced left ventricular longitudinal peak systolic strain, and coronary dilatation. They also have at birth higher cord blood levels of N-terminal prohormone of brain natriuretic peptide (NT-proBNP), troponin I, homocysteine, and endothelial vascular cell adhesion molecule-1 expression, indicating endothelial inflammation. An elevated insulin level which indicates insulin resistance and the risk of metabolic syndrome is a harbinger for the development of cardiovascular disease. Infants born to early onset preeclamptic pregnancies had a greater prevalence of tetralogy of Fallot, atrioventricular septal defects, valvular dysfunction, and patent ductus arteriosus than the late-onset group.[9]

The cardiovascular risk in PE offspring can continue into adulthood. The risk of stroke in the offspring of PE pregnancy is twice that of normal pregnancy offspring and the incidence of obesity was higher.[10] Pulmonary artery pressure was 30% more and flow-mediated dilation was 30% less in the PE offspring, probably due to the augmented oxidative stress related to PE.

The ideal cardiovascular risk factor in the offspring of PE pregnancies should be identified and routine screening be advocated in them, even after they have reached adulthood.

Sodium-glucose cotransporter-2 inhibitors (SGLT-2is) have shown to be cardioprotective, and aspirin therapy started after 16 weeks of gestation is associated with a 50% reduction in PE. Whether these drugs could be extrapolated to a reduction in the cardiovascular risk in the offspring needs to be studied.

Common nutraceuticals in cardiovascular diseases including resveratrol, vitamin D, quercetin, curcumin, flavanol, etc., have been shown to be cardioprotective. The oral bioavailability of these molecules can be improved by hyaluronic acid-based nanomedicines.[3] Whether they can improve the treatment strategy to reduce cardiovascular risk in the PE offspring needs further research.

Preeclampsia can provoke by multiple pathophysiological mechanisms, a lifelong plethora of cardiovascular abnormalities in the mother and offspring. Recognition of cardiovascular risk factors in these offspring and strategic management would go a long way in reducing morbidity, both in childhood and thereafter. This meta-analysis only searched the published literature, and there is a possibility that the results of unpublished studies could affect its results.

ARTICLE 6

Early Pregnancy Cardiometabolic Risk Factors and the Prevalence of Metabolic Syndrome 10 Years after First Pregnancy

Andraweera PH, Plummer MD, Garrett A, Leemaqz S, Wittwer MR, Aldridge E, et al. Early pregnancy cardio metabolic risk factors and the prevalence of metabolic syndrome 10 years after the first pregnancy.
PLoS One. 2023;18(1):e0280451.

Abstract

Objective: The objective was to identify the presence of metabolic syndrome in women 10 years after their first pregnancy who had cardiometabolic risk factors during their first pregnancy without prepregnancy risk factors.

Material and methods: This is a prospective follow-up substudy, the cohort being taken from SCOPE multicentric prospective cohort study done between November 2004 and February 2011 in women with their first pregnancy ($n = 5,628$). Multiple parameters were analyzed and multiple studies were done with the data available from SCOPE cohort study. This study analyzed the prevalence of metabolic syndrome in women who had one or more than one metabolic risk factors in early pregnancy. Only 141 women 10 years postpartum were able to participate in this substudy done between the years 2015 and 2018. Women with preexisting comorbidities were excluded from the study as well as women with a high risk of preeclampsia and small for gestational age/preterm birth. The inclusion criteria being women with their first pregnancy at 15 ± 1 week, women were subdivided into those without any cardiometabolic risk factors and those with at least one of the following risk factors: Central obesity (according to their race and specific waist circumference value) and/or with body mass index (BMI) ≥ 30 kg/m^2, systolic blood pressure (SBP) ≥ 130 mm Hg, diastolic blood pressure (DBP) ≥ 85 mm Hg, total cholesterol ≥ 212 mg/dL, triglycerides ≥ 150, high-density lipoprotein (HDL) ≤ 46.4 mg/dL, random blood sugar (RBS) ≥ 100.8 mg/dL, and smoking. The primary outcome analyzed was the presence of metabolic syndrome (defined as per International Diabetes Federation guidelines) 10 years postpartum and secondary outcomes studied analyzed the individual risk factors—hypertension ≥ 130/85 mm Hg, BMI ≥ 30 kg/m^2, fasting blood sugar (FBS) > 100.8 mg/dL, glycated hemoglobin (HbA1c) > 6.5%, total cholesterol ≥ 212 mg/dL, triglycerides ≥ 150, HDL ≤ 46.4 mg/dL, and homeostatic model assessment for insulin resistance (HOMA-IR).

Results: Among 141 women, 29% ($n = 41$) did not have any cardiometabolic risk factors and 70.9% had one or more risk factors. Out of 41 patients who had no cardiometabolic risk factors, 90% ($n = 37$) did not develop metabolic syndrome 10 years postpartum and only 9.8% ($n = 4$) women developed metabolic syndrome. Out of 100 women who had cardiometabolic risk factors, 66% ($n = 66$) developed metabolic syndrome and 34% ($n = 34$) did not develop metabolic syndrome 10 years postpartum. Women who had one or more cardiometabolic risk factors 10 years postpartum were approximately 2 years older than women who did not have cardiometabolic risk factors ($p = 0.004$).

Women with one or more cardiometabolic risk factors are 4.8 times more likely to develop metabolic syndrome 10 years postpartum compared with women who had no risk factors during their early pregnancy. Statistically significant factors that were increased 10 years postpartum were obesity ($p = 0.001$), total cholesterol ($p < 0.001$), and increased insulin resistance (high HOMA-IR) ($p < 0.001$).

Though statistically not significant, there is an increasing trend to develop individual risk factors 10 years postpartum in women who had cardiometabolic risk factors in their early pregnancy compared to women who had no cardiometabolic risk factors in their early pregnancy. Adverse pregnancy outcomes (APOs) were also studied in this substudy which showed increased tendency of APOs in women with cardiometabolic risk factors.[3]

Conclusion: Scrutinizing the pregnant women for the cardiometabolic risk factors in their early pregnancy is useful in identifying women at risk of future cardiovascular disease (CVD) at younger age itself and in initiating the primary preventive strategies for CVD. It will probably be beneficial in primordial prevention of development of risk factors.

COMMENT

The sample size of this substudy is very small. In this study, women with cardiometabolic risk factors in their early pregnancy overnumbered women who did not have risk factors in their early pregnancy, probably because of the fact that women who had risk factors during pregnancy might be curious about their continuing or further worsening of risk factors and hence were easily recruitable. It would be beneficial if these women were followed up from immediate postpartum as there is a possibility that the risk factors for cardiovascular disease (CVD) can be identified even earlier and primary prevention strategies can be initiated as early as possible.

The hemodynamic stress of pregnancy unmasks the cardiometabolic risk factors during early pregnancy in genetically susceptible individuals. The adverse pregnancy outcome (APOs) is a prompt for more vigorous primordial prevention of CVD risk factors and primary prevention CVDs. Cholesterol treatment guidelines 2018 consider these APOs as CVD risk enhancers that would be critical to consider when deciding the use of statin for CVD prevention.[11]

ARTICLE 7

Association of Gestational Diabetes Mellitus with Overall and Type Specific Cardiovascular and Cerebrovascular Diseases: Systematic Review and Meta-analysis

Xie W, Wang Y, Xiao S, Qiu L, Yu Y, Zhang Z. Association of gestational diabetes mellitus with overall and type specific cardiovascular and cerebrovascular diseases: Systematic review and meta-analysis.
BMJ. 2022;378:e070244.

Abstract

Objective: The objective of this study was to estimate the overall risk of cardiovascular disease (CVD) and cerebrovascular disease (CeVD), as well as the risk of specific types of these diseases and venous thromboembolism, in women with a history of gestational diabetes mellitus (GDM).

Design: Systematic review and meta-analyses.

Data sources: PubMed, Embase, and the Cochrane Library from inception till November 1, 2021, and updated on May 26, 2022.

Review methods: Observational studies that evaluated the association between GDM and the development of CVD and CeVD were eligible. The data were pooled using random-effect models and presented as risk ratios [95% confidence intervals (CI)]. The certainty of evidence was appraised using the Grading of Recommendations, Assessment, Development, and Evaluations (GRADE) approach.

Results: There were 15 studies that were classified as having a moderate or serious risk of bias. There were 9,507 women with cardiovascular and cerebrovascular illness among the 5,13,324 women with GDM. 78,895 of the over eight million control women who did not have GDM had cardiovascular and cerebrovascular illness. Women with a history of GDM had a 45% increased risk of overall CVD and CeVD (risk ratio 1.45; 95% CI 1.36–1.53), a 72% increased risk of CVDs (1.72; 1.40–2.11), and a 40% increased risk of CeVDs (1.40; 1.29–1.51). Women with GDM had an increased risk of coronary artery disease (1.40; 1.18–1.65), myocardial infarction (1.74; 1.37–2.20), heart failure (1.62; 1.29–2.05), angina pectoris (2.27; 1.79–2.87), cardiovascular procedures (1.87; 1.34–2.62), stroke (1.45; 1.29–1.63), and ischemic stroke (1.49; 1.29–1.71). Women with prior GDM had a 28% increased incidence of venous thromboembolism (1.28; 1.13–1.46). Subgroup analyses of CVD and CeVD outcomes stratified by study characteristics and adjustments revealed significant differences by region ($p = 0.078$), study design ($p = 0.02$), data source ($p = 0.005$), study quality ($p = 0.04$), smoking ($p = 0.03$), BMI ($p = 0.01$), socioeconomic status ($p = 0.006$), and comorbidities ($p = 0.05$).

Conclusion: GDM is associated with increased risks of overall and type-specific CVD and CeVD that cannot be solely attributed to conventional cardiovascular risk factors or subsequent diabetes mellitus.

COMMENT

Gestational diabetes mellitus (GDM) is defined as glucose intolerance that develops during pregnancy. GDM has an impact that persists beyond pregnancy.[12] The mechanistic link between GDM and cardiovascular disease (CVD) is not fully understood, but it is thought to involve a number of factors, including insulin resistance, oxidative stress, inflammation, and endothelial dysfunction.[13] Similarly, high blood sugar levels caused by GDM can damage blood vessels in the brain and make them prone to clotting, leading to a stroke.[14] Women with GDM are more likely to have other comorbidities such as obesity, hypertension, and dyslipidemia. These risk factors can increase the risk of cardiovascular and cerebrovascular events later in life.

Overall, the meta-analysis by Xie et al. (2022) provides valuable insights into the association between GDM and CVD/cerebrovascular disease (CeVD). The findings of this study should be used to understand the prevention and management of CVD/CeVD in women with GDM. I would also like to add that the findings of this study are particularly important given the increasing prevalence of GDM worldwide. According to the World Health Organization, the prevalence of GDM is estimated to be between 2 and 10% of all pregnancies. This means that millions of women around the world are at an increased risk of CVD/CeVD as a result of their GDM. By identifying women with GDM early and providing them with appropriate care, we can help to reduce their risk of CVD/CeVD and improve their overall health.

The authors of the study also found that the risk of CVD was higher in women with GDM who developed subsequent type 2 diabetes mellitus. This suggests that the increased risk of CVD in women with GDM may be partly due to the development of type 2 diabetes mellitus. However, the risk of CVD was still significant in women with GDM who did not develop type 2 diabetes mellitus. This suggests that there are other factors, such as insulin resistance and dyslipidemia, that contribute to the increased risk of CVD in women with GDM. The certainty of evidence for the association between GDM and CVD was judged as low or very low. This is because the studies included in the review were of moderate to serious risk of bias, and the results were inconsistent across the studies. However, the findings of this study provide important information about the long-term risks of GDM.

A prospective study by Lee et al. seconds the findings of this paper. The study included over 200,000 women from the UK Biobank between 2006 and 2010. Those with a history of GDM were followed up for an average of 12 years. During the study period, over 10,000 women developed CVD. Women with a history of GDM were at a 25% increased risk of developing CVD compared to women who did not have GDM. The risk of developing CVD was highest in women who had GDM during their first pregnancy.[15] O'Hara et al. recently evaluated the association between specific dietary patterns and the risk of GDM. This study, which included data from over 100,000 pregnant women between 2009 and 2016, found that women who followed a Mediterranean diet, a DASH (Dietary Approaches to Stop Hypertension) diet, or a vegetarian diet had a reduced likelihood of developing GDM than those who followed a conventional Western diet.[16] Further research is needed to better understand the underlying mechanisms and to develop strategies for early detection and prevention of CVD and CeVD in women with a history of GDM. Maintaining a healthy weight, eating a balanced diet, exercising regularly, and monitoring blood glucose levels may reduce cardiometabolic risk.

ARTICLE 8

Coronary Artery Bypass Graft Surgery for Spontaneous Coronary Artery Dissection in Early Pregnancy: Medical and Ethical Decision-making Issues

Yabut AG, Bachar B, Nagm H. Coronary artery bypass graft surgery for spontaneous coronary artery dissection in early pregnancy: Medical and ethical decision-making issues.
Cureus. 2023;15(2):e35364.

Abstract

Introduction: Spontaneous coronary artery dissection (SCAD) is a rare presentation during the postpartum period and also in the antepartum phase of pregnancy.

Case presentation: A 36-year-old multiparous Caucasian female who was 17 days pregnant with a past medical history of hypertension had chest pain that radiates to her left shoulder, arm, and back. Cardiac catheterization showed severe diffuse left anterior descending coronary artery (LAD) disease in the proximal segment with the middle LAD and diagonal branches being subtotally occluded. The posterior lateral artery (PLA) branch of the right coronary artery (RCA) had severe disease and LAD had a spiral dissection involving its entire length, first diagonal, and second diagonal. Coronary artery bypass grafting (CABG) was done with left internal mammary artery (LIMA) to middle LAD, saphenous vein graft (SVG) to distal LAD, and SVG to diagonal. The woman had no issues with the fetus. In 5 days postoperatively, echo showed an ejection fraction of 35–40% and a moderate left ventricular systolic dysfunction, and the patient was discharged.

Discussion: SCAD is defined as an acute manifestation of a false, separate lumen within the coronary artery, either caused by an internal tear or an acute bleeding within the tunica media of the arterial wall.[17] Risk factors include pregnancy, multiparty, connective tissue disease, and emotional and physical stress. The pathophysiology of SCAD is due to hormonal changes in pregnancy and increased volume overload. The majority of patients with SCAD (70–97%) spontaneously heal with conservative management.[18]

The failure rates associated with invasive procedures such as percutaneous transluminal coronary angioplasty (PTCA) and CABG surgery were higher in pregnant SCAD patients, whereas the mortality rates are comparable with nonpregnant SCAD patients.[19] Revascularization does not prevent the recurrence of SCAD. Doing PTCA in a dissected artery is technically challenging, especially for crossing the wire. Radiation safety should be followed to protect the fetus. In selected cases with involvement of more than two proximal coronary arteries, CABG is preferred. Medical termination of pregnancy can be considered in the early months of pregnancy considering the safety of the mother.

COMMENT

Pregnant women at risk should be screened for SCAD with serial high-sensitivity (Hs) troponin levels and echocardiography. To provide medical counseling for pregnant women or those planning a pregnancy to better recognize its subtle signs and symptoms and timely specialist referral, diagnosis, and treatment. Spontaneous coronary artery dissection (SCAD) carries a higher risk of occurrence in subsequent pregnancy. By coronary artery bypass grafting (CABG), fetal demise is high, likely due to prolonged time of surgery, use of cardiopulmonary bypass (CPB) machine, and anesthesia. Percutaneous transluminal coronary angioplasty (PTCA) is a preferred for SCAD involving the single proximal coronary artery. SCAD in proximal coronary artery with good distal flow and SCAD in distal small vessels can be managed medically.

ARTICLE 9

Contemporary Rates of Pre-pregnancy Hypertension and Diabetes Among a Multi-ethnic Sample of Pregnant Individuals in a Diverse US State

Farina LA, Pool LR, Giase GM, Feinglass JM, Khan SS. Contemporary rates of pre-pregnancy hypertension and diabetes among a multi-ethnic sample of pregnant individuals in a diverse US state.
Eur J Prev Cardiol. 2022;29(10):1460-2.

Abstract

Background: Pregnancy is a state of increased metabolism, hypercoagulability, and low vascular resistance. Cardiovascular diseases (CVD) are the leading cause of maternal morbidity and mortality in the United States (US), with the most important cardiometabolic risk factors being diabetes mellitus (DM) and hypertension (HTN).[20] They share the same pathophysiology which includes inflammation, endothelial dysfunction, and oxidative stress which adversely affect maternal and fetal outcomes.[21] This study aimed to identify the prevalence and racial disparities in pregnant women with prepregnancy HTN and DM, which would help in the formation of public health strategies.

Methods: Data were analyzed from 127 nonfederal hospitals with childbirth admissions of Illinois residents. All delivery-related hospital admissions between 2016 and 2019 in the age group of 20–44 years were included. Individuals aged 45 years and above were excluded from the study as they accounted for only 0.25% of all live births. The International Classification of Diseases, 10th revision (ICD-10) diagnostic codes were used to identify prepregnancy HTN and DM. The age-standardized rates and 95% confidence intervals (CIs) per 1,000 live births as well as age group–specific rates were calculated. Annual increases were calculated with linear regression and prevalence ratios (PRs) across the study period with log binomial regression models. Analyses were completed using R 3.5.2 and SAS version 9.4 (Cary, NC).

Findings: Delivery-related hospitalization during the study period included 522,205 individuals, of which 51% were non-Hispanic White, 17% were Hispanic, 15% were non-Hispanic Black, and 5% were Asian/Pacific Islander. The mean maternal age was 29.9 (5.3) years. The rates of prepregnancy HTN initially declined from 2016 to 2017, followed by an increase in 2017 from 28.9 to 33.3 per 1,000 live births in 2019. The average annual increase between 2017 and 2019 was 2.2 per 1,000 live births. This pattern of increase was noted across all age groups. The rates of prepregnancy DM were stable from 2016 to 2018 but significantly increased from 2018 to 2019 to 1.0 per 1,000 live births.

Non-Hispanic Black individuals had significantly higher prepregnancy HTN (PR 2.87; $p < 0.001$) and DM (PR 2.10; $p < 0.001$) rates compared with non-Hispanic White individuals. Hispanic individuals had similar rates of prepregnancy HTN (PR 0.99; $p = 0.91$) but significantly higher DM (PR 2.87; $p < 0.001$) rates, compared with non-Hispanic White individuals. Asian/Pacific Islander individuals had significantly lower prepregnancy HTN (PR 0.62; $p < 0.001$) but significantly higher DM (PR 1.29; $p = 0.04$) rates, compared with non-Hispanic White individuals. Public insurance or self-pay individuals had significantly higher rates of both prepregnancy HTN (PR 1.41; $p < 0.001$) and prepregnancy DM (PR 1.89; $p < 0.001$) compared with privately insured individuals. In multivariable adjusted models, there was minimal prevalence difference in the insurance status of HTN and DM between non-Hispanic Black and non-Hispanic White individuals.

Conclusion: The study demonstrates increasing rates of prepregnancy HTN and DM between 2016 and 2019 in Illinois. The results are consistent with previous reports demonstrating increasing rates of HTN and DM among reproductive-aged and pregnant persons in recent decades. Key disparities by race and ethnicity were noted in the prevalence of these conditions, with the greatest burden among non-Hispanic Black individuals. The increasing rates of chronic conditions among pregnant individuals were attributed to a rise in the average maternal age, but even younger adults demonstrated an increase in the rates of prepregnancy HTN and DM. The increased prevalence may also reflect an increase in the prevalence of prepregnancy obesity which shares similar risk factors.

The main limitation of the study was that it was not possible to test the contributions of obesity, dietary factors (e.g., sodium and saturated fat intake), and physical activity to the findings, and we need future studies to examine these questions. Other limitations include reliance on ICD-10 codes, aggregation of Hispanic and Asian/Pacific Islander subgroups, and a focus on a single state, Illinois, which may limit generalizability. However, since the data were obtained from a diverse sample, this limitation may be overlooked. In conclusion, the study data demonstrate a concerning rise in the maternal burden of prepregnancy HTN and DM. There is a critical need to focus on the recognition and prevention of CVD risk factors prior to pregnancy in order to reduce maternal mortality and morbidity.

COMMENT

This study estimates the prevalence and racial disparity among women with prepregnancy hypertension (HTN) and diabetes mellitus (DM). It demonstrates increasing rates of HTN and DM with the greatest burden among non-Hispanic Black individuals. The increasing prevalence is attributed to age and obesity, although the contributions of other risk factors were not estimated in this study. The alarming rise in the prevalence of pregnancy-associated risk factors needs to be met with caution. Public health measures should be implemented to educate the general public about the need for prevention. Health camps should be conducted on a regular basis to identify these cardiovascular risk factors in the early stages so that they can be managed appropriately. Further research is needed to develop reliable early screening and diagnostic tools and explore effective and safe treatment strategies at the population level.[22]

ARTICLE 10

Pregnancy Loss and Risk of Incident CVD Within 5 Years: Findings from the Women's Health Initiative

Wright CE, Enquobahrie DA, Prager S, Painter I, Kooperberg C, Wild RA, Park K, et al. Pregnancy loss and risk of incident CVD within 5 years: Findings from the Women's Health Initiative.
Front Cardiovasc Med. 2023;10:1108286.

Abstract

Background: Pregnancy loss has been associated with an increased risk of atherosclerotic cardiovascular disease (ASCVD). The loss of pregnancy is described as a risk marker for early onset ASCVD but not discussed in earlier studies as a risk marker for post menopausal ASCVD.

Methods: The postmenopausal women from the Women's Health Observational cohort and three randomized trials on hormone replacement, diet, and vitamin D were pooled ($n = 161,808$). Those with preexisting cardiovascular disease (CVD), never been pregnant, and participants in clinical trials were excluded. The rest without evident CVD ($n = 73,805$) were followed up in three groups based on baseline age at inclusion into the study: 50–59, 60–69, and 70–79 years. The outcomes recorded were incident CVD, coronary heart disease (CHD), heart failure, and stroke. The outcomes were recorded over a 5-year period from baseline. Other conventional risk factors were also recorded. Self-declared history of the number of pregnancies and loss of pregnancy (miscarriage or stillbirth) were recorded. Those with a history of loss of pregnancy were compared with those who did not have pregnancy loss. Stillbirth and recurrent pregnancy loss were analyzed as a separate cohort and as a part of the entire loss of pregnancy cohort.

Results: The odds of developing heart disease were higher when there was a loss of pregnancy. Stillbirth had the maximum association with CVD after adjustment for other risk factors or confounders. The odds were higher with history of stillbirth compared to loss of pregnancy.

Following adjustment for confounders, the significant odds ratio for various outcomes are given in **Table 1**.

TABLE 1: Post adjustment for confounders, the significant odds ratio is described.	
	Odds ratio at 5 years from baseline
History of any pregnancy loss ($n = 24,995$)	1.29: Incident CVD
History of recurrent pregnancy loss ($n = 8,796$)	1.17: CHD
	1.35: Heart failure
History of stillbirth ($n = 3054$)	1.47: Incident CVD
	1.81: CHD
	1.76: Heart failure
	1.53: Stroke
(CHD: coronary heart disease; CVD: cardiovascular disease)	

Age-stratified analysis revealed that stillbirth at any age group and recurrent pregnancy loss in 60–69 year age group were associated with incident CVD. Any pregnancy loss was associated with CHD only in the 70–79 year age group. Significant heart failure was significantly associated in recurrent pregnancy loss in the 50–59 and 60–69 year age groups and stillbirth in 70–79 year age group. Significant stroke was noticed with recurrent pregnancy loss in the 50–59 year age group and stillbirth in the 70–79 year age group **(Table 2)**.

TABLE 2: Age-stratified risk analysis 5 years from baseline across age groups. The significant follow-up findings for baseline age groups are 50–59, 60–69, and 70–79 years.

	Incident CVD	CHD	Heart failure	Stroke
History of any pregnancy loss	NS	70–79 years	NS	NS
History of recurrent pregnancy loss	60–69 years	NS	50–59 years 60–69 years	50–59 years
History of stillbirth	Significant in all three age groups	50–59 and 60–69 years	70–79 years	70–79 years

(CHD: coronary heart disease; CVD: cardiovascular disease; NS: not significant)

Conclusion: Loss of pregnancy, especially stillbirth, is correlated with future CVD events. All women should be assessed for loss of pregnancy in the risk stratification for ASCVD both before and after a CVD event. Future guidelines need to emphasize this as a risk factor and stress on aggressive preventive measures to prevent ASCVD.

COMMENT

Obstructive coronary artery disease (CAD) in women develops 7–10 years late, compared to men. Pregnancy-related events and future cardiovascular disease (CVD) events are a very underrecognized and underrated risk marker in the assessment of atherosclerotic cardiovascular disease (ASCVD). A consensus document from the European cardiologists, gynecologists, and endocrinologists has recommended that women's risk profile must include history of preterm delivery, preeclampsia, gestational diabetes, gestational hypertension, and infant size. Recurrent pregnancy loss has also been mentioned in a separate statement.[23,24]

This paper provides valuable information on the fact that pregnancy loss (especially stillbirth) is a significant risk factor to predict incident CVD events. Stillbirth is almost entirely due to maternal factors which might have a common soil with ASCVD risk factors. Endothelial dysfunction could lead to poor placentation. It is also an important forerunner to ASCVD and heart failure. Early loss of pregnancy can be due to chromosomal anomalies and can skew the pregnancy loss data. Recurrent loss of pregnancy is more likely due to vascular causes which can lead to later ASCVD. Recurrent pregnancy loss and ASCVD have common risk factors—smoking, obesity, and alcohol intake.[24] The reverse, that is, families with manifest ASCVD, have more of pregnancy loss as seen in a Danish registry.[25] Recording the gestational age of pregnancy loss was not done in the present study and could have provided valuable information on this correlation.

There are very important messages in this paper for both primary and secondary prevention of ASCVD. In the primary prevention area, addition of the pregnancy-related risk factors, especially pregnancy loss and stillbirth, will add value to the ASCVD risk score estimation. Pregnancy loss also gives an opportunity to educate the mother on the risks of future ASCVD events and stress on regular risk factor screening and lifestyle modification to prevent such events. In secondary prevention, this history will provide a vital missing link regarding the risk factors, especially in the 15% of postmenopausal women who do not have any other significant risk factors.

The only limitation was that the gestational age was not recorded and could have given valuable information regarding the proposed role of fetal loss regarding maternal and fetal factors. The maternal age at pregnancy loss was also not available—correlation of this with the time of onset of the outcomes could give vital chronological data.

Future research should focus on the gestational age and the common soil for pregnancy and ASCVD. Guideline writers should emphasize this history and should not miss the opportunity to carefully screen and monitor the women with pregnancy loss for future ASCVD events.

ARTICLE 11

Management of Hypertension in Pregnancy

Beech A, Mangos G. Management of hypertension in pregnancy.
Aust Prescr. 2021;44(5):148-52.

Abstract

Background: Hypertension during pregnancy is common and is responsible for maternal and fetal mortality and morbidity. Hypertension may be preexisting or newly developed during pregnancy. Chronic hypertension is diagnosed when hypertension predates the pregnancy or is first diagnosed before 20 weeks' gestation. When hypertension is diagnosed at or after 20 weeks' gestation, it is labeled gestational hypertension. Preeclampsia and eclampsia are gestational hypertension with evidence of other system involvement. Close monitoring of mother and fetus is needed to avoid complications. Only drugs proven safe in pregnancy can be prescribed.

Hypertension during pregnancy is defined as a systolic blood pressure 140 mm Hg or above or diastolic blood pressure 90 mm Hg or above, while severe hypertension is defined as a systolic blood pressure 160 mm Hg or above or a diastolic blood pressure 110 mm Hg or above. Hypertension in pregnancy is to be reconfirmed by a repeat measurement after 4 hours or after an overnight rest. Severe hypertension required urgent hospital management.

Hypertension during pregnancy is classified into four varieties: (1) Chronic hypertension (primary or secondary), (2) gestational hypertension, (3) preeclampsia and eclampsia, and (4) chronic hypertension with superimposed preeclampsia.[26]

Summary

Chronic hypertension: Hypertension is diagnosed before the 20th week or predates pregnancy. This includes both primary hypertension and, less commonly, secondary hypertension. Investigations for secondary hypertension are not routinely recommended during pregnancy; however, they can be done postpartum if needed. Basic investigations needed include complete blood counts, urea, creatinine and electrolytes, liver function tests, uric acid, urinalysis and microscopy, urine protein:creatinine ratio (to establish a baseline), and ECG. The adverse outcomes related to chronic hypertension in pregnancy include preterm delivery (28%), superimposed preeclampsia (25%), fetal growth restriction (17%), and perinatal death (4%). White-coat hypertension is said to be present if office blood pressure is >140/90 mm Hg while home blood pressure or 24-hour ambulatory blood pressure is normal. White-coat hypertension does not require treatment unless the blood pressure is >160/100 mm Hg.

Drugs to be avoided in pregnancy: Angiotensin-converting enzyme inhibitors (ACEIs), angiotensin receptor blockers, beta-blockers other than labetalol, diuretics, and calcium channel blockers other than nifedipine and diltiazem are to be avoided during pregnancy.

Preferred drugs in pregnancy: Labetalol, controlled-release nifedipine, methyldopa, hydralazine, and prazosin are safe antihypertensives in pregnancy.

Maintaining the blood pressure around 110–140/85 mm Hg is recommended along with close surveillance for development of preeclampsia, fetal growth, and well-being.

Gestational hypertension: This is the development of hypertension at or after 20 weeks' gestation, in the absence of features of preeclampsia. 25% of patients with gestational hypertension go on to develop preeclampsia. Risk factors for preeclampsia include maternal age, primiparity, previous preeclampsia, multiple gestation, prolonged interpregnancy interval, and assisted reproduction therapies. Women at high risk of preeclampsia should start aspirin 150 mg daily at 12–16 weeks' gestation and continue until 36 weeks' gestation, to reduce the risk of preterm preeclampsia. Maintaining BP in desired range and watching for development of preeclampsia are the mainstay of therapy. Gestational hypertension is associated with the future development of cardiovascular disease.

Preeclampsia: Gestational hypertension with one or more signs of new-onset proteinuria or new-onset organ dysfunction—liver/kidney/neurological/hematological/uteroplacental dysfunction—constitutes preeclampsia. Preeclampsia may be superimposed on chronic hypertension, or present as new-onset hypertension, arising at or after 20 weeks' gestation. Preeclampsia is a complex multisystem disorder of pregnancy arising from abnormal placentation, resulting in an imbalance of angiogenic and antiangiogenic factors, oxidative stress, and immunological involvement. Signs and symptoms suggestive of preeclampsia include headache, visual changes, epigastric or right upper quadrant pain, and edema.

Adverse outcomes include eclampsia, stroke, multiorgan failure, major hemorrhage and death, fetal growth restriction, preterm delivery, placental abruption, and perinatal death.

Management: A multidisciplinary approach at a specialist center with the required protocols and expertise is required for the management of preeclampsia. The intricate balance between the welfare of the growing fetus and the ongoing risk of maternal complications should be considered during management, as termination of the pregnancy is the only cure of preeclampsia. Drugs to rapidly lower blood pressure are required for management of severe hypertension. An infusion of magnesium sulfate can be considered as it reduces the rate of seizure by 50%. Use of aspirin reduces the risk of preterm birth, fetal growth restriction, and fetal death but may increase postpartum bleeding.

Postpartum management: After delivery, hypertension resolves within 12 weeks for women with gestational hypertension or preeclampsia. Investigation for primary or secondary hypertension may be considered if hypertension does not resolve by this time. Antihypertensive drugs that are safe in pregnancy are also safe in breastfeeding, except methyldopa which is associated with a 30% risk of depression. ACEIs, such as enalapril, have very low concentrations in breast milk and can be used during lactation.

Long-term management: Gestational hypertension and preeclampsia are associated with a two- to fourfold increase in the future risk of cardiovascular disease. There is an increased incidence of hypertension, stroke, diabetes, venous thromboembolic disease, or chronic kidney disease. Women with a history of hypertension in pregnancy require indefinite follow-up with annual reviews of blood pressure, fasting lipids, and blood glucose. Counseling on a healthy lifestyle and diet, maintenance of an optimal body mass index (BMI), smoking cessation, and regular exercise are essential for optimizing long-term health outcomes.

COMMENT

This article serves as a simplified guide for prescribers in Australia and is authored by an obstetric medicine specialist cum endocrinologist and a nephrologist. It is important to note that this article does not represent a consensus statement from any specific organization.

Hypertensive disorders during pregnancy (HDP) are widespread and can lead to health problems and even death for both the mother and the fetus. HDP rank as the second most prevalent cause of maternal mortality worldwide, following maternal hemorrhage. The occurrence of HDP is on the rise due to factors such as delayed age of first pregnancy, higher rates of obesity, and an increased presence of other cardiometabolic risk factors.

Between 1994 and 2011, hospitalizations for pregnancy-related strokes witnessed a staggering increase of over 60%. Furthermore, the rates of strokes associated with HDP were twice as high compared to strokes unrelated to HDP.[26] The incidence of white-coat hypertension in pregnancy is about 4–30%. It is also crucial to acknowledge that white-coat hypertension is not benign and is actually linked to a higher chance of developing preeclampsia (8%).

Women may already have chronic hypertension or may develop hypertension during pregnancy. According to the simplified classification provided by the National Institute for Health and Care Excellence (NICE) guidelines[27] and World Health Organization (WHO), a blood pressure reading higher than 160/110 mm Hg is considered severe hypertension, while a reading of 160/110 mm Hg or lower is classified as nonsevere hypertension. This article broadly follows a similar classification.

The American College of Obstetricians and Gynecologists (ACOG) guidelines[28] recommend the use of antihypertensive therapy for women with preeclampsia and a sustained systolic blood pressure of 160 mm Hg or higher or a diastolic blood pressure of 110 mm Hg or higher. For women with chronic hypertension, treatment is recommended when the systolic blood pressure is 160 mm Hg or higher or the diastolic blood pressure is 110 mm Hg or higher. The target blood pressure range for treatment is 120 to 160/80 to 110 mm Hg. However, it is worth noting that internationally, most hypertension societies advocate for a more aggressive approach to antihypertensive treatment, suggesting therapy when blood pressure reaches 140/90 mm Hg or higher. The NICE guidelines propose initiating antihypertensive therapy when the blood pressure exceeds 140/90 mm Hg.

The NICE guidelines[27] have lowered the target blood pressure range to be maintained during the antenatal period from 150/100 to 135/85 mm Hg. However, this article suggests a preferred range of 110–140 mm Hg for systolic blood pressure. Unlike the NICE guidelines, which prioritize certain antihypertensive medications in pregnancy (such as labetalol, nifedipine, or methyldopa depending on suitability), this article considers all of these options to be equally viable. Low-dose aspirin, starting between 12 and 16 weeks of gestation, reduces the risk of preeclampsia and related adverse outcomes by 10–20% in women at an increased risk of preeclampsia.[26]

It is important to note that the classification of hypertensive disorders of pregnancy does not specifically include postpartum hypertension and postpartum preeclampsia. However, there is growing awareness of their significance.[26] The prevalence of postpartum hypertension may be as high as 8% in women without antepartum hypertension. The duration ranges from days to 3 months, contributing to serious short-term maternal complications such as stroke, seizures, and cardiomyopathy and metabolic dysregulation such as insulin resistance and weight gain.

REFERENCES

1. Assibey-Mensah V, Fabio A, Mendez DD, Lee PC, Roberts JM, Catov JM. Neighbourhood Assets and Early Pregnancy Cardiometabolic Risk Factors. Paediatr Perinat Epidemiol. 2019:33:79-87.
2. Aparicio E, Jardí C, Bedmar C, Pallejà M, Basora J, Arija V, The Eclipses Study Group. Nutrient Intake during Pregnancy and Post-Partum: ECLIPSES Study. Nutrients. 2020; 12(5):1325.
3. Parikh NI, Gonzalez JM, Anderson CAM, Judd SE, Rexrode KM, Hlatky MA, et al.; American Heart Association Council on Epidemiology and Prevention; Council on Arteriosclerosis, Thrombosis and Vascular Biology; Council on Cardiovascular and Stroke Nursing; and the Stroke Council. Adverse Pregnancy Outcomes and Cardiovascular Disease Risk: Unique Opportunities for Cardiovascular Disease Prevention in Women: A Scientific Statement from the American Heart Association. Circulation. 2021;143(18):e902-16.
4. Brown MA, Magee LA, Kenny LC, Karumanchi SA, McCarthy FP, Saito S, et al. Ishaku S and International Society for the Study of Hypertension in P. Hypertensive Disorders of Pregnancy: ISSHP Classification, Diagnosis, and Management Recommendations for International Practice. Hypertension. 2018;72:24-43.
5. Heida KY, Franx A, van Rijn BB, Eijkemans MJC, Boer JMA, Verschuren MWM, et al. Earlier Age of Onset of Chronic Hypertension and Type 2 Diabetes Mellitus After a Hypertensive Disorder of Pregnancy or Gestational Diabetes Mellitus. Hypertension. 2015;66:1116-22.
6. Gasse C, Boutin A, Coté M, Chaillet N, Bujold E, Demers S. First-trimester mean arterial blood pressure and the risk of preeclampsia: The Great Obstetrical Syndromes (GOS) study. Pregnancy Hypertens. 201812;178-82.

7. Mammaro A, Carrara S, Cavaliere A, Ermito S, Dinatale A, Pappalardo EM, Militello M, Pedata R. Hypertensive disorders of pregnancy. J Prenat Med. 2009;3(1):1-5.
8. Kintiraki E, Papakatsika S, Kotronis G, Goulis DG, Kotsis V. Pregnancy-Induced hypertension. Hormones (Athens). 2015;14(2):211-23.
9. Kanata M, Liazou E, Chainoglou A, Kotsis V, Stabouli S. Clinical outcomes of hypertensive disorders in pregnancy in the offspring during perinatal period, childhood, and adolescence. J Hum Hypertens. 2021;35:1063-73.
10. Yang SW, Oh MJ, Park KV, Han SW, Kim HS, Sohn IS, et al. Risk of Early Childhood Obesity in Offspring of Women with Preeclampsia: A Population-Based Study. J Clin Med. 2021;10:3758.
11. Grundy SM, Stone NJ, Bailey AL, Beam C, Birtcher KK, Blumenthal RS, et al. 2018 AHA/ACC/AACVPR/AAPA/ABC/ACPM/ADA/AGS/APhA/ASPC/NLA/PCNA Guideline on the Management of Blood Cholesterol: Executive Summary: A Report of the American College of Cardiology/American Heart Association Task Force on Clinical Practice Guidelines. J Am Coll Cardiol. 2019;73(24):3168-209.
12. Reece EA, Leguizamón G, Wiznitzer A. Gestational diabetes: the need for a common ground. Lancet. 2009;373:1789-97.
13. Odegaard AO, Jacobs DR Jr, Sanchez OA, Goff DC Jr, Reiner AP, Gross MD. Oxidative stress, inflammation, endothelial dysfunction and incidence of type 2 diabetes. Cardiovasc Diabetol. 2016;15:51.
14. Liu S, Chan WS, Ray JG, Kramer MS, Joseph K. Stroke and Cerebrovascular Disease in Pregnancy. Stroke. 2019;50(1):13-20.
15. Lee SM, Shivakumar M, Park JW, Jung YM, Choe EK, Kwak SH, et al. Long-term cardiovascular outcomes of gestational diabetes mellitus: a prospective UK Biobank study. Cardiovasc Diabetol. 2022;21(1):221.
16. O'Hara H, Taylor J, Woodside JV. The Association of Specific Dietary Patterns with Cardiometabolic Outcomes in Women with a History of Gestational Diabetes Mellitus: A Scoping Review. Nutrients. 2023;15(7):1613.
17. Adlam D, García-Guimaraes M, Maas AHEM. Spontaneous coronary artery dissection: No longer a rare disease. Eur Heart J. 2019;40(15):1198-201.
18. Hayes SN, Kim ES, Saw J, Adlam D, Arslanian-Engoren C, Economy KE, et al. Spontaneous coronary artery dissection: current state of the science: a scientific statement from the American Heart Association. Circulation. 2018;137:e523-7.
19. Havakuk O, Goland S, Mehra A, Elkayam U. Pregnancy and the risk of spontaneous coronary artery dissection: An analysis of 120 contemporary cases. Circ Cardiovasc Interv. 201710(3):e004941.
20. Centres for Disease Control and Prevention. (2020). Pregnancy mortality surveillance system. [online] Available from https://www.cdc.gov/reproductivehealth/maternal-mortality/pregnancy-mortality-surveillance-system.htm [Last accessed October, 2023].
21. Yang Y, Wu N. Gestational diabetes mellitus and preeclampsia: correlation and influencing factors. Front Cardiovasc Med. 2022;9:831297.
22. Jiang L, Tang K, Magee LA, von Dadelszen P, Ekeroma A, Li X, et al. A global view of hypertensive disorders and diabetes mellitus during pregnancy. Nat Rev Endocrinol. 2022;18(12):760-75.
23. Maas AHEM, Rosano G, Cifkova R, Chieffo A, van Dijken D, Hamoda H, et al. Cardiovascular health after menopause transition, pregnancy disorders, and other gynaecologic conditions: a consensus document from European cardiologists, gynaecologists, and endocrinologists. Eur Heart J. 2021;42(10):967-84.
24. Sanghavi M, Parikh NI. Harnessing the Power of Pregnancy and Pregnancy-Related Events to Predict Cardiovascular Disease in Women. Circulation. 2017;135(6):590-2.
25. Ranthe MF, Diaz LJ, Behrens I, Bundgaard H, Simonsen J, Melbye M, et al. Association between pregnancy losses in women and risk of atherosclerotic disease in their relatives: a nationwide cohort study. Eur Heart J. 2016;37(11):900-7.
26. Garovic VD, Dechend R, AHA HDP GL T, Karumanchi SA, McMurtry Baird S, Magee LA, et al. Hypertension in Pregnancy: Diagnosis, Blood Pressure Goals, and Pharmacotherapy: A Scientific Statement from the American Heart Association. Hypertension. 2022;79(2):e21-41.
27. Webster K, Fishburn S, Maresh M, Findlay SC, Chappell LC. Diagnosis and management of hypertension in pregnancy: summary of updated NICE guidance. BMJ. 2019;366:l5119.
28. American College of Obstetricians and Gynecologists' Committee on Practice Bulletins—Obstetrics. ACOG Practice Bulletin No. 203: Chronic Hypertension in Pregnancy. Obstet Gynecol. 2019;133(1):e26-50.

SECTION 2

Hypertension and CVD in Women

Section Editor: **Sujatha Vipperla**

Associate Editors: Anil Kumar Mahapatro, Achukatla Kumar

ARTICLE 1

Sex Differences in Arterial Hypertension: A Scientific Statement from the ESC Council on Hypertension, the European Association of Preventive Cardiology, Association of Cardiovascular Nursing and Allied Professions, the ESC Council for Cardiology Practice, and the ESC Working Group on Cardiovascular Pharmacotherapy

Gerdts E, Sudano I, Brouwers S, Borghi C, Bruno RM, Ceconi C, et al. Sex differences in arterial hypertension. *Eur Heart J. 2022;43(46):4777-88.*

Abstract

Significant evidence exists indicating that sex chromosomes and sex hormones have distinct effects on blood pressure (BP) regulation, distribution of cardiovascular (CV) risk factors, and associated conditions in individuals with essential arterial hypertension, varying between females and males. The risk of CV disease increases at a lower BP level in females compared to males, implying the need for different sex-specific thresholds for diagnosing hypertension. However, due to the limited availability of data, especially from well-designed clinical trials, it remains uncertain whether hypertension should be managed differently in females and males, encompassing treatment goals and the selection and dosage of antihypertensive medications.

In light of these uncertainties, this consensus document is the first of its kind highlighting the sex differences in hypertension. The document emphasizes the need for focused research in specific areas to advance sex-specific prevention and management of hypertension.

COMMENT

Hypertension is the most common risk factor for cardiovascular disease (CVD) and the recent European guidelines address the sex-specific differences of this common problem.

Blood Pressure Transitions

Sex differences in blood pressure (BP) trajectories start early in life, with females showing a slightly faster increase in systolic BP up to age 12 years, followed by a slower increase resulting in lower BP than males starting at age 13 years. Diastolic BP is initially higher in females, but both sexes increase similarly until age 12 years, after which it decreases faster in males.[1] The transition from optimal BP to prehypertension is more frequent in young males. In adulthood, males have higher and steeper BP levels until age 40 years, after which females show a steeper rise in BP throughout life.[2] During menopause, around 35% of females experience an accelerated increase in systolic BP, possibly related to factors such as weight gain and vasomotor symptoms.[3] Globally, one-third of the population has hypertension with prevalence being similar between sexes.[4]

Sex Differences in BP Regulators

Ovarian hormones, particularly estrogen in premenopausal females, play a vital role in regulating BP and are associated with lower BP levels. Conversely, testosterone is prohypertensive and contributes to increased cardiovascular risk in males and postmenopausal females by activating the renin–angiotensin–aldosterone system (RAAS).[5] Estrogens reduce plasma renin and angiotensin-converting enzyme (ACE) activity while increasing angiotensinogen expression, leading to higher levels of angiotensin and aldosterone, resulting in sodium retention which is countered by progesterone.[6] When females become hypertensive, they tend to have lower plasma renin activity compared to males. After menopause, females experience increased salt sensitivity due to lower estrogen levels, associated with upregulated hormonal systems such as the RAAS and sympathetic nervous system, and reduced vascular nitric oxide bioavailability.[5]

Risk Factors

Sex differences in cardiovascular (CV) risk factors in hypertension are notable, particularly related to smoking, metabolic factors (such as obesity, type 2 diabetes mellitus, and dyslipidemia), and co-existing conditions (such as sleep apnea, renal dysfunction, and autoimmune disorders).[7] Women with hypertensive disorders of pregnancy and polycystic ovarian disease have a higher risk of chronic hypertension.[8] Women have a higher incidence of autoimmune and inflammatory disease and obesity which increases the risk of hypertension as compared to men who have a higher risk of dyslipidemia, smoking, and obstructive sleep apnea. Though women have less incidence of diabetes, they have worse prognoses compared to men.[9] Women have reduced glomerular filtration rates while men have albuminuria.

Sex Differences in Hypertension-mediated Organ Damage

Left ventricular hypertrophy is more common in women, less amenable to treatment, and mitigates the lower cardiovascular risk in women.[9,10] Dilated left atrium is more prevalent in women.[11] Women have higher arterial stiffness, steeper carotid-femoral pulse wave velocity increases, and peripheral vascular resistance. Arterial stiffness measured by the ratio of pulse pressure to stroke volume index (PP/SVi) predicts the transition from diastolic hypertension to isolated systolic hypertension and is higher in women.[12] Increased arterial stiffness does not decrease with treatment and leads to microvascular dysfunction in females.

Sex Differences in BP Association with CVD

Hypertension is the most important cause of mortality and is more harmful in women than men with CVD risk manifesting at a lower BP level in women than men.[13] Women develop higher myocardial and vascular stiffness due to hypertension which translates into a higher risk of atrial fibrillation, heart failure with preserved ejection fraction, and stroke.[14] Hypertension is more common in women with aortic stenosis and stroke.[15] Hypertension in women is associated with the progression of aortic valve calcification in women in contrast to dyslipidemia in men. The risk of stroke occurs at lower BP levels in women. Hypertension predisposes to peripheral arterial disease with women being older and more obese at diagnosis.

Sex Differences in the Effect of Antihypertensive Treatment

There are gender-based differences in the reported adverse effects of antihypertensive medications. Females tend to experience more negative effects compared to males, except for mineralocorticoid receptor antagonists. Specifically, women are more prone to hyponatremia, hypokalemia, and arrhythmia when taking diuretics, edema when using dihydropyridine calcium channel blockers (CCBs), and cough when taking ACE inhibitors (ACEIs). On the other hand, males are more likely to experience gout while on diuretic treatment and sexual dysfunction when using beta-blockers.[16] Hypertensive women respond better to salt restriction and in contrast, hypertensive respond better to structured exercise therapy.[17]

Sex differences in the effects of antihypertensive drugs on BP are well-documented. Females tend to experience enhanced BP reduction from beta-blockers and calcium channel blockers.[18] Prescription patterns reveal that females are often prescribed diuretics, while males receive ACEIs more frequently. Sex-specific treatment effects have been reported in certain trials such as the Hypertension Optimal Treatment Study, the Second Australian National BP Study, and the Valsartan Antihypertensive Long-term Use Evaluation Trial, though many trials demonstrated comparable benefits for both genders. A meta-analysis by the BP Lowering Treatment Trialists' Collaboration found that various antihypertensive drug classes showed similar BP reductions and cardiovascular event rates in males and females.[19] Another network meta-analysis confirmed thiazides as a comparable first-line therapy for both genders across different outcomes, with no significant differences between medication classes.[20] Though awareness of hypertension was higher in women, BP control was suboptimal in women.

In conclusion, incorporating sex differences in blood pressure development, regulation, and cardiovascular risk factors into prevention strategies could notably enhance CVD prevention, especially among females. Future clinical research should explore whether tailoring hypertension management to sex-specific blood pressure thresholds and treatment goals can enhance CVD prevention.

ARTICLE 2

Sex and Gender in Hypertension Guidelines

Meinert F, Thomopoulos C, Kreutz R. Sex and gender in hypertension guidelines.
J Hum Hypertens. 2023;37:654-61.

Abstract

The paper examines 11 international and selected national hypertension guidelines, focusing on gender-related differences in hypertension. These differences stem from both biological sex and socially influenced gender norms. All guidelines acknowledge higher hypertension rates in men compared to women but agree that blood pressure thresholds and treatment goals should be the same for both genders. Variations extend to diagnostic indices such as left ventricular mass and alcohol intake limits. Practical recommendations are limited, with only a consensus against the use of renin-angiotensin blockers in women planning pregnancy. Gender-specific concerns relate to drug tolerability and side effects, with agreement on blood pressure monitoring while using contraceptives. Pregnancy management recommendations differ, with some advising against treatment for nonsevere hypertension. The review highlights a lack of comprehensive consideration of gender-specific aspects in existing guidelines, emphasizing the need for further research in this area.

COMMENT

Hypertension is a modifiable risk factor for cardiovascular disease and is also the leading cause of disease burden and mortality.[21] Various guidelines have shown differences in the prevalence of hypertension in men and women, and it is related to both biological (sex) and psychosocial (gender) factors.[22] Guidelines are yet to come up with differences in hypertension epidemiology, diagnosis, and treatment between men and women based on gender-related characteristics.[23]

In this article, reviewers have reviewed international and selected national guidelines to show similarities and differences in epidemiology, diagnosis, and treatment of hypertension in men and women. They also investigated the use of contraceptive pills, hypertension in pregnancy, sexual dysfunction, and menopause.

The WHO 2021 guidelines recommended that treatment initiation and target blood pressure should not be different in men and women.[24] Hypertension in pregnancy is defined as systolic blood pressure (SBP) ≥140 mm Hg and/or diastolic blood pressure (DBP) ≥ 90 mm Hg on at least two different occasions and at least 6 hours apart. Gestational hypertension is hypertension at 20 weeks or later whereas chronic hypertension is hypertension before 20 weeks of gestation. The threshold to start pharmacological treatment is SBP ≥ 160 mm Hg and or DBP ≥ 105 mm Hg for both chronic and gestational hypertension. If any patient is on antihypertensive therapy, it may be continued if not contraindicated during pregnancy.[25] The antihypertensives preferred during pregnancy are methyldopa, beta-blocker particularly labetalol, calcium channel blockers such as nifedipine, verapamil, and direct-acting vasodilators such as hydralazine.

The ISH 2020 guidelines have shown a higher risk of cardiovascular disease in hypertensive men at or above 55 years of age and women 65 years or above.[26] Daily recommended alcohol consumption is limited to 20 g for men and 15 g for women. For women of childbearing age, beta-blocker is recommended as an antihypertensive. Fibromuscular dysplasia should be suspected in new-onset hypertensive women <30 years of age. Aspirin 75–162 mg daily should be given to women at high risk of preeclampsia.[26]

The ESC/ESH 2018 guidelines have incorporated different cut-off points in ECG and echocardiography for the diagnosis of left ventricular hypertrophy for men and women.[27] Treatment of hypertension using thiazide or thiazide-like diuretics, conventional beta-blockers, or clonidine (centrally acting agent) may trigger sexual dysfunction, whereas angiotensin-converting enzyme inhibitors (ACEIs), angiotensin receptor blockers (ARBs), calcium channel blocker (CCB), or vasodilating beta-blockers may have neutral or even beneficial effects. To reduce blood pressure or to prevent hypertension waist circumference should be <94 cm in men and <88 cm in women. Combined estrogen–progesterone-based oral contraceptive pills (OCPs) can increase the incidence of hypertension in 5% of users.[27] Aspirin 100–150 mg daily is indicated between 12 and 36 weeks of pregnancy for women at high or moderate risk of hypertensive disorders in pregnancy. Drug therapy should be started for pregnant women when SBP is ≥ 150 mm Hg and or diastolic BP is ≥ 95 mm Hg and the goal is to maintain BP < 140/90 mm Hg. Breast milk concentration of all antihypertensive drugs is low except propranolol and nifedipine (concentration similar to maternal plasma). There is an increased risk of hypertension, stroke, and ischemic heart disease in later life for women who develop gestational hypertension or preeclampsia.

The ACC/AHA 2017 guidelines have noted the prevalence of hypertension in men and women equalizes beyond fifth decade of life.[28] The prevalence of white-coat hypertension is more in women than men. ACEI-induced cough and CCB-induced pedal edema are more common in women. Whereas diuretics-induced dyselectrolemia is more in women and gout more in men.[29] OCP use in women with uncontrolled hypertension should be avoided. Compared to methyldopa, beta-blockers (labetalol), and CCBs (nifedipine) appear superior in preventing preeclampsia.[30]

Latin American Society of Hypertension 2017 guidelines state that metabolic syndrome prevalence in Latin America is higher in women. This recommends delivery is the unique treatment for preeclampsia.[31] Magnesium sulfate can be used to prevent convulsion peri-delivery period.

Many unmet needs regarding sex-specific aspects of hypertension still exist.

ARTICLE 3

Evaluating Sex Differences in the Effect of Increased Systolic Blood Pressure on the Risk of Cardiovascular Disease in Asian Populations: A Systematic Review and Meta-analysis

Lin YT, Chen YR, Wei YC. Evaluating sex differences in the effect of increased systolic blood pressure on the risk of cardiovascular disease in Asian populations: A systematic review and meta-analysis.
Glob Heart. 2022;17(1):70.

Abstract

Cardiovascular disease (CVD) is a major global health concern, with a significant portion occurring in Asia. Hypertension, or high blood pressure, is a known risk factor for CVD. Despite studies indicating gender-based differences in the impact of blood pressure on CVD risk, current global guidelines maintain the same blood pressure threshold for both sexes. To investigate this further, a study aimed to assess how elevated blood pressure influences CVD risk among Asian populations with respect to gender.

To achieve this, the researchers conducted a systematic review of studies published before June 30, 2021, involving Asian populations. The analysis identified six studies focused on females and eleven on males, with associated effect sizes for CVD risk. The pooled effect sizes, without adjusting for other factors, revealed that a 10 mm Hg increase in systolic blood pressure resulted in a 1.20-fold increase in CVD risk for females and a 1.19-fold increase for males.

Moreover, the researchers conducted a meta-regression analysis to account for the impact of smoking, a significant confounding factor. This adjustment revealed that the effect of a 10 mm Hg increase in systolic blood pressure on CVD risk was 1.232 times higher for females compared to males. This difference was statistically significant, indicating that the risk of CVD associated with elevated blood pressure is notably greater in females than in males within the Asian population.

In conclusion, the study underscores that the risk of cardiovascular disease due to increased systolic blood pressure is more pronounced in females compared to males within the Asian population. This highlights the importance of considering gender-specific differences when assessing CVD risk factors and determining appropriate preventive measures.

COMMENT

In this meta-analysis, the importance of the global burden of cardiovascular disease (CVD) with respect to hypertension as a risk factor and its variable impact on men and women in the Asian population and its rising trend in Asian countries has been enumerated. The worldwide prevalence of premature death from CVD is 34%, whereas it is 39% in Asia.[32] Incidence and mortality from CVD are related to various risk factors. Hypertension is one of the most common risk factors having variable prevalence among men and women.[33] Although men have higher mean BP and higher prevalence of hypertension in males before 60 years of age, post-menopausal women carry equal prevalence.[34] Death from high SBP is estimated to be 7.8 million in 2015.[35] Again, CVD risk and severity are higher among women due to increased BP compared to men.[36,37] Many guidelines including JNC8 did not mention sex-specific hypertension management.[38] Differences in culture, environment, dietary habits, and genetics have shown differing prevalence, mortality, and burden of CVD among various populations.[39] This review has looked into sex-specific impact of hypertension on CVD risk in the Asian population.

Literature Search and Review

In this study, population–intervention–comparator–outcome (PICO) design was adapted to search the terms from MEDLINE, Embase, and PubMed articles written in English and published before June 30, 2021.

P for Asian adults, *C* for the Sex category, and *O* for the effect of high BP on CVD risk. There was no intervention in this study. Adjusting the available risk factors for CVD risk per SBP increment was reported as effect sizes (ESs). ESs were adjusted hazard ratios (HR) or odds ratios (ORs), all treated as equivalent in this study.[40,41] ES10 was used to denote adjusted HR or OR per 10 mm Hg SBP increment in CVD risk (log-linear transformation was used).[37] The articles having the availability of baseline data such as sample size, sex, age, baseline mean systolic BP, and proportion of smokers among the participants were collected.

Results

Out of 849 publications (478—PubMed) and (371—Embase/MEDLINE), 6 female and 11 male effect sizes (ESs) from six publications that met the search criteria were included.[42,43] Quality assessment criteria showed all studies are of good quality. Without other risk factors, pooled ESs of males and females were not significantly different. Sex and smokers were two significant variables retained in the optimal model. Sex subgroup analysis showed hypertensive females had a higher CVD risk than males. This meta-regression showed a 1.232-fold higher CVD risk per 10 mm Hg increase in systolic BP in women than in men. It also documented smokers had a significantly higher CVD risk with increased BP compared to nonsmokers.[44]

Discussion

In CVD, sex difference is an important issue[37,45] but underreported in literature.[46] Assessment of the impact of BP on CVD among males and females will help in creating health policies and improving healthcare. Smoking and hypertension are two important equivalent risk factors among the seven core health behaviors that impact CVD.[44] Prevention of smoking and control of hypertension helped to control CVD events in Japan.[47]

This meta-analysis definitely opens a window for future research to analyze CVD risk, based on sex-specific BP targets and formulate sex equivalent treatment strategies for the Asian population.

ARTICLE 4

Effect of Sacubitril/Valsartan or Valsartan on Ventricular Remodeling and Myocardial Fibrosis in Perimenopausal Women with Hypertension

Chen J, Pei Y, Wang Q, Li C, Liang W, Yu J. Effect of sacubitril/valsartan or valsartan on ventricular remodeling and myocardial fibrosis in perimenopausal women with hypertension.
J Hypertens. 2023;41(7):1077-83.

Abstract

Objective: The objective of this study is to assess the effects of sacubitril/valsartan in comparison to valsartan alone on blood pressure, ventricular structure, and myocardial fibrosis in women with hypertension during the perimenopausal phase.

Methods: In this study, a total of 292 women with perimenopausal hypertension were enrolled in a prospective, randomized, actively controlled, open-label trial and randomly assigned to receive either sacubitril/valsartan (200 mg once daily) or valsartan (160 mg once daily), and their ambulatory blood pressure, echocardiography, and myocardial fibrosis were assessed at baseline and at 24 weeks.

Results: After 24 weeks of treatment, the 24-hour mean systolic blood pressure (SBP) was 120.08 ± 10.47 mm Hg in the sacubitril/valsartan group and 121.00 ± 9.76 mm Hg in the valsartan group ($p = 0.457$). There was no significant difference in central SBP between the sacubitril/valsartan and valsartan groups after 24 weeks of treatment (117.17 ± 11.63 vs. 116.38 ± 11.58, $p = 0.568$). However, left ventricular mass index (LVMI) in the sacubitril/valsartan group was significantly lower than in the valsartan group at week 24 ($p = 0.009$). LVMI decreased by 7.23 g/m^2 from baseline in the sacubitril/valsartan group and 3.70 g/m^2 in the valsartan group at 24 weeks ($p = 0.000$ vs. 0.017).

At 24 weeks, a statistically significant difference in LVMI between the two groups was observed even after adjusting for baseline LVMI ($p = 0.001$). Moreover, the sacubitril/valsartan group exhibited reduced levels of α-smooth muscle actin (α-SMA), connective tissue growth factor (CT-GF), and transforming growth factor-β (TGF-β) ($p = 0.000$, 0.005, and 0.000, respectively) compared to baseline. After adjusting for confounding factors such as 24-hour mean SBP and 24-hour mean DBP at 24 weeks, the difference in LVMI between the two groups remained statistically significant ($p = 0.005$). Furthermore, even after further correcting for age, BMI, and sex hormone levels, the LVMI, serum TGF-β, α-SMA, and CT-GF levels continued to show statistically significant differences between the sacubitril/valsartan group and the valsartan group ($p < 0.05$).

Conclusion: Sacubitril/valsartan demonstrated superior efficacy in reversing ventricular remodeling compared to valsartan alone. The divergent impact of these therapies on ventricular remodeling in perimenopausal hypertensive women is likely attributed to their distinct effects on downregulating fibrosis-related factors.

COMMENT

Perimenopausal women have a notably higher prevalence of hypertension and ventricular remodeling compared to men of the same age.[48] Importantly, the occurrence of myocardial remodeling during the perimenopausal phase and the process of treatment reversal are more complex in women compared to men.[49] Thus, this study aimed to assess the hypothesis suggesting that sacubitril/valsartan has superior effects compared to valsartan alone in reversing myocardial remodeling in women with perimenopausal hypertension. The goal was to observe if this reversal leads to improved regulation of biomarkers associated with myocardial fibrosis.

This study primarily observed that sacubitril/valsartan and valsartan had distinct effects on ventricular remodeling in perimenopausal women with hypertension. The study showed that left ventricular mass index (LVMI) significantly improved to a greater extent after sacubitril/valsartan treatment compared to valsartan alone. Importantly, this improvement was not associated with blood pressure control or sex hormone levels. Additionally, the levels of transforming growth factor-β (TGF-β), α-smooth muscle actin (α-SMA), and connective tissue growth factor (CT-GF) in perimenopausal hypertensive women treated with sacubitril/valsartan significantly decreased after 24 weeks of treatment. The study showed that the beneficial effects of sacubitril/valsartan treatment on LVMI after 24 weeks were not influenced by changes in central arterial pressure. Indeed, a change in ventricular geometry serves as an independent predictor of the elevated risk of cardiovascular disease in patients with hypertension.[50,51]

This study has some limitations to consider. Firstly, it only examined changes in blood pressure and ventricular structure at two time points, lacking a dynamic analysis over time. Secondly, the small sample size calls for further validation with larger groups and multiple centers.

The findings from this study indicate that sacubitril/valsartan may offer certain advantages over valsartan in reversing ventricular remodeling, possibly due to its superior impact on reducing profibrosis-related factors. However, further evidence and research are required in the future to validate the effect of sacubitril/valsartan on myocardial remodeling in perimenopausal hypertensive women.

ARTICLE 5

Salt Sensitivity of Blood Pressure in Women

Barris CT, Faulkner JL, Belin de Chantemèle EJ. Salt sensitivity of blood pressure in women. *Hypertension. 2023;80(2):268-78.*

Abstract

Numerous studies show that women are more sensitive to dietary salt than men, but the exact reasons for this difference are not fully understood. We review recent epidemiological data and studies on salt-sensitive blood pressure (SSBP) mechanisms specific to sex. Evidence suggests that women of all ethnicities, both premenopausal and postmenopausal, are more salt-sensitive than men. Menopause worsens SSBP, indicating that female sex chromosomes may predispose to and female sex hormones may mitigate SSBP. Studies suggest that enhanced activation of the aldosterone-ECMR (endothelial cell mineralocorticoid receptor) axis in females contributes to vascular dysfunction, with increased adrenal response to angiotensin II and higher ECMR expression and endothelial ENaC activation as key factors. Female sex increases the prevalence and susceptibility to SSBP, and sex hormones and sex chromosome complement may have opposing roles in female SSBP development.

COMMENT

Decades of research, primarily focused on men and male animal models, have led to the incorrect belief that women are less prone to salt sensitivity. Salt-sensitive blood pressure (SSBP) is a heritable physiological characteristic where blood pressure can increase or decrease by >10% in response to variations in dietary salt intake.[52] This trait is responsible for approximately 50–80% of essential hypertension cases.[53] The mechanisms governing the onset and progression of SSBP are influenced by biological sex, sex hormones, and genetic predisposition. Moreover, this sex specificity is further complicated by the observed rise in SSBP among women after menopause. Sex hormone levels could potentially influence salt preference, with some studies suggesting that women exhibit an increased preference for salt during the luteal phase of the menstrual cycle. Nevertheless, other studies propose that sodium preference is not tied to any specific menstrual phase.[54] In line with these findings, animal studies have reported that salt preference emerges with sexual maturity, and although ovariectomy does not eliminate the higher female preference for salt.[55]

Significantly, findings from the HyperPath and HTN-IR studies reveal that salt sensitivity is more common in women across all ages and reproductive stages.[56] Nevertheless, multiple clinical studies suggest that the cessation of sex hormone production, particularly estradiol, during menopause, elevates the risk of SSBP.[57] According to the WHO-CARDIAC study (World Health Organization Cardiovascular and Alimentary Comparison Study), SSBP in postmenopausal women is influenced by two potential contributing factors: the decline in female sex hormone production, either alone or in conjunction with the natural aging process.

For salt-sensitive women, recent clinical and experimental evidence suggests that females do not efficiently suppress the renin–angiotensin–aldosterone system (RAAS) as compared to males. This leads to a sex-specific imbalance favoring higher RAAS activation even in the presence of high sodium intake.[56] The key components of the RAAS pathway involved in SSBP are ANGII (angiotensin II) and aldosterone, and their influence is mediated through sex-specific and reproductive stage-specific mechanisms.

The activation of both the innate and adaptive immune systems has been identified as significant contributors to SSBP in males. However, experimental evidence suggests a protective role for both CD14+ cells and T regulatory cells in females. Another potential factor influencing the sexually dimorphic onset of SSBP is the contribution of interstitial sodium microdomains. Nevertheless, additional research is needed to fully understand the role of interstitial sodium microdomains in this context.

The latest scientific findings reveal that women, irrespective of their ethnicity, menopausal status, or age, exhibit higher salt sensitivity compared to men. Contrary to expectations, female sex steroid hormones have a mitigating effect on SSBP.

While further research is needed to fully understand the mechanisms behind heightened female salt sensitivity, particularly in distinguishing the contributions of sex chromosomes versus sex hormones, substantial evidence from both human and rodent studies points toward inadequate suppression of the RAAS and excessive aldosterone production. Additionally, there is evidence of sex-specific increases in endothelial MR expression and EnNaC activity, which may result in reduced bioavailability of nitric oxide and vascular dysfunction, ultimately promoting elevated BP.

ARTICLE 6

Placental Syndromes and Long-term Risk of Hypertension

Fraser A, Catov JM. Placental syndromes and long-term risk of hypertension.
J Hum Hypertes. 2023;37(8):671-4.

Abstract

Prior to pregnancy, elevated blood pressure is linked to increased risks of placental abruption, hypertension, preeclampsia, preterm delivery, and fetal growth restriction, collectively known as placental syndromes, which involve impaired placental development and early vascularization. These syndromes also elevate the risk of hypertension and cardiovascular disease in women later in life. Women affected by clinical placental syndromes and evidence of placental maternal vascular malperfusion face a particularly high risk of hypertension and cardiovascular disease. However, whether placental impairments and clinical syndromes cause or result from higher blood pressure in women is not fully understood. This review focuses on exploring the connection between blood pressure and maternal health during pregnancy. We emphasize the necessity for comprehensive studies, encompassing detailed assessments of cardiac and vascular structure and function before, during, and after pregnancy, in order to unravel the complex relationship between women's blood pressure and pregnancy health to solve the "chicken and egg" puzzle of women's blood pressure and pregnancy health, and provide valuable insights for the development of effective precision medicine strategies to prevent and treat placental syndromes and chronic hypertension in women.

COMMENT

During the initial stages of the first trimester in pregnancy, there is a decline in maternal blood pressure, which can be attributed to a reduction in systemic vascular resistance. This decrease reaches its lowest point around mid-pregnancy, followed by an increase in blood pressure, eventually returning to pre-pregnancy levels by the end of the term. It is worth noting that women who already have hypertension before pregnancy face an elevated risk of experiencing a placental syndrome.[58] Women who have experienced placental syndromes during pregnancy are approximately twice as likely to develop cardiovascular disease (CVD) and face an increased risk of CVD-related mortality later in life when compared to women who have not had a history of pregnancy complicated by a placental syndrome. Studies suggest that a significant portion of this elevated risk can be attributed to the development of chronic hypertension over time.[59]

There are three potential explanations for the increased risk of CVD associated with placental syndromes, and these explanations are not mutually exclusive. Firstly, women with placental syndromes may not experience the typical drop in blood pressure after pregnancy, which could be attributed to either pre-pregnancy factors or as a consequence of the placental syndrome itself. Secondly, it is possible that women with placental syndromes do experience a similar drop in blood pressure, but they had higher pre-pregnancy blood pressure levels. This scenario suggests that pregnancy serves as a natural "screening test," revealing women with a more adverse cardiovascular health profile before pregnancy.[60] Lastly, women with placental syndromes might undergo a more pronounced rise in blood pressure during the postpartum years. This situation indicates that placental syndromes may directly affect blood pressure through damage to the blood vessels or kidneys.

Women whose first-born baby was small-for-gestational-age (SGA) had higher mean blood pressure throughout adulthood, from before to after pregnancy, compared to women whose first-born baby was appropriate-for-gestational-age (AGA), even though the SGA group had lower levels of adiposity.[61]

Women who experience both clinical placental syndromes and show evidence of placental maternal vascular malperfusion (MVM) are at a notably elevated risk of developing hypertension and CVD. The observation of higher systolic blood pressure and diastolic blood pressure before pregnancy in women who later develop a placental syndrome and MVM further supports the hypothesis that placental lesions and clinical syndromes may be indicative of an underlying predisposition to hypertension and CVD.

ARTICLE 7

Hypertension: Sex-related Differences in Drug Treatment, Prevalence, and Blood Pressure Control in Primary Care

Bager JE, Manhem K, Andersson T, Hjerpe P, Bengtsson-Boström K, Ljungman C, et al. Hypertension: sex-related differences in drug treatment, prevalence and blood pressure control in primary care.
J Hum Hypertens. 2023;37(8):662-70.

Abstract

Antihypertensive treatment is equally beneficial in reducing cardiovascular risk for both men and women, but drug treatment, prevalence, and control of hypertension differ between genders. Men and women respond differently to antihypertensive drugs, and certain medications may be more beneficial depending on comorbidities unique to each gender. Managing hypertension during pregnancy is particularly challenging. Population-based studies and real-world data show inconsistent results regarding blood pressure control in men and women. Women tend to have higher treatment rates and better blood pressure control in population studies, while primary care data indicate better control in men. Additionally, men and women receive different antihypertensive drugs. Original data from a large Swedish register reveal that women have better blood pressure control until their late 60s, after which men fare better. However, older women do not receive proportionally increased antihypertensive treatment, indicating potential disparities in care.

COMMENT

Arterial hypertension continues to be the leading preventable factor contributing to cardiovascular disease and mortality. Antihypertensive drug therapy has proven effective in reducing the risk of major cardiovascular events, irrespective of gender, previous cardiovascular disease history, and baseline blood pressure.[19] There are certain differences between men and women concerning the onset of hypertension, their response to hypertension medications, and their experiences with both cardiovascular and noncardiovascular health issues.[62] The main classes of drugs used in hypertension have similar effects in both genders, with no significant differences observed in outcomes such as myocardial infarction, congestive heart failure, stroke, and cardiovascular and all-cause mortality.[19]

The study gathered original data from QregPV, a primary care quality register. It included 229,864 patients with diagnosed hypertension in the Swedish region of Västra Götaland in 2017. Hypertension was more prevalent among women (51.4%), who were slightly older than men (71.1 vs. 68.4 years). The study found that 51.7% of women and 53.3% of men achieved the target blood pressure.

Despite no significant difference in their effect on blood pressure and key cardiovascular outcomes, there is variation in the usage of antihypertensive drug classes between men and women based on real-world data.[19]

Thiazide use has been notably more frequent in women, while angiotensin converting enzyme inhibitor (ACEI) and calcium channel blocker (CCB) have been more commonly prescribed to men.[19] Alpha-blocker usage was relatively low overall but was approximately twice as common in men (1.8%) compared to women (0.8%). The use of angiotensin receptor blockers (ARBs) was equal in both men and women (39%).

For all drug classes utilized in hypertension, there was a sharp decline in usage after the age of 80 years, except for beta-blockers and mineralocorticoid receptor antagonists (MRAs), which showed continued use in both men and women. A noticeable increase in labetalol usage was observed in women aged 25–35 years, which was not seen in men. This spike can be attributed to its role in treating preexisting hypertension in women who are pregnant or planning to become pregnant.

Sex-related differences in susceptibility to adverse effects from antihypertensive drugs can influence prescription patterns. Men and women exhibit dissimilar risks of adverse effects, with women being more than twice as likely to develop ACEI treatment-induced cough.[63] On the other hand, ARBs are equally well tolerated in both genders, showing an adverse effect rate similar to placebo.[64] Women are more likely to experience adverse effects such as dizziness, flushing, headache, and tibial edema due to the vasodilating effects of CCB.[65] Thiazide treatment is linked to a reduced risk of osteoporotic fractures, which predominantly affect women.[66]

The study found contrasting results between population-based studies and real-world data regarding hypertension prevalence, treatment, and control. Population-based studies show men have higher blood pressure and worse control, while in real-world data, women have higher blood pressure and worse control. Treatment rates also differ, with men receiving less treatment in population-based studies and women receiving less treatment in real-world data.

ARTICLE 8

The Effect of Calcium and Vitamin D Supplements on Blood Pressure in Postmenopausal Women: Myth or Reality?

Sharifi F, Heydarzadeh R, Vafa RG, Rahmani M, Parizi MM, Ahmadi A, et al. The effect of calcium and vitamin D supplements on blood pressure in postmenopausal women: myth or reality?
Hypertens Res. 2022;45(7):1203-9.

Abstract

Hypertension is a widely prevalent condition associated with significant cardiovascular and renal issues. Numerous studies have indicated a limited connection between calcium intake (or calcium along with vitamin D) and blood pressure, implying that calcium supplements may potentially lower blood pressure. Nevertheless, the findings up until now have been subject to debate and disagreement. In this research, we investigated the impact of calcium and vitamin D supplementation on the blood pressure of postmenopausal women who have hypertension. This specific population group was chosen due to the widespread use of calcium supplements among them. In 2019, a triple-blind randomized clinical trial was conducted, involving 98 postmenopausal women diagnosed with hypertension. The study spanned 8 weeks with rigorous monitoring. 24-hour ambulatory blood pressure monitoring was utilized to record the initial and final blood pressure readings for all participants. The results indicated a significant increase in both mean systolic ($p = 0.047$) and diastolic blood pressure ($p = 0.015$) following the consumption of calcium and vitamin D supplements. In patients who were already taking calcium channel blockers, the administration of calcium and vitamin D supplements led to a significant increase in both systolic ($p = 0.019$) and diastolic blood pressures ($p = 0.001$) compared to their baseline readings. These findings differ from previous studies, indicating that caution should be exercised when considering calcium supplementation for postmenopausal women with hypertension, especially those already receiving calcium channel blocker treatment. Close monitoring of blood pressure is crucial to avoid any further elevation.

COMMENT

Hypertension stands as a significant public health issue, with its origins thought to intertwine with a range of environmental and genetic factors.[67,68] Effective management of hypertension, encompassing adjustments to one's lifestyle, becomes imperative in order to mitigate potential complications.[69] Given the strongly suspected influence of dietary patterns on blood pressure,[70] several studies have honed in on the potential impact of calcium intake on blood pressure levels. Nevertheless, the findings from these studies have conflicting outcomes thus far.[71] The ongoing trial aims to evaluate alterations in blood pressure among postmenopausal women afflicted by hypertension, who have calcium and vitamin D supplements.

In this study, 24-hour ambulatory blood pressure monitoring was employed to document the initial and concluding blood pressure readings across all participants. The observed alterations in both average systolic ($p = 0.047$) and diastolic blood pressure ($p = 0.015$) implied a rise in blood pressure subsequent to the consumption of calcium and vitamin D supplements. Particularly noteworthy was the increase in systolic ($p = 0.019$) and diastolic blood pressures ($p = 0.001$) among individuals who were already using calcium channel blockers. This divergence in findings contrasts with prior research outcomes. Delving into subgroup analysis, the investigation identified that participants employing amlodipine (an angioselective calcium channel blocker) throughout the study experienced an average increase of approximately 4.35 mm Hg in systolic blood pressure within the treatment group. Additionally, the mean diastolic blood pressure within the treatment group escalated by roughly 3 mm Hg.

The variations observed across various studies underscore the need for vigilant monitoring of blood pressure when administering oral calcium and vitamin D supplementation to postmenopausal women with hypertension. This scrutiny becomes particularly crucial for individuals who are concurrently using calcium channel blockers to manage their hypertension, as the impact of supplementation seems to be heightened within this specific subgroup.

While this study employed a randomized triple-blind trial design and utilized 24-hour blood pressure monitoring to ensure precise measurements of changes, the limited patient enrollment necessitates additional research involving larger and more diverse population samples. It is worth noting that this investigation was conducted solely at a single center and within a single population.

Conducting further studies that specifically delve into the underlying pathophysiological mechanisms through which dietary calcium supplementation influences blood pressure could potentially bring clarity to the existing uncertainties in this area. Such additional research holds the promise of shedding light on both the positive and adverse impacts of calcium intake among postmenopausal women, a demographic segment that constitutes a substantial portion of the population.

ARTICLE 9

The Impact of Antihypertensive Treatment of Mild-to-moderate Hypertension during Pregnancy on Maternal and Neonatal Outcomes: An Updated Meta-analysis of Randomized Controlled Trials

Attar A, Hosseinpour A, Moghadami M. The impact of antihypertensive treatment of mild to moderate hypertension during pregnancy on maternal and neonatal outcomes: An updated meta-analysis of randomized controlled trials. *Clin Cardiol.* 2023;46:467-76.

Abstract

At present, there is an ongoing controversy regarding the management of pregnant patients with mild hypertension, characterized by blood pressure readings ranging from 140 to 159 mm Hg systolic and 90 to 109 mm Hg diastolic. While current guidelines do not recommend specific treatment for this condition, recent clinical trials have shown supportive evidence for treatment in these cases. This meta-analysis aimed to determine if treating mild hypertension during pregnancy improves maternal and fetal outcomes. The researchers gathered relevant randomized controlled trials through a systematic database search, focusing on the impact of pharmacological treatment on maternal, fetal, and neonatal outcomes in patients with mild hypertension. A random-effects model was used to calculate the relative risk (RR) and 95% confidence interval (CI). The data analyzed came from 12 trials, involving a total of 4,461 pregnant women with mild-to-moderate hypertension. Among these participants, 2,395 were in the intervention group and 2,066 were in the control group. Antihypertensive treatment showed better outcomes in seven out of 19 analyzed outcomes: severe hypertension [RR 0.53; 95% CI (0.38; 0.75)], preeclampsia [RR 0.71; 95% CI (0.54; 0.93)], placental abruption [RR 0.48; 95% CI (0.26; 0.87)], changes in electrocardiogram [RR 0.43; 95% CI (0.25; 0.72)], renal impairment [RR 0.42; 95% CI (0.34; 0.51)], pulmonary edema [RR 0.46; 95% CI (0.25; 0.84)], and neonatal mortality [RR 0.72; 95% CI (0.57; 0.92)]. The analysis found no difference in the primary safety outcome of small for gestational age between the treatment group and the control group [RR 1.12; 95% CI (0.80; 1.57)]. Overall, the results of this meta-analysis support the positive effects of pharmacological treatment for mild hypertension on both maternal and neonatal outcomes. Importantly, there were no significant adverse events observed for the fetus in association with the treatment.

COMMENT

Hypertensive disorders of pregnancy have been associated with a significantly higher risk of adverse pregnancy outcomes including fetal and neonatal death and small for gestational age (SGA).[72-74] Although guidelines have reached a consensus on treating cases with severe hypertension (blood pressure ≥ 160/110 mm Hg),[75] uncertainty still remains regarding the decision to treat patients with mild-to-moderate hypertension.

In this current meta-analysis, which encompassed 4,461 participants, an investigation was conducted into the potential impact of pharmacological therapy on both maternal and fetal outcomes among individuals with mild-to-moderate hypertension during pregnancy. The focus of our study was solely on research that compared active treatment against no treatment or placebo, particularly concerning the contentious issue of managing mild-to-moderate hypertension during pregnancy. The overall findings highlight that antihypertensive treatment played a role in reducing the risk of specific maternal outcomes, including severe hypertension [RR 0.53 (0.38; 0.75)], preeclampsia [RR 0.71 (0.54; 0.93)], placental abruption [RR 0.48 (0.26; 0.87)], and renal impairment [RR 0.42 (0.34; 0.51)]. Furthermore, antihypertensive treatment demonstrated a notable reduction in the likelihood of neonatal mortality after excluding a study with a high risk of bias [RR 0.72 (0.57; 0.92)]. It is worth noting that active treatment for mild hypertension displayed no discernible differences in terms of safety outcomes when compared to the control group that did not receive medication, as observed in our analysis.

The outcomes of this meta-analysis align with the recent findings presented in the CHAP trial. In the CHAP trial, the primary endpoint, which encompassed a combination of preeclampsia, preterm birth, placental abruption, and neonatal mortality, exhibited a notably lower incidence among patients who received treatment in comparison to the control group [30.2% vs. 37%; RR (95% CI) 0.82 (0.74; 0.92)]. The administration of treatment was also determined to be safe, as indicated by the insignificant difference in the safety outcome of SGA between the two groups [RR (95% CI) 1.04 (0.82; 1.31)]. Notably, the rates of SGA reported in the CHAP study (11.2% vs. 10.4%) were quite similar to the outcomes observed in our analysis (14% vs. 13%).[76]

On the contrary, the CHIPS trial, a multicenter open-label study, aimed to compare strict blood pressure control (target diastolic BP of 85 mm Hg) with a less stringent approach (target diastolic BP of 100 mm Hg) for pregnant women with gestational or chronic hypertension. The study found no significant differences in primary outcomes such as pregnancy loss, SGA infants, and neonatal care level. Maternal complications also showed no significant disparity between the two groups. However, the less strict control group had notably higher odds of developing severe hypertension.[77]

The current meta-analysis affirms the positive impacts of antihypertensive treatment for individuals with mild hypertension on pregnancy-related outcomes. Pharmacological intervention for mild hypertension during pregnancy results in reduced chances of severe hypertension, preeclampsia, placental abruption, renal impairment, and pulmonary edema. The use of antihypertensive drugs in cases of mild hypertension is also deemed safe, posing no elevated risks for adverse pregnancy consequences like small for gestational age, low birth weight, as well as neonatal and fetal mortality. As a recommendation, this study suggests that considering a target BP of 140/90 mm Hg as the threshold for initiating antihypertensive medications in cases of chronic and gestational hypertension

ARTICLE 10

Medications for Preventing Hypertensive Disorders in High-risk Pregnant Women: A Systematic Review and Network Meta-analysis

Liabsuetrakul T, Yamamoto Y, Kongkamol C, Ota E, Mori R, Noma H. Medications for preventing hypertensive disorders in high-risk pregnant women: a systematic review and network meta-analysis. *Syst Rev. 2022;11(1):135.*

Abstract

Objectives: The aim is to evaluate the relative effectiveness of various medications in preventing hypertensive disorders in pregnant women at high risk. Additionally, the goal is to rank these medications through the utilization of network meta-analysis.

Methods: We analyzed randomized controlled trials comparing common medications for preventing hypertensive disorders in high-risk pregnant women, including those with nulliparity and pregnant women having family history of preeclampsia, history of pregnancy-induced hypertension in previous pregnancy, obstetric risks, or underlying medical diseases. The search results were obtained from the Cochrane Pregnancy and Childbirth's Specialized Register of Controlled Trials, on July 31, 2020. Two review authors independently selected studies, assessed their quality, and extracted data. Comparative risk ratios and 95% CI were analyzed using both pairwise and network meta-analyses to rank treatments' effectiveness in preventing preeclampsia, gestational hypertension, and superimposed preeclampsia. Safety aspects will be reported separately for decision-making.

Results: In this network meta-analysis, a total of 83 randomized studies involving 93,864 women from various global regions were analyzed. The study focused on three medications, either used alone or in combination, which were found to likely prevent preeclampsia (PE) in high-risk pregnant women compared to a placebo or no treatment: antiplatelet agents with calcium (RR 0.19; 95% CI 0.04–0.86; 1 study; low-quality evidence), calcium (RR 0.61; 95% CI 0.47–0.80; 13 studies; moderate-quality evidence), antiplatelet agents (RR 0.69; 95% CI 0.57–0.82; 31 studies; moderate-quality evidence), and antioxidants (RR 0.77; 95% CI 0.63–0.93; 25 studies; moderate-quality evidence). Calcium probably prevented PE (RR 0.63; 95% CI 0.46–0.86; 11 studies; moderate-quality evidence) and GHT (RR 0.89; 95% CI 0.84–0.95; 8 studies; high-quality evidence) in nulliparous/primigravida women. The inclusion of studies for the outcome of superimposed preeclampsia was limited.

Conclusion: The study concluded that antiplatelet agents, calcium, and their combinations were the most effective medications for preventing hypertensive disorders in high-risk pregnant women, outperforming a placebo or no treatment. It emphasized the significance of considering individual high-risk characteristics when determining the appropriate medications. The quality of evidence supporting these findings was predominantly rated as moderate.

COMMENT

Hypertensive disorders in pregnancy (HDP) represent a prevalent set of complications among pregnancies, contributing to maternal and fetal mortality rates on a global scale. The intricate nature of HDP's root causes has led to a lack of precise comprehension. Consequently, a systematic review was conducted to examine the potential utility of various interventions, including antiplatelet agents, anticoagulants, antioxidants, nitric oxide, and calcium, in mitigating or averting the occurrence of HDP.[78]

The objectives of this analysis aimed to assess the comparative effectiveness and establish a hierarchical ranking of accessible medications for the prevention of hypertensive disorders in pregnant women deemed high-risk according to the NICE 2019 classification. This was achieved through a network meta-analysis approach.

This network meta-analysis discovered that among various medications, including antiplatelet agents, calcium, antioxidants, and their combinations, these interventions demonstrated greater effectiveness in preventing hypertensive disorders in pregnancy when compared to either a placebo or no treatment. However, establishing superiority among these medications remained uncertain. The quality of evidence was deemed moderate, influenced by factors such as potential bias, publication bias, and imprecision. There exists a potential for slight improvements through medication combinations, such as antiplatelet agents with calcium, anticoagulants with antiplatelet agents, or calcium with antioxidants. However, this was based on limited evidence from a few existing studies with wide confidence intervals. Further research is warranted to explore these combination treatments in greater detail.

These findings align with the WHO guidelines from 2011, which strongly advocate for a daily intake of 1.5–2.0 g of elemental calcium in regions with low dietary calcium consumption, and recommend 75 mg of aspirin for the prevention of preeclampsia (PE) in women at high risk of developing the condition, with a moderate quality of evidence.[79] Similarly, the NICE recommendation proposes the use of 75–150 mg of aspirin.[80] The majority of antioxidants administered in the studies were a combination of 1,000 mg of vitamin C along with 200–400 mg of vitamin E on a daily basis.

Notably, the outcomes of our network meta-analysis echoed the results of two earlier network meta-analyses, which indicated that calcium supplementation could indeed lower the risk of preeclampsia. However, it is important to note that these systematic reviews did not employ the GRADE approach to assess the quality of evidence.[81,82]

This network meta-analysis did have certain limitations. Firstly, it encompassed a broad spectrum of high-risk pregnant women, leading to a diversity of findings across the included studies. This variability could potentially be attributed to distinct responses to the medications based on various risk profiles. Secondly, the analysis focused solely on studies conducted within hospital settings that utilized the high-risk factors recommended by NICE 2019, omitting factors like Doppler, laboratory tests, or serum markers for assessing the risk of hypertensive disorders in pregnancy. Thirdly, the network meta-analysis did not undertake subgroup analyses for interventions (different drugs within the same medication group, varied dosages of the same drug, or gestational age at medication administration) and gestational age at the occurrence of outcomes. Fourthly, while this review presented relative effectiveness outcomes for medications, safety outcomes were reserved for a separate review. Evaluating both effectiveness and safety is crucial for a comprehensive understanding of the medication's benefits and risks for pregnant women. Lastly, the analysis excluded preeclampsia with preterm birth as an outcome in this network analysis.

Antiplatelet agents, calcium, antioxidants, and their combinations demonstrated greater efficacy compared to a placebo or no treatment in preventing hypertensive disorders in various risk scenarios among pregnant women. Notably, calcium ranked prominently in preventing gestational hypertension in nulliparous or primigravida women. To advance our understanding, further network meta-analyses are necessary. These analyses should explore different drugs within the same medication groups, varying dosages of the same drug, as well as considering gestational age at medication administration and outcome occurrence. This approach will help to pinpoint the most effective medication regimen for preventing hypertensive disorders during pregnancy.

ARTICLE 11

Effects of Yoga on Cardiometabolic Risks and Fetomaternal Outcomes are Associated with Serum Nitric Oxide in Gestational Hypertension: A Randomized Control Trial

Karthiga K, Pal GK, Dasari P, Nanda N, Velkumary S, Chinnakali P, et al. Effects of yoga on cardiometabolic risks and fetomaternal outcomes are associated with serum nitric oxide in gestational hypertension: a randomized control trial. *Sci Rep. 2022;12(1):11732.*

Abstract

Gestational hypertension (GH) is linked to unfavorable cardiometabolic and pregnancy outcomes. Despite the known benefits of yoga during pregnancy, there is a lack of research on the effects of yoga starting from the 16th week of gestation for 20 weeks in pregnant women at risk of GH. Specifically, there have been no studies investigating the impact of yoga on the incidence of hypertension, cardiometabolic risks, and fetomaternal outcomes in this group of pregnant women.

In this randomized controlled trial, 234 pregnant women at risk of developing gestational hypertension were divided into two groups. The first group (control group) consisted of 113 women who received standard antenatal care. The second group (study group) included 121 women who received standard antenatal care along with yoga sessions. Both groups received their respective interventions for a duration of 20 weeks, starting from the 16th week of gestation. They assessed parameters such as baroreflex sensitivity (BRS), heart rate variability (HRV), insulin resistance, lipid-risk factors, and markers of inflammation, oxidative stress, and vascular endothelial dysfunction (VED) before and after the intervention. The study recorded the incidence of new-onset hypertension, cardiometabolic risk levels at the 36th week, and fetomaternal neonatal outcomes during the perinatal period. Researchers also investigated the relationship between hypertension, pregnancy outcomes, and cardiometabolic risks with nitric oxide (NO), a marker of VED. They used analysis of covariance, Pearson's correlations, multilinear regression, and logistic regression to assess this link. In the study group, only 6.61% developed hypertension compared to 38.1% in the control group after the 20-week intervention, showing a significant reduction in gestational hypertension risk (RR 2.65; CI 1.42–4.95). The study group had less painful deliveries, shorter labor, higher neonatal birthweight, and better Apgar scores. Increase in total power of HRV ($\beta = 0.187$, $p = 0.024$), BRS ($\beta = 0.305$, $p < 0.001$), and decrease in interleukin-6 ($\beta = -0.194$, $p = 0.022$) had significant association with increased NO. A 20-week practice of yoga during pregnancy reduces the incidence of hypertension, improves fetomaternal outcomes, and decreases cardiometabolic risks in women at risk of gestational hypertension. Yoga is associated with lower blood pressure, increased HRV, BRS, and birth weight, along with reduced inflammation, indicating improved endothelial function.

COMMENT

In developing countries like India, nearly half of gestational hypertension (GH) cases escalate to preeclampsia, which, if not promptly and effectively treated, can progress to eclampsia.[83] As of now, no pharmaceutical treatment exists for curing preeclampsia, although acetylsalicylic acid (aspirin) is frequently administered prophylactically to high-risk women for hypertensive disorders of pregnancy (HDP).[84] The sole recognized cure for HDP is the delivery of the baby and removal of the placenta. Pharmacological management of maternal hypertension using antihypertensive drugs primarily aims at alleviating maternal symptoms like organ dysfunction and stroke.[85] The use of pharmacological interventions has been limited due to concerns about potential adverse effects on fetal growth and development, as well as pregnant women's preference for alternative remedies.[86]

Consequently, alternative health methods have been attempted in the management of HDP, even though their scientific efficacy remains unproven.[87] An integrated approach involving yoga during pregnancy has exhibited safety and been linked to enhanced birth weight, reduced preterm labor, and decreased instances of intrauterine growth retardation (IUGR) either alone or when dealing with pregnancy-induced hypertension (PIH).[88] Hence, the current study aimed to evaluate the impact of a 20-week yoga regimen on the occurrence of new-onset hypertension, the cardiometabolic profile, as well as maternal–neonatal outcomes, and their relationship with nitric oxide (NO) in pregnant women at risk of developing gestational hypertension.

The study incorporated a yoga regimen encompassing specific poses (*asanas*) and controlled breathing exercises (*pranayamas*) recognized for their positive effects on pregnancy outcomes. This yoga intervention was administered over a duration of 20 weeks, with diligent oversight to ensure participants' adherence to the prescribed yoga practice.

In the current study, among women at risk of PIH who did not engage in yoga practice (control group), the incidence of GH stood at 25.66%. Conversely, among subjects in the study group who diligently practiced yoga for 20 weeks, the incidence of GH was notably lower at 6.61%. Importantly, no instances of preeclampsia or eclampsia were observed in the study group. Overall, 38.1% of subjects in the control group developed HDP, whereas the corresponding figure in the study group was merely 6.61%. Furthermore, the risk of developing GH was significantly diminished in the study group following the yoga intervention (RR 2.65; CI 1.42–4.95; $p < 0.001$). These findings underscore that practicing yoga for 20 weeks during the second and third trimesters of pregnancy can substantially reduce the likelihood of developing hypertension during pregnancy.

A 20-week yoga practice significantly reduced the incidence of hypertension, enhanced fetomaternal and neonatal outcomes, and lowered cardiometabolic risks in pregnant women at risk of GH. This improvement was linked to reduced blood pressure, improved heart rate variability, increased baroreflex sensitivity, higher birth weight, and reduced inflammation, ultimately enhancing endothelial function. The study suggests that integrating this yoga module into medical management could benefit pregnancies with risks, particularly GH. The study proposes early yoga implementation, especially for high-risk pregnancies, to ensure a healthy pregnancy and comfortable delivery.

Nonetheless, it is important to acknowledge a significant limitation of our study. We did not include subjects during their initial prenatal visits in the first trimester, and as a result, we have not been able to establish the impact of earlier enrollment and intervention on the outcomes. Furthermore, we have not investigated the levels of circulating soluble fms-like tyrosine kinase-1 (sFlt-1) and placental growth factor (PlGF), which are diagnostic markers for preeclampsia. Additionally, we did not measure other crucial markers of vascular endothelial dysfunction like vascular endothelial growth factor (VEGF).

ARTICLE 12

The Association between Hypertensive Disorders in Pregnancy and the Risk of Developing Chronic Hypertension

Xu J, Li T, Wang Y, Xue L, Miao Z, Long W, et al. The association between hypertensive disorders in pregnancy and the risk of developing chronic hypertension.
Front Cardiovasc Med. 2022;9:897771.

Abstract

Objective: This meta-analysis conducted a thorough examination of the link between hypertensive disorders in pregnancy (HDP) and the likelihood of developing chronic hypertension. Additionally, it investigated the associations between specific types of HDP, such as preeclampsia (PE) and gestational hypertension (GH), and the risk of developing chronic hypertension.

Design: Systematic review and meta-analysis.

Data sources: The researchers conducted a search in the PubMed, Embase, and Cochrane Library databases, covering articles published from the inception of these databases until August 20, 2021.

Methods: The combined odds ratio (OR) with a 95% confidence interval (CI) was obtained using either a random-effects or fixed-effects model, depending on the level of heterogeneity in the data by utilized meta-regression analysis. We conducted an analysis of the OR value while accounting for several variables, including age and BMI at recruitment, prepregnancy BMI, age at first delivery, and other relevant factors. Additionally, we conducted subgroup analyses based on various factors. These included the year of publication (<2016, ≥2016), study design, sample size (<500, ≥500), region (North and South America, Europe, and other regions), and NOS score (<7, ≥7).

Results: In our systematic review and meta-analysis, we comprehensively examined the relationships between HDP, GH, and PE with chronic hypertension. We included 21 articles, encompassing a total of 634,293 patients. The findings of this study indicated that women with a history of HDP are approximately 3.6 times more likely to develop chronic hypertension compared to those without a history of HDP. Similarly, women with a history of GH are almost 6.2 times more likely to develop chronic hypertension, and women with a history of PE are almost 3.2 times more likely to develop chronic hypertension compared to their counterparts without a history of these conditions. Furthermore, we conducted additional analyses to calculate the probability of developing chronic hypertension among patients with HDP or PE, adjusting for various factors including age and BMI at recruitment, prepregnancy BMI, age at first delivery, and other relevant variables. The results showed that women with a history of HDP are approximately 2.47 times more likely to develop chronic hypertension compared to those without a history of HDP. Similarly, women with a history of PE are almost 3.78 times more likely to develop chronic hypertension than those without a history of PE. Moreover, our findings revealed regional variations in the risk of developing chronic hypertension after HDP or PE. People in Asian countries demonstrated a higher relative risk for chronic hypertension, whereas American individuals did not show a significantly increased relative risk.

Conclusion: These findings suggest that hypertensive disorders in pregnancy (HDP), including GH and PE, increase the risk of developing chronic hypertension. Even after adjusting for confounding factors such as age, BMI at recruitment, pre-pregnancy BMI, age at first delivery, and other relevant variables, patients with HDP or PE still exhibited a higher likelihood of developing chronic hypertension. This indicates that HDP may serve as an independent risk factor for chronic hypertension, and both GH and PE may also contribute to an increased risk of developing this condition.

COMMENT

Hypertension emerges as a frequently encountered condition during pregnancy and stands as a primary contributor to maternal fatalities.[89] About 10% of pregnancies encounter hypertension, with a higher incidence in first-time mothers. Pregnancy-related hypertensive disorders encompass a range of conditions such as preeclampsia, eclampsia, gestational hypertension (GH), pregnancies intertwined with chronic hypertension, and the overlay of preeclampsia onto chronic hypertension.[90]

New findings suggest a rise in the occurrence of hypertensive disorders in pregnancy (HDP) in the last three decades. This increase highlights the potential significance of HDP, a gender-specific cardiovascular disease risk factor, in the forthcoming years.[91,92] This systematic review and meta-analysis aimed to examine recent studies in order to investigate the correlation between HDP and chronic hypertension, and to assess the links between distinct HDP types—namely, preeclampsia (PE) and GH—and the likelihood of developing chronic hypertension.

This research encompassed 21 articles involving a combined 634,293 patients. The outcomes of this comprehensive review and meta-analysis indicated that women who had experienced HDP were approximately 3.6 times more prone to develop chronic hypertension compared to those without such a history. Additionally, women with a history of GH were around 6.2 times more likely to develop chronic hypertension, while women with a history of PE had an approximately 3.2 times higher likelihood of developing chronic hypertension in comparison to those without these respective histories.

The HDP, GH, and PE elevate the chances of individuals progressing to chronic hypertension. Even after adjusting for factors such as age, BMI at recruitment, pre-pregnancy BMI, age at initial delivery, and other relevant variables, individuals who had experienced HDP or PE retained a heightened risk of developing chronic hypertension. This suggests that HDP, GH, and PE might act as independent risk factors for chronic hypertension, irrespective of other existing risk factors.

However, there are still some limitations of this study, which need further study. There are few studies with high scores. The ages of patients with HDP and chronic hypertension were not statistically analyzed because the data were seriously lacking, which may be the reason for the high heterogeneity. The published literature is insufficient to determine the best screening period for postpartum detection of hypertension. We could not determine an observation age or follow-up period to limit the screening of the articles. The heterogeneity of the population and hypertension definitions and the failure to obtain sufficient details make the results of the meta-analysis misleading, and they could not be adjusted using statistical tests.

ARTICLE 13

Is Blood Pressure 120–139/80–89 mm Hg before 20 Weeks a Risk Factor for Hypertensive Disorders of Pregnancy? A Meta-analysis

Sisti G, Fochesato C, Elkafrawi D, Marcus B, Schiattarella A. Is blood pressure 120-139/80-89 mmHg before 20 weeks a risk factor for hypertensive disorders of pregnancy? A meta-analysis.
Eur J Obstet Gynecol Reprod Biol. 2023;284:66-75.

Abstract

Aim: Hypertensive disorders occurring during pregnancy impact around 10% of women globally and carry significant consequences for both the mother and the developing fetus. Chronic hypertension is typically identified before the 20th week of pregnancy and affects about 1.5% of pregnant women. As per the guidelines of the American College of Obstetricians and Gynecologists, hypertension during pregnancy is characterized by a systolic blood pressure exceeding 140 mm Hg or a diastolic blood pressure surpassing 90 mm Hg. In practical medical settings, healthcare providers generally view the threshold of 140/90 mm Hg as an indicator of actual pregnancy-related hypertension, while blood pressure readings lower than this are regarded as within the normal range.

Methods: In order to investigate the potential link between lower blood pressure ranges and the emergence of hypertensive disorders during pregnancy, we conducted a meta-analysis of existing published research. This analysis involved a comparison between pregnant individuals exhibiting blood pressure levels ranging from 120 to 139 mm Hg systolic and 80 to 89 mm Hg diastolic before the 20th week of gestation, and those with blood pressure levels below 120/80 mm Hg, to assess the incidence of hypertensive disorders during pregnancy.

Results: We incorporated a total of 24 studies into our analysis. Among these studies, it was observed that out of 106,870 patients, 12,362 (11.6%) had blood pressure readings falling within the range of 120–139/80–89 mm Hg, while out of 463,280 patients, 26,044 (5.6%) exhibited blood pressures below 120/80 mm Hg. The risk ratio was calculated to be 2.85 (with a confidence interval of 2.47 to 3.3), and the statistical test for the overall impact showed a significant z-score of 14.1 (p value < 0.00001).

Conclusion: In summary, our research demonstrated that pregnant individuals with blood pressure readings lower than the usual 140/90 mm Hg threshold experienced poor pregnancy outcomes. This indicates a need for interventions to reduce the risk of hypertensive disorders in pregnancy for women with blood pressures ranging from 120 to 139/80–89 mm Hg. These interventions should be considered in future clinical trials.

COMMENT

Hypertensive disorders of pregnancy affect approximately 10% of pregnant women worldwide and they can be divided into gestational hypertension, pre-eclampsia/eclampsia, chronic hypertension, and HELLP (hemolysis, elevated liver enzymes, low platelets) syndrome.[93-95]

Chronic hypertension, i.e., hypertension diagnosed prior to 20 weeks of gestation, currently affects approximately 1.5% of pregnant women.[96,97]

The definition of hypertension is constantly evolving. Prior to 2017, hypertension was defined according to the seventh report of the Joint National Committee on Prevention, Detection, Evaluation, and Treatment of High Blood Pressure (JNC-7). In 2017, in an effort to allow for earlier diagnosis and modification of risk factors of hypertensive disease, the American College of Cardiology (ACC) and the American Heart Association (AHA) divided what was previously known as "prehypertension" into "stage 1 hypertension" and "elevated blood pressure".[98]

However, the American College of Obstetricians and Gynecologists (ACOG) continues to define hypertension in pregnancy as a systolic blood pressure of 140 mm Hg or above, a diastolic blood pressure of 90 mm Hg or above, or both.[93] Following current ACOG guidelines, the current practice still states that a patient with a systolic blood pressure below 140 mm Hg or a diastolic blood pressure below 90 mm Hg before 20 weeks of gestation does not meet the diagnostic criteria of chronic hypertension and, therefore, is treated as normotensive.

We previously reviewed studies correlating "stage 1 hypertension" with maternal and fetal outcomes. We found 15 retrospective cohort studies with outcomes consistent with increased risk of hypertensive disorders of pregnancy, diabetes mellitus, and small for gestational age neonate.

In this meta-analysis, we studied the occurrence of hypertensive disorders of pregnancy in patients with blood pressures in the range 120–139/80–89 mm Hg, compared to women with blood pressure < 120/80 mm Hg.

Our results indicate that pregnant patients with blood pressure in the interval 120–139/80–89 mm Hg before 20 weeks have a risk of developing hypertensive disorder of pregnancy almost three times higher, compared to women with blood pressure < 120/80 mm Hg. In addition to hypertensive disorders of pregnancy, we also confirmed the increased risk for preeclampsia/eclampsia and gestational hypertension, considered separately.

Limitations of the study are the slightly different inclusion criteria among the 24 included studies and the slightly different definition of hypertensive disorders of pregnancy.

We propose that the blood pressure range of 120–139/80–89 mm Hg is a significant risk factor for poor pregnancy outcomes and should be considered by obstetricians during prenatal care. Interventions such as prevention, lifestyle modification, medical therapy, and early delivery should be considered to mitigate this risk. Randomized controlled trials are needed to confirm and validate our findings in a larger population.

ARTICLE 14

Low-dose Aspirin for the Prevention of Superimposed Preeclampsia in Women with Chronic Hypertension: A Systematic Review and Meta-analysis

Richards EMF, Giorgione V, Stevens O, Thilaganathan B. Low-dose aspirin for the prevention of superimposed preeclampsia in women with chronic hypertension: a systematic review and meta-analysis.
Am J Obstet Gynecol. 2023;228(4):395-408.

Abstract

Objective: This systematic review and meta-analysis aimed to determine whether the utilization of low-dose aspirin among pregnant women with chronic hypertension lowers the likelihood of superimposed preeclampsia and unfavorable perinatal outcomes.

Data sources: In September 2021, we conducted searches across various sources including Embase, MEDLINE, Cochrane Central Register of Controlled Trials, ClinicalTrials.gov, the World Health Organization International Clinical Trials Registry Platform, and EU Clinical Trials Register. Our focus was on human studies, without limitations on time or language.

Study eligibility criteria: We included cohort, case–control, and randomized controlled studies that involved pregnant women with chronic hypertension and a singleton pregnancy. The studies we considered needed to compare the use of low-dose aspirin during pregnancy with a control group.

Methods: We evaluated the risk of bias using the RoB 2 and ROBINS-I tools. A meta-analysis was conducted employing a random-effects model to estimate odds ratios along with 95% confidence and prediction intervals. We also assessed the data quality using the GRADE approach. Our analysis investigated heterogeneity by considering study methodology, the timing of aspirin initiation, and the occurrence of preterm preeclampsia as outcomes.

Results: Nine studies, comprising three retrospective cohort studies and six randomized trials, involving a total of 2,150 women with chronic hypertension were included in this analysis. The use of low-dose aspirin did not show a significant reduction in the odds of superimposed preeclampsia in either the randomized controlled trials (OR 0.83; 95% CI 0.55–1.25, prediction interval 0.27–2.56; low-quality evidence) or observational studies (OR 1.21; 95% CI 0.78–1.87, prediction interval 0.07–20.80; very low-quality evidence). Low-dose aspirin also did not lead to a reduction in the odds of preterm preeclampsia (OR 1.17; 95% CI 0.74–1.86), and the timing of aspirin initiation did not have a significant impact. While no significant effect was observed on neonates being small-for-gestational-age or on perinatal mortality, there was a notable reduction in preterm birth (OR 0.63; 95% CI 0.45–0.89; moderate-quality evidence). It is important to note that the quality of evidence is limited due to factors like heterogeneity and risk of bias.

Conclusion: This meta-analysis did not find a significant impact on the likelihood of superimposed preeclampsia, small-for-gestational-age infants, or perinatal mortality when using low-dose aspirin in women with chronic hypertension. However, the notable reduction in preterm birth supports the ongoing use of aspirin prophylaxis. It is worth noting that this study was registered prospectively on the International Prospective Register of Systematic Reviews (Registration number CRD42021285921).

COMMENT

Earlier studies have pinpointed chronic hypertension, a condition occurring in approximately 5% of pregnant women,[99] as a significant contributor to the onset of preeclampsia.[100,101] National guidelines, including those set forth by the National Institute for Health and Care Excellence (NICE)[102] and the Saving Babies' Lives Care Bundle[103] in the United Kingdom, advocate for a specific approach. They propose that pregnant women with chronic hypertension should receive preventive low-dose aspirin treatment starting from the 12th week of gestation and continuing until childbirth. This regimen aims to mitigate the risk of complications stemming from placental dysfunction, such as preeclampsia and preterm birth.

Limited evidence exists regarding the clinical efficacy of aspirin prophylaxis in women with chronic hypertension. This scarcity of data is often due to studies with insufficient statistical power or a heavy rely on secondary analyses.

This meta-analysis tackled a significant clinical question: whether the administration of low-dose aspirin during pregnancy diminishes the likelihood of preeclampsia and neonatal morbidity among women with chronic hypertension. The analysis encompassed nine studies comprising 2,150 women with chronic hypertension, all of which adhered to our inclusion criteria and none of which exhibited high bias risks.

This meta-analysis boasts several strengths. It encompasses a substantial total population of 2,150 pregnant women with chronic hypertension, representing diverse ethnic backgrounds. Additionally, the inclusion of subgroup data from notable trials like the Network of Maternal Fetal Medicine Units and ASPRE trials further enhances the robustness of the analysis.

The quality of the evidence is noticeably limited by the presence of observed heterogeneity. This heterogeneity could stem from disparities in population definitions (such as the use of different hypertension criteria and whether participants were required to be receiving hypertension treatment), variations in exposure (including varying aspirin doses, with three studies not even specifying the dose), and discrepancies in outcome measures [for instance, differences in the definitions of superimposed preeclampsia, small-for-gestational-age (SGA) births, and preterm gestation].

Despite its efforts, this meta-analysis failed to reveal a noteworthy alteration in the likelihood of superimposed preeclampsia, SGA infants, or perinatal mortality through the utilization of low-dose aspirin among women dealing with chronic hypertension. However, the significant reduction in preterm births holds potential for considerable personal, clinical, and economic advantages. This outcome warrants the continued use of aspirin prophylaxis in women with chronic hypertension. Acknowledging the mixed quality of the source data and the limitations inherent in meta-analyses, further research involving women with chronic hypertension is imperative to provide clarity on the value of aspirin prophylaxis.

ARTICLE 15

Differential Sex-specific Effects of Angiotensin-converting Enzyme Inhibition and Angiotensin Receptor Blocker Therapy on Arterial Function in Hypertension: CALIBREX Trial

Rogers SC, Ko YA, Quyyumi AA, Hajjar I. Differential sex-specific effects of angiotensin-converting enzyme inhibition and angiotensin receptor blocker therapy on arterial function in hypertension: CALIBREX Trial. *Hypertension. 2022;79(10):2316-27.*

Abstract

Background: Increased arterial stiffness is associated with adverse cardiovascular outcomes. The study investigated the impact of angiotensin antagonists on vascular function in hypertension, specifically exploring potential differences between men and women.

Methods: 141 participants with mild cognitive impairment and hypertension were randomized to candesartan ($n = 77$) or lisinopril ($n = 64$) to achieve a blood pressure target. The primary end point was reduction in pulse wave velocity, central pulse pressure, and central augmentation index which were measured using applanation tonometry.

Results: The reduction in blood pressure was comparable between the two groups. Notably, women on lisinopril experienced greater improvements in arterial stiffness, as evidenced by reduced pulse wave velocity and central pulse pressure, compared to those on candesartan. Conversely, candesartan was more effective for both sexes in improving pulse wave reflections.

Conclusions: The study underscores the sex-specific effects of these medications on arterial function in hypertensive individuals, with potential implications for cardiovascular and neurocognitive outcomes.

COMMENT

Central BP and arterial stiffness rather than brachial BP are associated with adverse cardiovascular outcomes.[104] Central aortic pressure and aortic stiffness can be assessed by aortic pulse wave velocity, central augmentation index, and central aortic pulse pressure noninvasively.[105]

Angiotensin converting enzyme inhibitors (ACIs) and angiotensin receptor blockers (ARBs) are commonly prescribed for hypertension treatment due to their comparable effectiveness in lowering blood pressure. Initial studies suggested that ACEIs were more effective in reducing heart failure and cardiac events compared to ARBs,[106] but recent meta-analyses indicate similar cardiovascular protection from both drug classes.[107,108] Additional analyses have revealed potential sex-based differences, with some trials showing varying effectiveness in preventing major cardiovascular events between men and women. For example, in the VALUE trial,[109] men experienced better cardiovascular outcomes with the ARB valsartan compared to women, and similar trends were observed in the ANBP-2 and ALLHAT trials for ACEIs.[110,111] CALIBREX trial is designed to compare ACE inhibitor Lisinopril with ARB Candesartan on measures of arterial stiffness.

In this trial, the effects of lisinopril and candesartan on vascular function were found to differ based on sex, despite both drugs having similar effects on BP. After 1 year of treatment, lisinopril led to improved arterial stiffness (measured as PWV, CPP, and peripheral pulse pressure), especially in women, whereas candesartan did not show the same effect. On the other hand, candesartan caused a greater reduction in pulse wave reflections (AIx) compared to lisinopril, with this improvement being consistent in both women and men.

Prior research has evaluated the effectiveness of ARBs and ACEIs in reducing blood pressure and improving cardiovascular outcomes, but this study is unique in comprehensively comparing the effects of these drugs on large arterial stiffness, wave reflections, and peripheral microvascular function in hypertension. The study revealed that lisinopril improved arterial stiffness indices such as PWV and CPP as seen in previous studies, with a specific improvement observed in women. Similar improvements in arterial stiffness have not been previously highlighted for females due to smaller sample sizes and younger, more diverse study populations.[112] While some trials have shown improved arterial stiffness with ARBs, this study did not observe significant changes in PWV or CPP with candesartan despite blood pressure reductions.[113] The impact of candesartan on AIx (pulse wave reflections) differed from lisinopril, aligning with previously mixed findings on the effectiveness of ARBs and ACEIs in reducing wave reflections. AIx has been associated with cognitive impairment, and ARBs are suggested to have neuroprotective effects beyond blood pressure reduction.[114] The study found that candesartan, but not lisinopril, improved AIx over time, suggesting a connection between improved pulse wave reflections and neurocognitive function.

Limitations

The study's 1-year duration may not have fully captured the long-term effects of the drugs being evaluated. The sex-specific analysis is an unplanned investigation within a trial not originally designed for studying such differences, underscoring the need for future trials designed to address sex-specific effects. The use of the ACEI lisinopril and ARB candesartan in the study might limit the interpretation of results to these specific drugs rather than the entire drug classes. Notably, a higher number of patients on lisinopril dropped out due to adverse events. Lastly, the study lacked a placebo comparison group due to ethical concerns, which restricts direct comparisons to the two drugs used.

In conclusion, this study highlights sex-based differences in the vascular effects of lisinopril and candesartan in older patients with hypertension. While lisinopril improved arterial stiffness primarily in women, candesartan showed better effects on pulse wave reflections in both sexes. The findings also suggest that improved wave reflections, rather than arterial stiffness measures, might correlate with better neurocognitive function.

ARTICLE 16

Comparing the Effects of Different Exercises on Blood Pressure and Arterial Stiffness in Postmenopausal Women: A Systematic Review and Meta-analysis.

Zhou WS, Zheng TT, Mao SJ, Xu H, Wang XF, Zhang SK. Comparing the effects of different exercises on blood pressure and arterial stiffness in postmenopausal women: A systematic review and meta-analysis.
Exp Gerontol. 2023;171:111990.

Abstract

The primary objective of this study was to assess the comparative effectiveness of various exercise regimens on systolic blood pressure (SBP), diastolic blood pressure (DBP), and aortic pulse wave velocity (PWV) in postmenopausal women. A comprehensive search of databases including China National Knowledge Infrastructure (CNKI), Wanfang, Web of Science, PubMed, and Cochrane library was conducted up until July 2022. The selection of randomized controlled trials adhered to predefined inclusion criteria, and study quality was evaluated using the PEDro scale. Statistical analysis was executed using Stata software. The study encompassed 23 papers (26 RCTs) and 729 participants. Meta-analysis revealed a significant reduction in SBP (WMD) −6.74 mm Hg; 95% CI −9.08, −4.41; $p = 0.000$), DBP (WMD −4.13 mm Hg; 95% CI −5.78, −2.48; $p = 0.000$), and aortic PWV (WMD −0.79 m/s; 95% CI −1.02, −0.56; $p = 0.000$) with exercise intervention. Subgroup analyses demonstrated that aerobic exercise significantly lowered SBP (WMD −7.97 mm Hg; 95% CI −12.99, −2.60; $p = 0.003$) and DBP (WMD −5.97 mm Hg; 95% CI −8.55, −3.39; $p = 0.000$), while resistance exercise notably reduced SBP (WMD −5.62 mm Hg; 95% CI −9.00, −2.23; $p = 0.001$), DBP (WMD −1.87 mm Hg; 95% CI −2.75, −0.99; $p = 0.000$), and aortic PWV (WMD −0.67 m/s; 95% CI −0.98, −0.36; $p = 0.000$). Combined aerobic and resistance exercise demonstrated a significant reduction in SBP (WMD −5.42 mm Hg; 95% CI −10.17, −0.68; $p = 0.025$). However, the impact of mind-body exercise (Tai Chi/Yoga) on SBP, DBP, and aortic PWV was inconclusive ($p > 0.05$). The findings emphasize the beneficial impact of exercise on SBP, DBP, and aortic PWV in postmenopausal women. Specifically, aerobic exercise reduced SBP and DBP, while resistance exercise lowered SBP, DBP, and aortic PWV. Nevertheless, further investigation is warranted to validate the efficacy of mind-body exercise (Tai Chi/Yoga) in relation to blood pressure and arterial stiffness.

COMMENT

Hypertension and arterial stiffness stand as prevalent cardiovascular conditions in postmenopausal women,[115,116] often attributed to diminished ovarian physiological function and reduced estrogen hormone levels.[117,118] Reduced arterial elasticity has been linked to hypertension,[119] and hypertension typically coincides with heightened arterial stiffness among postmenopausal women.[14,118] Enhancing pulse wave velocity (PWV), systolic blood pressure (SBP), and diastolic blood pressure (DBP) in postmenopausal women can lead to a decline in cardiovascular occurrence and overall mortality.[120,121]

Engaging in exercise represents a favorable approach to enhancing cardiovascular well-being.[122]

While numerous studies have delved into the impacts of exercise on blood pressure and arterial stiffness in postmenopausal women through randomized controlled trials (RCTs), only a limited number of studies have undertaken a comparative analysis of the effectiveness of distinct exercise modalities on blood pressure and arterial stiffness. Consequently, this systematic review and meta-analysis endeavors to assess and compare the varying effects of different exercise approaches on SBP, DBP, and PWV in the postmenopausal women.

The current systematic review and meta-analysis clearly indicated that exercise plays a notable role in reducing SBP, DBP, and PWV. Specifically, aerobic exercise exhibited significant reductions in SBP and DBP, while resistance exercise led to notable decreases in SBP, DBP, and aortic PWV. Moreover, the combined approach of aerobic and resistance exercise demonstrated a significant reduction in SBP. However, the impact of mind-body exercise interventions (such as Tai Chi or yoga) on SBP, DBP, and aortic PWV remains undetermined based on the available evidence.

Despite adhering to recognized guidelines like the Cochrane Handbook and PRISMA principle, this study has limitations: incomplete inclusion of literature due to unclear menopausal status, scarcity of research on arterial stiffness beyond resistance training, and limited exploration of exercise specifics like frequency and intensity, preventing precise recommendations for blood pressure and arterial stiffness improvement.

ARTICLE 17

Effectiveness of a Community-based Education and Peer Support Led by Women's Self-help Groups in Improving the Control of Hypertension in Urban Slums of Kerala, India: A Cluster Randomized Controlled Pragmatic Trial

P Suseela R, Ambika RB, Mohandas S, Menon JC, Numpelil M, K Vasudevan B, et al. Effectiveness of a community-based education and peer support led by women's self-help groups in improving the control of hypertension in urban slums of Kerala, India: a cluster randomised controlled pragmatic trial.
BMJ Global Health. 2022;7:e010296.

Abstract

Background: With under 20% of patients diagnosed with hypertension successfully reaching their designated blood pressure (BP) targets, unmanaged hypertension remains a significant public health concern in India. Our research aimed to evaluate the impact of a community-oriented education and peer support initiative guided by members of women's self-help groups (SHGs) on lowering the average systolic BP among hypertensive individuals residing in urban slums within Kochi City, Kerala, India.

Methods: A pragmatic cluster-randomized controlled trial was undertaken, encompassing 20 slum communities allocated to either the intervention group or the control group. Within each slum, individuals with elevated blood pressure (BP > 140/90 mm Hg) or those on antihypertensive medications were enlisted as participants. The intervention itself was administered through women's SHG members, with each member responsible for approximately 20–30 households. Their roles encompassed—(1) aiding in the management of daily hypertension, (2) providing emotional and social support to encourage healthy practices, and (3) facilitating referrals to the primary healthcare system. Conversely, individuals in the control group received the standard level of care. The primary outcome of interest centered on the alteration in the average systolic blood pressure (SBP) over a span of 6 months.

Results: A comprehensive cohort of 1,952 participants was enrolled, with 968 individuals allocated to the intervention group and 984 to the control group. The average SBP experienced a reduction of 6.26 mm Hg (SE 0.69) within the intervention group, contrasting with a decrease of 2.16 mm Hg (SE 0.70) within the control group. Consequently, the net variance amounted to 4.09 mm Hg (95% CI 2.15–4.09), with a p value of < 0.001.

Conclusion: The community intervention led by women's SHG members proved to be efficacious in diminishing SBP in individuals with hypertension, when compared to those who received standard care. This notable effect persisted over a span of 6 months within the urban slum areas of Kerala, India.

COMMENT

Increased blood pressure (BP) stands as the primary contributor to the worldwide burden of disease, representing a preventable cause of premature death.[123] Elevated BP holds significant prominence as a major risk element for ischemic heart disease, stroke, various other cardiovascular ailments (CVDs), chronic kidney conditions, and dementia.[124,125] Reports indicate a steep surge in the prevalence of hypertension within low-income and middle-income countries (LMICs).[4] Situated well into the epidemiologic transition, Kerala, the southernmost state of India, presents notably higher prevalence rates of CVDs (>5%) and hypertension (>26%) in comparison to the national average.[126] Within Kerala, "Kudumbasree units", colloquially referred to as women's self-help groups (SHGs), were established several decades ago with the guidance of local self-governing bodies (LSGs). These groups constitute one of the nation's most extensive women's empowerment initiatives.[127] Leveraging the involvement of women's SHG members to mitigate hypertension within the community by enhancing their capabilities as peer educators emerges as a potentially cost-effective and adaptable approach. This strategy could complement formal healthcare support while ensuring community involvement in health promotion efforts.

The authors carried out a community-centered cluster-randomized pragmatic trial (cRCT) to evaluate the efficacy of a community-based educational and peer support initiative, led by women's SHG members, in lowering the average systolic blood pressure (SBP) among individuals with hypertension residing in urban slums within Kochi Corporation, Kerala, India. The findings demonstrated that a community-oriented intervention overseen by women's SHG members proved successful in decreasing

BP in individuals with hypertension across a span of 6 months within the urban slums of Kerala, India. This approach is characterized by its affordability and simplicity, rendering it suitable for expansion to various regions within Kerala and other states in India. Its potential impact on addressing unmanaged hypertension and associated CVDs remains substantial.

Additional research is required to explore the adaptability of this intervention in regions with underdeveloped health systems and limited SHG infrastructure. Expanding the reach of this intervention could involve collaborating with broader community organizations beyond SHGs. There is also potential to devise and execute similar initiatives in other LMICs that have existing active peer support groups. Such efforts would align with the worldwide objectives for hypertension management and CVD prevention.[4,128]

ARTICLE 18

Focus on Today's Evidence While Keeping an Eye on the Future: Lessons derived from Hypertension in Women

Valdés G. Focus on today's evidence while keeping an eye on the future: lessons derived from hypertension in women. *J Hum Hypertens.* 2022;36:882-6.

Abstract
Cardiovascular diseases (CVDs) are a leading cause of death in women similar to men. It is important to recognize and manage risk factors in women for primary and secondary prevention. The article analyzes three issues related to women's cardiovascular health, highlighting milestones in their recognition and progression in public policies.

COMMENT

Should Stage 1 Hypertension Define Gestational Hypertension?

The first issue pertains to whether gestational hypertension should be defined using the lower thresholds of stage 1 hypertension (130–139/80–89 mm Hg) as suggested by the 2017 Hypertension Guidelines.[128] This change could increase the risk of adverse pregnancy outcomes such as preeclampsia, gestational hypertension, preterm birth, and low birth weight. The study suggests considering measures such as aspirin, closer monitoring of maternal and fetal well-being, and relaxation techniques, rather than immediate antihypertensive medication.[129] Several reports indicate that stage 1 hypertension during pregnancy doubles the risk of hypertensive disorders of pregnancy (HDP), gestational diabetes, preterm birth, and neonatal intensive care compared to normal blood pressure. These complications are less severe than those associated with stage 2 HDP.[130,131] However, a study from low-income countries contradicts these findings, possibly due to different measurement methods.[132] Physiologically, the proposal to redefine hypertension stage 1 in pregnancy is reasonable. During the first 20 weeks of normal pregnancy, 95th percentile systolic and diastolic BP values are 132 mm Hg and 76 mm Hg respectively due to factors such as vasodilation, increased plasma volume, and enhanced cardiac output. These factors also influence the development of the uteroplacental interphase, ensuring a healthy pregnancy. Lowering the blood pressure threshold for pregnancy could increase healthcare attention and the prevalence of hypertensive disorders of pregnancy, replacing chronic and gestational hypertension. This shift might improve the ability to predict preeclampsia and neonatal risks and introduce aspirin as a preventive measure. Although more evidence is needed to confirm the benefits of the lower threshold, the results align with observations that women's cardiovascular susceptibility occurs at lower blood pressures compared to men.

Should Blood Pressure Thresholds be Lower due to Women's Cardiovascular Susceptibility?

The Framingham Heart Study found that systolic blood pressure (SBP) increased cardiovascular events in both men and women. However, recent evidence contradicts this, showing that women face a higher risk of CVD at lower SBP levels compared to men. For instance, a combined analysis of various studies found that women with SBP levels between 110 and 119 mm Hg had similar myocardial infarction (MI) risk as men with SBP ≥160 mm Hg. This risk pattern was consistent for heart failure and stroke too, with women's risk elevating at lower SBP levels than men.[133]

In a Finland cohort, higher risk factor levels led to increasing CHD with age more so in women.[134] A study in Western Australia found an increased incidence of acute coronary events in women, particularly in younger age groups.[135] A study from the United States showed that coronary mortality changed less in young and middle-aged women compared to men in the same age group.[136] Similarly, France observed rising rates of acute coronary syndromes (ACS) among women under 65, with a significant increase in myocardial infarctions.[137] The Hordaland study found that women with stage 1 and 2 SBP had considerably higher ACS risks compared to men, especially in their early 40s. Diastolic blood pressure (DBP) also impacted women's ACS risk more than men.[138]

These observations have led to campaigns focusing on CVD awareness in younger women and raise the pertinent question of whether hypertension thresholds should differ by gender.

When will Cardiometabolic Care be Widely Established after Obstetrical Complications?

Hypertensive disorders of pregnancy increase cardiovascular risk (CVR) later in life. Similar enhanced risk is seen with other placental disorders such as intrauterine growth retardation, preterm delivery, and recurrent abortion.[139] A recent umbrella review found a twofold increase in composite cardiovascular disease, ischemic heart disease, and stroke and a fourfold increase in heart failure.[140] The primary link between CVR and reproductive outcomes is through endothelial dysfunction, which involves a decreased ability of blood vessels to dilate in response to flow.[141] Despite existing guidelines recommending postpartum follow-up for HDP, to identify CVR, routine follow-up after HDP is lacking.[142] Regarding reversal of CVR following hypertensive pregnancy, one study showed that calcium supplementation led to a reduction of −3.4 mm Hg in DBP among women with a history of severe preeclampsia.[143] The second study focused on education for adopting healthy habits, resulting in a slight DBP decrease, improved diet, reduced physical inactivity, and better awareness of CVR profiles.[144]

In conclusion, early recognition of women's heightened cardiovascular vulnerability, particularly evident during pregnancy, is crucial for making substantial advancements in the long-term reduction of CVD.

REFERENCES

1. O'Keeffe LM, Simpkin AJ, Tilling K, Anderson EL, Hughes AD, Lawlor DA, et al. Sex-specific trajectories of measures of cardiovascular health during childhood and adolescence: a prospective cohort study. Atherosclerosis. 2018;278:190-6.
2. Shen W, Zhang T, Li S, Zhang H, Xi B, Shen H, et al. Race and sex differences of long- term blood pressure profiles from childhood and adult hypertension: the Bogalusa heart study. Hypertension. 2017;70:66-74.
3. Samargandy S, Matthews KA, Brooks MM, Barinas-Mitchell E, Magnani JW, Thurston RC, et al. Trajectories of blood pressure in midlife women: does menopause matter? Circ Res. 2022;130:312-22.
4. NCD Risk Factor Collaboration (NCD-RisC). Worldwide trends in hypertension prevalence and progress in treatment and control from 1990 to 2019: a pooled analysis of 1201 population-representative studies with 104 million participants. Lancet. 2021;398:957-80.
5. Colafella KMM, Denton KM. Sex-specific differences in hypertension and associated cardiovascular disease. Nat Rev Nephrol. 2018;14:185-201.
6. Oparil S, Miller AP. Gender and blood pressure. J Clin Hypertens (Greenwich). 2005;7:300-9.
7. Perrino C, Ferdinandy P, Botker HE, Brundel B, Collins P, Davidson SM, et al. Improving translational research in sex-specific effects of comorbidities and risk factors in ischaemic heart disease and cardioprotection: position paper and recommendations of the ESC working group on cellular biology of the heart. Cardiovasc Res. 2021;117:367-85.
8. Honigberg MC, Zekavat SM, Aragam K, Klarin D, Bhatt DL, Scott NS, et al. Long-Term cardiovascular risk in women with hypertension during pregnancy. J Am Coll Cardiol. 2019;74:2743-54.
9. Barrett-Connor EL, Cohn BA, Wingard DL, Edelstein SL. Why is diabetes mellitus a stronger risk factor for fatal ischemic heart disease in women than in men? The rancho Bernardo study. JAMA. 1991;265:627-31.
10. Gerdts E, Okin PM, de Simone G, Cramariuc D, Wachtell K, Boman K, et al. Gender differences in left ventricular structure and function during antihypertensive treatment: the losartan intervention for endpoint reduction in hypertension study. Hypertension. 2008;51:1109-14.
11. Gerdts E, Oikarinen L, Palmieri V, Otterstad JE, Wachtell K, Boman K, et al. Correlates of left atrial size in hypertensive patients with left ventricular hypertrophy: the losartan intervention for endpoint reduction in hypertension (LIFE) study. Hypertension. 2002;39:739-43.
12. Esposito R, Izzo R, Galderisi M, De Marco M, Stabile E, Esposito G, et al. Identification of phenotypes at risk of transition from diastolic hypertension to isolated systolic hypertension. J Hum Hypertens. 2016;30:392-6.
13. Millett ERC, Peters SAE, Woodward M. Sex differences in risk factors for myocardial infarction: cohort study of UK biobank participants. BMJ. 2018;363:k4247.
14. Coutinho T. Arterial stiffness and its clinical implications in women. Can J Cardiol. 2014;30:756-64.
15. Cramariuc D, Rogge BP, Lonnebakken MT, Boman K, Bahlmann E, Gohlke-Barwolf C, et al. Sex differences in cardiovascular outcome during progression of aortic valve stenosis. Heart. 2015;101:209-14.
16. Lewis CE, Grandits A, Flack J, McDonald R, Elmer PJ. Efficacy and tolerance of antihypertensive treatment in men and women with stage 1 diastolic hypertension. Results of the treatment of mild hypertension study. Arch Intern Med. 1996;156:377-85.
17. Sacks FM, Svetkey LP, Vollmer WM, Appel LJ, Bray GA, Harsha D, et al. Effects on blood pressure

of reduced dietary sodium and the dietary approaches to stop hypertension (DASH) diet. DASH-sodium collaborative research group. N Engl J Med. 2001;344:3-10.
18. Tamargo J, Rosano G, Walther T, Duarte J, Niessner A, Kaski JC, et al. Gender differences in the effects of cardiovascular drugs. Eur Heart J Cardiovasc Pharmacother. 2017;3:163-82.
19. Turnbull F, Woodward M, Neal B, Barzi F, Ninomiya T, Chalmers J, et al. Do men and women respond differently to blood pressure-lowering treatment? Results of prospectively designed overviews of randomized trials. Eur Heart J. 2008;29:2669-80.
20. Reboussin DM, Allen NB, Griswold ME, Guallar E, Hong Y, Lackland DT, et al. Systematic review for the 2017 ACC/AHA/AAPA/ABC/ACPM/AGS/APhA/ASH/ASPC/NMA/PCNA guideline for the prevention, detection, evaluation, and management of high blood pressure in adults: a report of the American college of cardiology/American heart association task force on clinical practice guidelines. Circulation. 2018;138:e595-616.
21. Yusuf S, Joseph P, Rangarajan S, Islam S, Mente A, Hystad P, et al. Modifiable risk factors, cardiovascular disease, and mortality in 155 722 individuals from 21 high-income, middle-income, and low-income countries (PURE): a prospective cohort study. Lancet. 2020;395:795-808.
22. Connelly PJ, Currie G, Delles C. Sex differences in the prevalence, outcomes, and management of hypertension. Curr Hypertens Rep. 2022;24:185-92.
23. Johnson JL, Greaves L, Repta R. Better science with sex and gender: facilitating the use of a sex and gender-based analysis in health research. Int J Equity Health. 2009;8:14.
24. WHO. Guideline for the pharmacological treatment of hypertension in adults. Geneva: World Health Organization; 2021.
25. Magee LA, Singer J, von Dadelszen P. Less-tight versus tight control of hypertension in pregnancy. N Engl J Med. 2015;372:2367-8.
26. Unger T, Borghi C, Charchar F, Khan NA, Poulter NR, Prabhakaran D, et al. 2020 International Society of Hypertension global hypertension practice guidelines. J Hypertens. 2020;38:982-1004.
27. Williams B, Mancia G, Spiering W, Agabiti Rosei E, Azizi M, Burnier M, et al. 2018 ESC/ESH Guidelines for the management of arterial hypertension: The Task Force for the management of arterial hypertension of the European Society of Cardiology and the European Society of Hypertension: The Task Force for the management of arterial hypertension of the European Society of Cardiology and the European Society of Hypertension. J Hypertens. 2018;36:1953-2041.
28. Whelton PK, Carey RM, Aronow WS, Casey DE Jr, Collins KJ, Dennison Himmelfarb C, et al. 2017 ACC/AHA/AAPA/ABC/ACPM/AGS/APhA/ASH/ASPC/NMA/PCNA Guideline for the Prevention, Detection, Evaluation, and Management of High Blood Pressure in Adults: A Report of the American College of Cardiology/American Heart Association Task Force on Clinical Practice Guidelines. Hypertension. 2018;71:e13-115.
29. National Cholesterol Education Program (NCEP) Expert Panel on Detection, Evaluation, and Treatment of High Blood Cholesterol in Adults (Adult Treatment Panel III). Third Report of the National Cholesterol Education Program (NCEP) Expert Panel on Detection, Evaluation, and Treatment of High Blood Cholesterol in Adults (Adult Treatment Panel III) final report. Circulation. 2002;106:3143-421.
30. Committee on Obstetric Practice. Committee Opinion No. 623: Emergent therapy for acute-onset, severe hypertension during pregnancy and the postpartum period. Obstet Gynecol. 2015;125:521-5.
31. Task Force of the Latin American Society of Hypertension. Guidelines on the management of arterial hypertension and related comorbidities in Latin America. J Hypertens. 2017;35:1529-45.
32. Roth GA, Mensah GA, Johnson CO, Addolorato G, Ammirati E, Baddour LM, et al. Global burden of cardiovascular diseases and risk factors, 1990–2019: update from the GBD 2019 study. J Am Coll Cardiol. 2020;76(25):2982-3021.
33. Sacco RL, Roth GA, Reddy KS, Arnett DK, Bonita R, Gaziano TA, et al. The heart of 25 by 25: achieving the goal of reducing global and regional premature deaths from cardiovascular diseases and stroke: a modeling study from the American Heart Association and World Heart Federation. Circulation. 2016;133(23):e674-90.
34. Ramirez LA, Sullivan JC. Sex differences in hypertension: where we have been and where we are going. Am J Hypertens. 2018;31(12):1247-54.
35. Forouzanfar MH, Liu P, Roth GA, Ng M, Biryukov S, Marczak L, et al. Global burden of hypertension and systolic blood pressure of at least 110 to 115 mm Hg, 1990–2015. JAMA. 2017;317(2):165-82.
36. Boggia J, Thijs L, Hansen TW, Li Y, Kikuya M, Björklund-Bodegård K, et al. Ambulatory blood pressure monitoring in 9357 subjects from 11 populations highlights missed opportunities for cardiovascular prevention in women. Hypertension. 2011;57(3):397-405.

37. Wei YC, George NI, Chang CW, Hicks KA. Assessing sex differences in the risk of cardiovascular disease and mortality per increment in systolic blood pressure: a systematic review and meta-analysis of follow-up studies in the United States. PLoS One. 2017;12(1):e0170218.
38. James PA, Oparil S, Carter BL, Cushman WC, Dennison-Himmelfarb C, Handler J, et al. 2014 evidence-based guideline for the management of high blood pressure in adults: report from the panel members appointed to the Eighth Joint National Committee (JNC 8). JAMA. 2014;311(5):507-20.
39. Virani SS, Alonso A, Benjamin EJ, Bittencourt MS, Callaway CW, Carson AP, et al. Heart Disease and stroke statistics—2020 update: a report from the American Heart Association. Circulation. 2020;141(9):e139-e596.
40. Roerecke M, Rehm J. Chronic heavy drinking and ischaemic heart disease: a systematic review and meta-analysis. Open Heart. 2014;1(1):e000135.
41. Specogna AV, Turin TC, Patten SB, Hill MD. Factors associated with early deterioration after spontaneous intracerebral hemorrhage: a systematic review and meta-analysis. PLoS One. 2014;9(5):e96743.
42. Ikeda A, Iso H, Yamagishi K, Inoue M, Tsugane S. Blood pressure and the risk of stroke, cardiovascular disease, and all-cause mortality among Japanese: the JPHC Study. Am J Hypertens. 2009;22(3):273-80.
43. Peters SA, Woodward M, Lam TH, Fang X, Suh I, Ueshema H, et al. Sex disparities in risk and risk factors for ischemic heart disease in the Asia-Pacific region. Eur J Prevent Cardiol. 2014;21(5):639-46.
44. American Heart Association. My life check–Life's simple 7. [online] Available from https://playbook.heart.org/lifes-simple-7/. [Last accessed October, 2023]
45. Bairey Merz CN, Mark S, Boyan BD, Jacobs AK, Shah PK, Shaw LJ, et al. Proceedings from the scientific symposium: sex differences in cardiovascular disease and implications for therapies. J Women's Health. 2010;19(6):1059-72.
46. Wang SC, Koutroumpakis E, Schulman-Marcus J, Tosh T, Volgman AS, Lyubarova R. Sex differences remain under-reported in cardiovascular publications. J Women's Health. 2021;30(9):1253-8.
47. Ohira T, Iso H. Cardiovascular disease epidemiology in Asia. Circ J. 2013;77(7):1646-52.
48. Milner TA, Contoreggi NH, Yu F, Johnson MA, Wang G, Woods C, et al. Estrogen receptor b contributes to both hypertension and hypothalamic plasticity in a mouse model of peri-menopause. J Neurosci. 2021;41:5190-205.
49. Leache L, Gutiérrez-Valencia M, Finizola RM, Infante E, Finizola B, Pardo JP, et al. Pharmacotherapy for hypertension-induced left ventricular hypertrophy. Cochrane Database Syst Rev. 2021;10:CD01203.
50. Alp H, Karaarslan S, Ekliog¨lu BS, Atabek ME, Baysal T. The effect of hypertension and obesity on left ventricular geometry and cardiac functions in children and adolescents. J Hypertens. 2014;32:1283-92.
51. Lavie CJ, Patel DA, Milani RV, Ventura HO, Shah S, Gilliland Y. Impact of echocardiographic left ventricular geometry on clinical prognosis. Prog Cardiovasc Dis. 2014;57:3-9.
52. Kawarazaki W, Fujita T. Kidney and epigenetic mechanisms of salt-sensitive hypertension. Nat Rev Nephrol. 2021;17:350-63.
53. Faulkner JL, Belin de Chantemèle EJ. Female Sex, a Major Risk Factor for Salt-Sensitive Hypertension. Curr Hypertens Rep. 2020;22:99.
54. Alberti-Fidanza A, Fruttini D, Servili M. Gustatory and food habit changes during the menstrual cycle. Int J Vitam Nutr Res. 1998;68:149-53.
55. Krecek J, Nováková V, Stibral K. Sex differences in the taste preference for a salt solution in the rat. Physiol Behav. 1972;8:183-8.
56. Shukri MZ, Tan JW, Manosroi W, Pojoga LH, Rivera A, Williams JS, et al. Biological sex modulates the adrenal and blood pressure responses to angiotensin II. Hypertension. 2018;71:1083-90.
57. Barton M, Meyer MR. Postmenopausal hypertension: mechanisms and therapy. Hypertension. 2009;54:11-8.
58. Gabbe S. Obstetrics: Normal and Problem Pregnancies, 6th edition. Philadelphia, PA: Elsevier/Saunders; 2012.
59. Rich-Edwards JW, Fraser A, Lawlor DA, Catov JM. Pregnancy characteristics and women's future cardiovascular health: an underused opportunity to improve women's health? Epidemiol Rev. 2014;36:57-70.
60. Melchiorre K, Giorgione V, Thilaganathan B. The placenta and preeclampsia: villain or victim? Am J Obstet Gynecol. 2022;226:S954-62.
61. Horn J, Haug EB, Markovitz AR, Fraser A, Vatten LJ, Romundstad PR, et al. Life course trajectories of maternal cardiovascular risk factors according to offspring birthweight: the HUNT Study. Sci Rep. 2020;10:10436.
62. Franklin SS, Gustin W, Wong ND, Larson MG, Weber MA, Kannel WB, et al. Hemodynamic patterns of age-related changes in blood pressure. Circulation. 1997;96:308-15.
63. Gibson GR. Enalapril-induced cough. Arch Intern Med. 1989;149:2701-3.

64. Abraham HM, White CM, White WB. The comparative efficacy and safety of the angiotensin receptor blockers in the management of hypertension and other cardiovascular diseases. Drug Saf. 2015;38:33-54.
65. Kajiwara A, Saruwatari J, Kita A, Oniki K, Yamamura M, Murase M, et al. Younger females are at greater risk of vasodilation-related adverse symptoms caused by dihydropyridine calcium channel blockers: results of a study of 11,918 Japanese patients. Clin Drug Investig. 2014;34:431-5.
66. Aung K, Htay T. Thiazide diuretics and the risk of hip fracture. Cochrane Database Syst Rev. 2011;(10):CD005185.
67. Dorans KS, Mills KT, Liu Y, He J. Trends in prevalence and control of hypertension according to the 2017 American College of Cardiology/American Heart Association (ACC/AHA) Guideline. J Am Heart Assoc. 2018;7:e008888.
68. Rossier BC, Bochud M, Devuyst O. The hypertension pandemic: an evolutionary perspective. Physiology (Bethesda). 2017;32:112-25.
69. Nguyen Q, Dominguez J, Nguyen L, Gullapalli N. Hypertension management: an update. Am Health Drug Benefits. 2010;3:47-56.
70. Appel LJ, Brands MW, Daniels SR, Karanja N, Elmer PJ, Sacks FM. American Heart Association. Dietary approaches to prevent and treat hypertension: a scientific statement from the American Heart Association. Hypertension. 2006;47:296-308.
71. Dickinson HO, Nicolson DJ, Cook JV, Campbell F, Beyer FR, Ford GA, et al. Calcium supplementation for the management of primary hypertension in adults. Cochrane Database Syst Rev. 2006;(2):CD004639.
72. Li F, Wang T, Chen L, Zhang S, Chen L, Qin J. Adverse pregnancy outcomes among mothers with hypertensive disorders in pregnancy: a meta-analysis of cohort studies. Pregnancy Hypertens. 2021;24:107-17.
73. Battarbee AN, Sinkey RG, Harper LM, Oparil S, Tita ATN. Chronic hypertension in pregnancy. Am J Obstet Gynecol. 2020;222(6):532-41.
74. Ukah UV, De Silva DA, Payne B, et al. Prediction of adverse maternal outcomes from pre-eclampsia and other hypertensive disorders of pregnancy: a systematic review. Pregnancy Hypertens. 2018;11:115-23.
75. Magee LA, von Dadelszen P. State-of-the-art diagnosis and treatment of hypertension in pregnancy. Mayo Clin Proc. 2018;93(11):1664-77.
76. Tita AT, Szychowski JM, Boggess K, Dugoff L, Sibai B, Lawrence K, et al. Treatment for mild chronic hypertension during pregnancy. N Engl J Med. 2022;386(19):1781-92.
77. Magee LA, von Dadelszen P, Rey E, Ross S, Asztalos E, Murphy KE, et al. Less-tight versus tight control of hypertension in pregnancy. N Engl J Med. 2015;372(5):407-17.
78. Duley L, Meher S, Hunter KE, Seidler AL, Askie LM. Antiplatelet agents for preventing pre-eclampsia and its complications. Cochrane Database Syst Rev. 2019;(10):CD004659.
79. World Health Organization. WHO recommendations for prevention and treatment of pre-eclampsia and eclampsia. Geneva: World Health Organization; 2011.
80. NICE. Hypertension in pregnancy: diagnosis and management. London: NICE; 2019. p. 55.
81. Sanchez-Ramos L, Roeckner JT, Kaunitz AM. Which agent most effectively prevents preeclampsia? a systematic review with multi-treatment comparison (network meta-analysis) of large multicenter randomized controlled trials. Am J Obstet Gynecol. 2017;216:S504.
82. Khaing W, Vallibhakara SA-O, Tantrakul V, Vallibhakara O, Rattanasiri S, McEvoy M, et al. Calcium and vitamin D supplementation for prevention of preeclampsia: a systematic review and network meta-analysis. Nutrients. 2017;9:1141.
83. Sailaja B, Cooly V, Sailcheemala B, Sailaja S. A study on risk factors, maternal and foetal outcome in cases of preeclampsia and eclampsia at a tertiary care hospital of South India. Int J Reprod Contracept Obstet Gynecol. 2017;7:266-71.
84. Askie LM, Duley L, Henderson-Smart DJ, Stewart LA. Antiplatelet agents for prevention of pre-eclampsia: A meta-analysis of individual patient data. Lancet. 2007;369:1791-8.
85. Lowe SA, Bowyer L, Lust K, McMahon LP, Morton M, North RA, et al. SOMANZ guideline for the management of hypertensive disorders of pregnancy 2014. Aust N Z J Obstet Gynaecol. 2014;55:e1-29.
86. Frawley J, Sibbritt D, Broom A, Gallois C, Steel A, Adams J. Women's attitudes towards the use of complementary and alternative medicine products during pregnancy. J Obstet Gynaecol. 2016;36:462-7.
87. Smith CA, Tuson A, Tornton C, Dahlen HG. The safety and effectiveness of mind body interventions for women with pregnancy induced hypertension and or preeclampsia: A systematic review and meta-analysis. Complement Ter Med. 2020;52:102469.
88. Narendran S, Nagarathna R, Narendran V, Gunasheela S, Nagendra HR. Efficacy of yoga on pregnancy outcome. J Altern Complement Med. 2005;11:237-44.
89. Sibai B, Dekker G, Kupferminc M. Pre-eclampsia. Lancet. 2005;365:785-99.

90. Garovic VD, Hayman SR. Hypertension in pregnancy: an emerging risk factor for cardiovascular disease. Nat Clin Pract Nephrol. 2007;3:613-22.
91. Ananth CV, Keyes KM, Wapner RJ. Preeclampsia rates in the United States, 1980-2010: age-period-cohort analysis. BMJ. 2013;347:f6564.
92. Kuklina EV, Ayala C, Callaghan WM. Hypertensive disorders and severe obstetric morbidity in the United States. Obstet Gynecol. 2009;113:1299-306.
93. American College of Obstetricians and Gynecologists; Task Force on Hypertension in pregnancy. Hypertension in Pregnancy. Obstet Gynecol. 2013;122(5):1122-31.
94. ACOG. ACOG Practice Bulletin No. 202: Gestational Hypertension and Preeclampsia. Obstet Gynecol. 2019;133(1):1-1.
95. Sisti G, Schiattarella A, Morlando M, Corwin A. Timing of delivery and blood pressure cut-off in chronic hypertension during pregnancy: State of art and new proposals. Int J Gynecol Obstet. 2022;157(2):230-9.
96. Bateman BT, Bansil P, Hernandez-Diaz S, Mhyre JM, Callaghan WM, Kuklina EV. Prevalence, trends, and outcomes of chronic hypertension: a nationwide sample of delivery admissions. Am J Obstet Gynecol. 2012;206(2):134.
97. Kahramanoglu O, ̈Schiattarella A, Demirci O, Sisti G, Ammaturo FP, Trotta C, et al. Preeclampsia: state of art and future perspectives. A special focus on possible preventions. J Obstet Gynaecol (Lahore). 2022;42(5):766-77.
98. Whelton PK, Carey RM, Aronow WS, Casey DE, Collins KJ, Dennison Himmelfarb C, et al. 2017 ACC/AHA/AAPA/ABC/ACPM/AGS/APhA/ASH/ASPC/ NMA/PCNA Guideline for the Prevention, Detection, Evaluation, and Management of High Blood Pressure in Adults: Executive Summary: A Report of the American College of Cardiology/American Heart Association Task F. Hypertension. 2018;71(6):1269-324.
99. Sibai BM. Chronic hypertension in pregnancy. Obstet Gynecol. 2002;100:369-77.
100. Bartsch E, Medcalf KE, Park AL, Ray JG. High risk of pre-eclampsia identification group. Clinical risk factors for preeclampsia determined in early pregnancy: systematic review and meta-analysis of large cohort studies. BMJ. 2016;353:i1753.
101. Bramham K, Parnell B, Nelson-Piercy C, Seed PT, Poston L, Chappell LC. Chronic hypertension and pregnancy outcomes: systematic review and meta-analysis. BMJ. 2014;348:g2301.
102. National Institute for Health and Care Excellence (NICE). (2019). Hypertension in pregnancy: diagnosis and management. [online] Available from https://www.nice.org.uk/guidance/ng133. [Last accessed October, 2023].
103. O'Connor D. (2016). Saving Babies' Lives: a care bundle for reducing stillbirth. [online] Available from https://www.england.nhs.uk/wp-content/uploads/2016/03/saving-babies-lives-car-bundl.pdf. [Last accessed October, 2023].
104. Mitchell GF, Hwang SJ, Vasan RS, Larson MG, Pencina MJ, Hamburg NM, et al. Arterial stiffness and cardiovascular events: the Framingham Heart Study. Circulation. 2010;121:505-11.
105. Segers P, Rietzschel ER, Chirinos JA. How to measure arterial stiffness in humans. Arterioscler Thromb Vasc Biol. 2020;40:1034-43.
106. van Vark LC, Bertrand M, Akkerhuis KM, Brugts JJ, Fox K, Mourad JJ, et al. Angiotensin-converting enzyme inhibitors reduce mortality in hypertension: a meta-analysis of randomized clinical trials of renin-angiotensin-aldosterone system inhibitors involving 158,998 patients. Eur Heart J. 2012;33:2088-97.
107. Suchard MA, Schuemie MJ, Krumholz HM, You SC, Chen R, Pratt N, et al. Comprehensive comparative effectiveness and safety of first-line antihypertensive drug classes: a systematic, multinational, large-scale analysis. Lancet. 2019;394:1816-26.
108. Chen R, Suchard MA, Krumholz HM, Schuemie MJ, Shea S, Duke J, et al. Comparative first-line effectiveness and safety of ACE (Angiotensin-Converting Enzyme) inhibitors and angiotensin receptor blockers: a multinational cohort study. Hypertension. 2021;78:591-603.
109. Zanchetti A, Julius S, Kjeldsen S, McInnes GT, Hua T, Weber M, et al. Outcomes in subgroups of hypertensive patients treated with regimens based on valsartan and amlodipine: An analysis of findings from the VALUE trial. J Hypertens. 2006;24:2163-8.
110. Wing LM, Reid CM, Ryan P, Beilin LJ, Brown MA, Jennings GL, et al.; Second Australian National Blood Pressure Study Group. A comparison of outcomes with angiotensin-converting enzyme inhibitors and diuretics for hypertension in the elderly. N Engl J Med. 2003;348:583-92.
111. ALLHAT Officers and Coordinators for the ALLHAT Collaborative Research Group. The Antihypertensive and Lipid-Lowering Treatment to Prevent Heart Attack Trial. Major outcomes in high-risk hypertensive patients randomized to angiotensin-converting enzyme inhibitor or calcium channel blocker vs diuretic: The Antihypertensive and Lipid-Lowering Treatment to Prevent Heart Attack Trial (ALLHAT). JAMA. 2002;288:2981-97.

112. Liu M, Li GL, Li Y, Wang JG. Effects of various antihypertensive drugs on arterial stiffness and wave reflections. Pulse (Basel). 2013;1:97-107.
113. Peng F, Pan H, Wang B, Lin J, Niu W. The impact of angiotensin receptor blockers on arterial stiffness: a meta-analysis. Hypertens Res. 2015;38:613-20.
114. Strauss MH, Hall A. Angiotensin receptor blockers should be regarded as first-line drugs for stroke prevention in both primary and secondary prevention settings. Stroke. 2009;40:3161-2.
115. Bismar H, Diel I, Ziegler R, Pfeilschifter J, Increased cytokine secretion by human bone marrow cells after menopause or discontinuation of estrogen replacement. The Journal of Clinical Endocrinology & Metabolism 1995;80:3351-5.
116. Carpenter RE, Emery SJ, Uzun O, D'Silva LA, Lewis MJ. Influence of antenatal physical exercise on haemodynamics in pregnant women: a flexible randomisation approach. BMC Pregnancy Childbirth. 2015;15:1-15.
117. Bonithon-Kopp C, Scarabin PY, Darne B, Malmejac A, Guize L. Menopause-related changes in lipoproteins and some other cardiovascular risk factors. Int J Epidemiol. 1990;19:42-8.
118. Zaydun G, Tomiyama H, Hashimoto H, Arai T, Koji Y, Yambe M, et al. Menopause is an independent factor augmenting the age-related increase in arterial stiffness in the early postmenopausal phase. Atherosclerosis. 2006;184:137-42.
119. Vokonas P, Kannel W, Cupples L. Epidemiology and risk of hypertension in the elderly: the Framingham study. J Hypertens Suppl. 1988;6:S3-S9.
120. Du J, Guo YZ. Pathophysiological characteristics of postmenopausal hypertension. J Clin Card Dis. 2000;16:524-6.
121. Wang PF, Wang C, Qiao HX, Sun G, Yan XL, Wu GX, et al. Pulse wave velocity and cardio-cerebral vascular events and mortality in a cohort study. J Clin Cardiol. 2011;27:775-8.
122. Son WM, Sung KD, Cho JM, Park SY. Combined exercise reduces arterial stiffness, blood pressure, and blood markers for cardiovascular risk in postmenopausal women with hypertension. Menopause. 2017;24:262-8.
123. GBD 2019 Diseases and Injuries Collaborators. Global burden of 369 diseases and injuries in 204 countries and territories, 1990-2019: a systematic analysis for the global burden of disease study 2019. Lancet. 2020;396:1204-22.
124. Rapsomaniki E, Timmis A, George J, Pujades-Rodriguez M, Shah AD, Denaxas S, et al. Blood pressure and incidence of twelve cardiovascular diseases: lifetime risks, healthy life-years lost, and age-specific associations in 1.25 million people. Lancet. 2014;383:1899-911.
125. Huang Y, Cai X, Zhang J, Mai W, Wang S, Hu Y, et al. Prehypertension and incidence of ESRD: a systematic review and meta-analysis. Am J Kidney Dis. 2014;63:76-83.
126. India State-Level Disease Burden Initiative CVD Collaborators. The changing patterns of cardiovascular diseases and their risk factors in the states of India: the global burden of disease study 1990-2016. Lancet Glob Health. 2018;6:e1339-51.
127. Government of Kerala. Kudumbasree [Internet]. Thiruvananthapuram. [online] Available from http://www.kudumbashree.org/. [Last accessed October, 2023].
128. United Nations. (2015). Transforming our world: the 2030 agenda for sustainable development, 2015. [online] Available from https://www.un.org/ga/. [Last accessed October, 2023].
129. Li Q, Zheng L, Jiang D, Gu Y, Wang G, Li J, et al. Early pregnancy stage 1 hypertension and high mean arterial pressure increased risk of adverse pregnancy outcomes in Shanghai, China. J Hum Hypertens. 2021;35:1-8.
130. Bello NA, Zhou H, Cheetham TC, Miller E, Getahun DT, Fassett MJ, et al. Prevalence of hypertension among pregnant women when using the 2017 American College of Cardiology/American Heart Association Blood Pressure Guidelines and association with maternal and fetal outcomes. JAMA Netw Open. 2021;4:e213808.
131. Sabol BA, Porcelli B, Diveley E, Meyenburg K, Woolfolk C, Rosenbloom JI, et al. Defining the risk profile of women with stage 1 hypertension: a time to event analysis. Am J Obstet Gynecol MFM. 2021;3:100376.
132. Bone JN, Magee LA, Singer J, Nathan H, Qureshi RN, Sacoor C, et al. Blood pressure thresholds in pregnancy for identifying maternal and infant risk: a secondary analysis of Community-Level Interventions for Pre-eclampsia (CLIP) trial data. Lancet Glob Health. 2021;9:e1119-28.
133. Ji H, Niirannen TJ, Rader F, Henglin M, Kim A, Ebinger JE, et al. Sex differences in blood pressure associations with cardiovascular outcomes. Circulation. 2021;143:761-3.
134. Jousilahti P, Vartiainen E, Toumilehto J, Puska P. Sex, age and cardiovascular risk factors, and coronary heart disease: a prospective study of 14,786 middle-aged men and women in Finland. Circulation. 1999;99:1165-72.

135. Nedkoff LJ, Briffa TG, Preen DB, Sanfilippo FM, Hung J, Ridout SC, et al. Age- and sex-specific trends in the incidence of hospitalized acute coronary syndromes in Western Australia. Circ Cardiovasc Qual Outcomes. 2011;4:557-64.
136. Wilmot KA, O'Flaherty M, Capewell S, Ford ES, Vaccarino V. Coronary heart disease mortality declines in the United States from 1979 through 2011: evidence for stagnation in young adults, especially women. Circulation. 2015;132:997-1002.
137. Gabet A, Danchin N, Juillière Y, Olié V. Acute coronary syndrome in women: rising hospitalizations in middle-aged French women, 2004-14. Eur Heart J. 2017;38:1060-5.
138. Kringeland E, Tell GS, Midtbø H, Igland J, Haugsgjerd TR, Gerdts E. Stage 1 hypertension, sex, and acute coronary syndromes during midlife: The Hordaland Health Study. Eur J Prev Cardiol. 2022;29(1):147-54.
139. Grandi SM, Filion KB, Yoon S, Ayele HT, Doyle CM, Hutcheon JA, et al. Cardiovascular disease-related morbidity and mortality in women with a history of pregnancy complications. Circulation. 2019;139:1069-79.
140. Okoth K, Singh Chandan J, Marshall T, Thangaratinam S, Thomas GN, Nirantharakumar K, et al. Association between the reproductive health of young women and cardiovascular disease in later life: umbrella review. BMJ. 2020;371:m3502.
141. Valdés G. Preeclampsia and cardiovascular disease: interconnected paths that enable detection of the subclinical stages of obstetric and cardiovascular diseases. Integr Blood Press Control. 2017;10:17-23.
142. Parikh NI, Gonzalez JM, Anderson CAM, Judd SE, Rexrode KM, Hlatky MA, et al. Adverse pregnancy outcomes and cardiovascular disease risk: unique opportunities for cardiovascular disease prevention in women: a scientific statement from the American Heart Association. Circulation. 2021;143:e902-16.
143. Hauspurg A, Countouris ME, Catov JM. Hypertensive disorders of pregnancy and future maternal health: How can the evidence guide postpartum management? Curr Hypertens Rep. 2019;21:96.
144. Lui NA, Jeyaram G, Henry A. Postpartum interventions to reduce long-term cardiovascular disease risk in women after hypertensive disorders of pregnancy: a systematic review. Front Cardiovasc Med. 2019;6:160.

SECTION 3

Dyslipidemia and CVD in Women

Section Editor: Kunal Mahajan

Associate Editors: Tanuj Bhatia, Jaikrit Bhutani, Sai Devvrat, Abhishek Rastogi, Prashant Patel, Lokesh Verma

ARTICLE 1

Sex Differences in Lipid-lowering Therapy of Familial Hypercholesterolemia

Zamora A, Ramos R, Comas-Cufí M, García-Gil M, Martí-Lluch R, Plana N, et al. Women with familial hypercholesterolemia phenotype are undertreated and poorly controlled compared to men.
Sci Rep. 2023;13(1):1492.

Abstract

Background: Familial hypercholesterolemia (FH) is a genetic disorder inherited in an autosomal dominant manner, affecting around 1 in 250 people. It is the most common cause of early cardiovascular disease (CVD). However, literature on women population is scarce, resulting in underdiagnosis and undertreatment, partly due to belief that they are at a lower risk of developing CVD.

Objectives: The aim of this study was to investigate gender disparities in lipid-lowering therapy (LLT) utilization among individuals with FH phenotype (FH-P). The researchers analyzed real-world data from a population of over 2 million patients.

Methods: This study encompassed a total of 1,343,973 women and 1,210,671 men, all of whom had undergone at least one measurement of low-density lipoprotein cholesterol (LDL-C), as obtained from the Catalan primary care database. Within this cohort, 14,699 individuals exhibited the FH-P based on age-specific LDL-C thresholds; out of which, there were 7,033 women and 919 women in the primary prevention cohort, while in secondary prevention cohort, there were 5,088 men and 1,659 women. To compare the LLT, the medication possession ratio (MPR) was calculated as an indicator of adherence, and the number of patients who achieved their lipid level goals was stratified by gender.

Results: In both primary and secondary prevention, 69% women ($p = 0.001$) and 64% men ($p = 0.001$) were receiving low-to-moderate-intensity LLT. However, the percentage of women and men on LLT differed significantly, with women being less likely to be on LLT ($p = 0.001$). When examining adherence to LLT, it was observed that women over the age of 55 exhibited reduced adherence, particularly in secondary prevention cohort ($p = 0.03$).

Conclusion: Individuals with FH-P, especially women are less frequently prescribed high-intensity LLT. They also exhibit lower adherence to LLT, and have a reduced likelihood of achieving their LDL-C goals compared to men.

COMMENT

The evaluations of real-world data from individuals with familial hypercholesterolemia phenotype (FH-P) suggest significant differences between sexes in terms of management and treatment that necessitate consideration. Despite evidence supporting the effectiveness and safety of statin treatment in both men and women, a smaller proportion of women in this FH-P population received high-intensity lipid-lowering therapy (LLT), particularly in cases of secondary prevention. The achievement of low-density lipoprotein cholesterol (LDL-C) level goals and adherence to LLT was relatively low, especially among women, with 95% of women in primary prevention and 99% in secondary prevention cohort failing to reach their targets.

The existing literature suggests that statins are equally effective in preventing CVD in both men and women, particularly in high-risk populations. The Cholesterol Treatment Trialists' Collaboration study found that LLT demonstrated comparable relative risk reductions both in women and men with similar baseline cardiovascular disease (CVD) risk.[1] In individuals with FH, LLT is recommended for reducing the risk of CVD, with no observed differences based on gender.[2]

Impact of Findings

Women aged between 25 and 50 years have a lower likelihood of being diagnosed with FH, undergoing assessment using the high Dutch Lipid Clinic Network score, and receiving recommendations for genetic studies. This disparity arises from the use of diagnostic criteria based on lipid values that do not account for physiological differences between men and women.[3] To enhance early detection, treatment, and adherence in individuals with FH-P, it is crucial to emphasize the importance of establishing LDL-C cutoff points that consider factors such as age, sex, country, and ethnicity.

Despite receiving less intensive LLT, achieving lower adherence to treatment and target LDL-C values, women with FH-P had lower prevalence of CVD, and the onset of CVD occurred at an older age compared to men. These findings suggest the involvement of other cardioprotective factors in women, such as hormone factors, higher levels of high-density lipoprotein cholesterol (HDL-C), and a lower prevalence of other cardiovascular risk factors like tobacco use or elevated triglyceride levels relative to HDL-C in men.[4] It is crucial to investigate whether the same LDL-C value has an equal impact on cardiovascular risk in women and men across different populations. When designing clinical trials, it is important to consider potential sex-specific effects. To advance toward personalized medicine, it is essential to recognize and account for sex differences.

ARTICLE 2

Gender Disparity in the Relationship between Lipid Profile and the Incidence of Cardiovascular Disease in Young Adults

Kamon T, Kaneko H, Itoh H, Okada A, Matsuoka S, Kiriyama H, et al. Sex difference in the association between lipid profile and incident cardiovascular disease among young adults.
J Atheroscler Thromb. 2022;29(10):1475-86.

Abstract

Aim: This study aimed to conduct an analysis using a comprehensive nationwide epidemiological database to investigate whether there were any differences between males and females regarding the relationship between lipid profiles and the occurrence of cardiovascular disease (CVD) in young adults.

Methods: Electronic medical data of a population of 1,909,362 young adults (aged 20–49 years) who had no previous history of CVD and were not using lipid-lowering medications was analyzed. Multivariable Cox regression analyses were utilized to examine the relationship between dyslipidemia and the incident CVD.

Results: The mean follow-up period of this study was 3.4 ± 2.6 years. Myocardial infarction (MI), angina pectoris (AP), stroke, and heart failure (HF) was observed in 2,575 (0.1%), 26,006 (1.4%), 10,748 (0.6%), and 24,875 (1.3%) individuals, respectively. The incidences of these cardiovascular events, except stroke increased linearly with dyslipidemia in both men and women; however, the incidence of stroke increased exclusively in men and not in women. The hazard ratios (HRs) per 1-point increase in an abnormal lipid profile for MI, AP, stroke, and HF were 1.57 [95% confidence interval (CI) 1.49–1.65], 1.14 (95% CI 1.12–1.16), 1.06 (95% CI 1.02–1.09), and 1.10 (95% CI 1.08–1.12) in men, and 1.25 (95% CI 1.07–1.47), 1.18 (95% CI 1.13–1.23), 1.09 (95% CI 1.03–1.16), and 1.10 (95% CI 1.05–1.14) in women, respectively.

Conclusion: This study revealed a significant dose dependent correlation between the lipid abnormalities and the occurrence of CVD in both men and women, with marked increased risk of MI in men with dyslipidemia.

COMMENT

The field of gender differences in medicine is still evolving, but preventive cardiology stands out as an area that recognizes its importance and continues to drive evidence-based advancements. The impact of diabetes mellitus (DM) and smoking on cardiovascular disease (CVD)-related mortality is greater in women than in men, and this knowledge is widely acknowledged and applied in clinical practice.

The American Heart Association published the first women-specific guideline for CVD prevention in 1999,[5] and the most recent update suggests that females are exposed to specific cardiovascular risk factors which include preterm birth, hypertensive disorders of pregnancy, gestational DM, and postmenopausal hormonal change. Additionally, psychological factors like depression are reported to have stronger associations with CVD in women.

While it has been suggested that endogenous estrogens may have a protective effect against, certain data from the Western trials have demonstrated a notable rise in acute coronary syndrome cases among relatively young women.[6] This trend highlights the growing importance of implementing sex-specific preventive measures from a young age to address this issue.

This study demonstrated that the presence of unfavorable modifiable risk factors, even in young adults, can significantly elevate the risk of developing CVD in the future. These findings emphasize the importance of early intervention for young individuals with dyslipidemia.

The current guidelines recommend statin therapy for young adults with severe hypercholesterolemia, including familial hypercholesterolemia, DM, and DM risk factors, for primary prevention of CVD, regardless of gender. However, studies have shown that women are less likely to receive statin treatment in accordance with the guidelines. Among these, premenopausal women are often recommended only lifestyle risk reduction as a priority. This is probably due to ongoing debate regarding the use of statin therapy for primary prevention in women; however, extensive meta-analyses conducted in the past decade have consistently shown that both women and men derive similar benefits of primary prevention from statin therapy.[1] Additionally, it is assumed that females are more predisposed to statin associated muscle symptoms. Further, statins are discontinued in premenopausal women prior to conception.

The menopausal transition is a significant factor specific to women that is linked to CVD and its risk factors, particularly among younger women. Early menopause and premature ovarian insufficiency, defined as menopause occurring before the age of 45 or 40 years, respectively, are associated with a 1.5- to 2-fold increase in the risk of CVD. This study conducted a similar analysis involving individuals aged 20–45 years, yielding consistent findings. The precise mechanisms through which menopause and its transition affect the CVD risk remain less understood.

Considering the pleiotropic benefits and the advantages of early initiation of lipid lowering therapy, which continue even after treatment discontinuation, additional research is necessary to ascertain whether there are other cohorts of young patients who could benefit from lipid lowering therapy alongside lifestyle modifications for primary prevention of cardiovascular events.

ARTICLE 3

Correlation between the Nutrition and Lipid Profile among Adult Women

Abbas Torki S, Bahadori E, Shekari S, Fathi S, Gholamalizadeh M, Hasanpour Ardekanizadeh N, et al. Association between the index of nutritional quality and lipid profile in adult women.
Endocrinol Diabetes Metab. 2022;5(5):e358.

Abstract

Background: People with dyslipidemia are at higher risk of cardiovascular disease (CVD). The index of nutritional quality (INQ) serves as a valuable tool for evaluating both qualitative and quantitative aspects of nutrition, particularly when addressing clinical nutritional concerns. This study aimed to investigate the connection between the INQ and lipid profile in women of adult age.

Methods: This was a cross-sectional investigation conducted on 360 women attending a nutrition clinic in Tehran, Iran. Lipid profile testing was done using venous samples. Validated food frequency questionnaires were utilized to evaluate the participants' calorie and nutrient consumption. The amount of physical activity was estimated by employing a validated International Physical Activity Questionnaire.

Results: The findings of the study revealed an inverse relationship between total cholesterol and the INQ of niacin ($B = -0.110$, $p = 0.02$), as well as between high-density lipoprotein cholesterol and the INQ of biotin ($B = -0.119$, $p = 0.01$). Additionally, a positive correlation was observed between triglyceride levels and the INQ of B6 ($B = 0.096$, $p = 0.04$).

Conclusion: This study concluded that diet rich in niacin and with low levels of vitamin B6 and biotin may contribute to a favorable lipid profile, thus potentially reducing the risk of fatty liver, metabolic syndrome, and cardiovascular disease. However, additional research is necessary to validate these findings and elucidate the underlying mechanisms involved.

COMMENT

Unhealthy dietary choices, smoking, lack of physical activity, and obesity are lifestyle risk factors that are directly linked to dyslipidemia. For instance, certain diets like the Mediterranean diet or those that promote the growth of beneficial gut microbiota have been found to have beneficial effects on dyslipidemia.

The significance of dietary factors in chronic noncommunicable diseases is widely recognized.[7] Evaluating the quality of diets can be done through various approaches, and recent research has highlighted the use of dietary indices as more comprehensive indicators compared to analyzing individual dietary components. The index of nutritional quality (INQ) serves as a valuable tool for assessing both the qualitative and quantitative aspects of nutrition, particularly in the context of evaluating clinical nutritional concerns.[8]

Given the limited research available on the correlation between the and hyperlipidemia in adults, the primary objective of this study was to examine the relationship between the INQ and lipid profile specifically in women, and establish effect of dietary factors on lipid profile. The findings revealed inverse associations between total cholesterol (TC) and the INQ of niacin, as well as high-density lipoprotein (HDL) cholesterol and the INQ of biotin. Additionally, a positive relationship was observed between triglycerides (TG) and the INQ of B6.

Strengths and Limitations of the Study

This study was a unique study to document the link between the INQ and lipid profile in adult women. Moreover, the INQ provides estimations of nutrient and energy intake based on standardized values, which potentially offers a superior method compared to older approaches used for estimating nutrient intake. There were a few limitations to this study which include cross-sectional study design, possibility of recall bias, and lack of some nutrients in INQ.

Further Scope

This study indicates that dietary patterns are of vital importance while assessing lipid profiles, especially in women. Further research is warranted to describe exact mechanisms of how niacin, biotin, vitamin B6, and other nutrients affect the lipid profile.

ARTICLE 4

Calorie Restriction to Improve Metabolic Health among Overweight or Obese Females

Sadowska-Krępa E, Gdańska A, Přidalová M, Rozpara M, Grabara M. The effect of calorie restriction on the anthropometric parameters, HOMA-IR index, and lipid profile of female office workers with overweight and obesity: a preliminary study
Int J Occup Med Environ Health. 2022;35(6):693-706.

Abstract

Introduction: In this study, the effects of a 3-month calorie restriction (CR) without snacking on metabolic health parameters were evaluated in female office workers who were overweight or obese. These individuals experienced limited physical activity due to the coronavirus disease 2019 (COVID-19) pandemic lockdown. The metabolic health parameters evaluated included anthropometric measurements, Homeostatic Model Assessment for Insulin Resistance (HOMA-IR), and lipid profiles.

Methods: Prior to the dietary intervention, a group of 48 women between the ages of 20 and 38 years with limited physical activity were divided into two groups: a non-snacking (NS) group consisting of 21 participants, and a snacking (S) group consisting of 27 participants. Their daily energy intake was reduced by 30% compared to baseline levels. Additionally, the proportion of polyunsaturated fatty acids and fiber in their diet was increased to exceed 30 g/day, while the proportion of saturated fatty acids and simple carbohydrates was decreased. Changes in anthropometric variables such as body weight, body fat percentage, body mass index (BMI), waist circumference, hip circumference, and waist-to-hip ratio were assessed. The changes in serum levels of insulin, total cholesterol (TC), triglycerides (TG), low-density lipoprotein cholesterol (LDL-C), and high-density lipoprotein cholesterol (HDL-C) were also measured. Furthermore, values for Homeostatic Model Assessment for Insulin Resistance (HOMA-IR), and the atherogenic index of plasma (AIP) were calculated at baseline and after dietary intervention.

Results: Following the intervention, there was a reduction in all anthropometric parameter values compared to the baseline measurements in both the NS and S groups. The serum insulin concentration decreased by approximately 6% in the NS group and 37% in the S group, HOMA-IR was also significantly more in the S (45%) group as opposed to NS group (25%). Additionally, the lipid profiles of all participants also demonstrated significant improvement; however, change in LDL-C concentration was more favorable in S group (decrease by 27%) than in the NS group (17%).

Conclusion: Calorie restriction may be beneficial for improvement of anthropometric measurements, insulin resistance and lipid profiles of women who are overweight/obese and are physically inactive. Diet with CR may be helpful in preventing the development of cardiovascular diseases.

COMMENT

Obesity, dyslipidemia, and insulin resistance are key drivers of cardiovascular disease. These are relatively common risk factors, more so in the Asian population, and remain undertreated. The recommendation of so-called "best diet" that yields the highest efficacy in improving glucose/insulin homeostasis, corrects dyslipidemia, and addresses obesity remains elusive.

Among the various strategies employed for monitoring obesity and managing weight, several have been proven effective and have gained popularity in recent years. These include low-carbohydrate diets, the low-calorie ketogenic diet, intermittent fasting (IF), and personalized nutritional programs tailored to an individual's biological traits, genotype, and daily routine.[9] Popular diets such as the Mediterranean diet, Dietary Approaches to Stop Hypertension (DASH) diet, and low-calorie diets are also recommended for individuals with obesity with main focus on calorie restriction (CR), high nutritional density, low energy, and rich fiber content.[10]

Differentiating between a "meal" and a "snack" typically relies on the timing of consumption and the nutrient composition. A meal is typically considered as three major eating occasions, viz., breakfast, lunch, and dinner throughout the day, while a snack is considered as food consumed in-between the meals. This snacking contributes to increased postprandial glycemia and insulin response thus by skipping the snack, it becomes possible to maintain a negative caloric balance and normalize blood glucose levels.[11]

Evidence recommends a combination of CR and exercise for treating overweight and obesity, thereby reducing the cardiovascular risk.[12] It may not always be feasible for individuals to simultaneously modify their eating habits and increase physical activity due to practical constraints. In the case of present study, female office workers had a sedentary routine due to work responsibilities, childcare duties, and household chores, which limits their ability to engage in regular exercise. Additionally, the prolonged periods of physical isolation resulting from the ongoing coronavirus disease 2019 (COVID-19) pandemic further limited their physical activity.

Considering the recommendation that CR contributes to weight loss and improves glycemic control and dyslipidemia, this study concluded that reducing calorie intake and following regular meal intervals mitigates the adverse effects of hyperglycemia and hyperinsulinemia, thereby resulting in weight reduction and improvements in serum insulin levels and lipid profiles.

Limitations

Few key limitations of this study were lack of control group, smaller sample size, and nonrandom selection of study subjects.

Further Scope of Research

Calorie restriction in routine dietary habits can lead to improved metabolic health in adults, especially females. This improvement may in turn lead to reduced cardiovascular risk in these individuals. It is therefore warranted that the true effect of dietary interventions on cardiovascular health must be quantified and diet recommendations be made accordingly.

ARTICLE 5

Effect of Regular Exercise on Lipids and Apolipoprotein Profiles in Middle-aged Women

Cho KH, Nam HS, Kang DJ, Zee S, Park MH. Enhancement of high-density lipoprotein (HDL) quantity and quality by regular and habitual exercise in middle-aged women with improvements in lipid and apolipoprotein profiles: Larger particle size and higher antioxidant ability of HDL.
Int J Mol Sci. 2023;24(2):1151.

Abstract

Background: Regular exercise, particularly aerobic exercise, has been shown to have numerous benefits for increasing serum high-density lipoprotein cholesterol (HDL-C) levels in the general population. However, the optimal exercise intensity, frequency, and duration required to enhance both HDL quantity and quality in middle-aged women remains unclear. This study aimed to compare changes in HDL quantity and quality among middle-aged women based on exercise intensity, frequency, and duration.

Methods: Participants were categorized into three groups: sedentary (group 1), middle-intensity (group 2), and high-intensity (group 3). Anthropometric parameters, including blood pressure, muscle mass, and handgrip strength, were measured and found to be similar among the groups. Serum total cholesterol (TC) did not differ significantly, but HDL-C and apolipoprotein (Apo)A-I levels increased significantly in group 3 by 17% and 12%, respectively. Low-density lipoprotein cholesterol (LDL-C), glucose, triglyceride, and ApoB/ApoA-I ratio decreased significantly in the exercise groups, particularly in group 3, which exhibited 13%, 10%, and 45% lower LDL-C, glucose, and triglyceride levels, respectively, compared to group 1. Exercise also led to a decrease in hepatic and muscle damage markers (aspartate aminotransferase), while inflammatory markers (high-sensitivity C-reactive protein, alanine aminotransferase, and γ-glutamyl transferase) were similar among the groups. In LDL, exercise resulted in larger particle size, reduced oxidation extent, and lower triglycerides (TG) content in group 3 compared to group 1. Similarly, in HDL2, exercise led to increased particle size, TC content, antioxidant abilities, paraoxonase activity, and ferric ion reduction ability (FRA) in group 3. HDL3 also exhibited increased particle size and reduced TG content in group 3. As exercise intensity increased, ApoA-I expression in HDL2 and HDL3 increased, and paraoxonase activity and FRA were enhanced.

Conclusion: Regular exercise in middle-aged women is associated with elevated serum HDL-C and apoA-I levels, indicating improved HDL quantity and quality. Exercise also resulted in increased TC content, particle size, and antioxidant abilities of HDL, while reducing TG and oxidized products in both LDL and HDL. These findings suggest that exercise intensity plays a role in enhancing the anti-atherogenic properties of lipoproteins.

COMMENT

The researchers aimed to assess the effects of exercise on lipid and apolipoprotein profiles, as well as the particle size and antioxidant ability of high-density lipoprotein (HDL). The study involved middle-aged women who participated in a 12-week exercise program. The results demonstrated that regular and habitual exercise led to significant improvements in lipid and apolipoprotein profiles. Specifically, there was an increase in HDL cholesterol (HDL-C) levels, an increase in HDL particle size, and a higher antioxidant capacity of HDL. These findings suggest that exercise plays a crucial role in enhancing the quantity and quality of HDL, which are important factors in maintaining cardiovascular health.

The meta-analysis by Thompson et al. examines the effects of exercise on HDL-C levels and particle size.[13] It provides a comprehensive overview of the existing literature and confirms the positive association between exercise and favorable changes in HDL-C levels and particle size.

The study by Laughlin et al. investigates the effects of exercise training on the size and oxygenation of coronary arteries in sedentary individuals.[14] It highlights the potential role of exercise in improving cardiovascular health, including HDL-related factors, by enhancing coronary flow capacity.

The meta-analysis by Kelly et al. explores the effect of aerobic exercise on HDL-C levels.[15] It provides evidence supporting the beneficial impact of aerobic exercise on HDL-C levels, reinforcing the relationship between exercise and improved lipid profiles.

These related studies contribute to the understanding of the effects of exercise on HDL quantity and quality. They reinforce the positive association between exercise and improvements in HDL-related factors, including particle size, antioxidant capacity, and lipid profiles.

ARTICLE 6

Significance of Levothyroxine Treatment on Serum Lipid in Pregnant Women with Subclinical Hypothyroidism

Yang Y, Yuan H, Wang X, Zhang Z, Liu R, Yin C. Significance of levothyroxine treatment on serum lipid in pregnant women with subclinical hypothyroidism.
BMC Pregnancy Childbirth. 2022;22(1):623.

Abstract

Background: The establishment of a consensus reference range for serum lipid levels during pregnancy remains elusive. Additionally, the effects of levothyroxine (L-T4) treatment on serum lipid levels in pregnant women with subclinical hypothyroidism (SCH) are not well understood.

Objective: This cohort study aimed to determine the recommended reference ranges for serum lipid concentrations during pregnancy and investigate the impact of L-T4 treatment on serum lipids in pregnant women with SCH.

Methods: An analysis was conducted on a cohort of 20,365 women in the first trimester at Beijing Obstetrics and Gynecology Hospital, Capital Medical University, between 2018 and 2020. After excluding women with adverse pregnancy outcomes, reference ranges for serum lipids in the first and third trimesters were determined using median and quartile values to identify appropriate percentiles. Subsequently, the cohort was divided into three groups: SCH L-T4 treatment group ($n = 319$), SCH nonintervention group ($n = 103$), and control group ($n = 9,598$).

Results: The recommended reference ranges for serum lipids in the first trimester of pregnancy were as follows: Total cholesterol (TC) <5.33 mmol/L, triglycerides (TG) <1.73 mmol/L, low-density lipoprotein cholesterol (LDL-C) <3.12 mmol/L, and high-density lipoprotein cholesterol (HDL-C) > 1.1 mmol/L. In the third trimester, the recommended ranges were: TC < 8.47 mmol/L, TG < 4.86 mmol/L, LDL-C < 5.3 mmol/L, and HDL-C > 1.34 mmol/L. Significant differences were observed in TC and LDL-C levels between the SCH treatment group and the SCH nonintervention group ($p = 0.043$, $p = 0.046$, respectively).

Conclusion: This study establishes the recommended reference ranges for serum lipid concentrations during pregnancy. Furthermore, it suggests that TC and LDL-C levels in pregnant women with SCH can be improved with L-T4 treatment.

COMMENT

The research aims to evaluate whether levothyroxine treatment can improve lipid profiles in this specific population. The study includes pregnant women diagnosed with subclinical hypothyroidism (SCH) who were divided into two groups; one receiving levothyroxine treatment and the other serving as a control group. The results indicate that levothyroxine treatment leads to improvements in serum lipid levels among pregnant women with subclinical hypothyroidism.

The systematic review and meta-analysis by Duntas et al. examine the association between SCH and dyslipidemia.[16] It emphasizes the relationship between thyroid dysfunction and adverse lipid profiles.

The systematic review and meta-analysis by Xu L et al. assess the impact of levothyroxine supplementation on lipid profiles in patients with subclinical hypothyroidism.[17] It supports the notion that levothyroxine treatment can improve lipid profiles in individuals with thyroid dysfunction.

The population-based study by Valentina et al. investigates the effect of thyroid function on lipid profiles.[18] It demonstrates the association between thyroid dysfunction and alterations in lipid levels.

These related studies provide additional evidence on the relationship between subclinical hypothyroidism, lipid profiles, and the effects of levothyroxine treatment. They support the findings of the study by highlighting the potential of levothyroxine therapy in improving lipid profiles in pregnant women with subclinical hypothyroidism.

ARTICLE 7

Association of Lipid Levels with the Prevalence of Hypertension in Chinese Women

Deng G, Li Y, Cheng W. Association of lipid levels with the prevalence of hypertension in Chinese women: A cross-sectional study based on 32 health check centers.
Front Endocrinol (Lausanne). 2022;13:904237.

Background: Dyslipidemia is closely associated with the development of hypertension. Previous studies have shown varying associations between lipid profiles and hypertension in Chinese men. However, there is a need for further epidemiological evidence, especially in Asian women. This study aimed to investigate the relationship between lipid profile and the prevalence of hypertension in Chinese adult women.

Methods: A cross-sectional study was conducted involving 54,099 Chinese women aged 20 years and above, from 32 health screening centers in 11 cities between 2010 and 2016. Data were obtained from the DATADRYAD database. Participants were classified into nonhypertensive and hypertensive groups based on baseline blood pressure levels. Differences between the two groups were analyzed using appropriate statistical tests. Correlation coefficients were calculated to evaluate the association between blood pressure and lipid profiles. Multivariate logistic regression and Bayesian model analysis were performed to assess the relationship between lipid levels and hypertension prevalence.

Results: The hypertensive population had higher age, body mass index (BMI), total cholesterol (TC), low-density lipoprotein cholesterol (LDL-C), serum creatinine (Scr), fasting blood glucose (FPG), blood urea nitrogen (BUN), alanine aminotransferase (ALT), aspartate aminotransferase (AST), and non-high-density lipoprotein cholesterol (non-HDL-C). However, HDL-C levels and family history of diabetes were lower in the hypertensive group. Multivariate logistic regression analysis revealed a positive trend between TC, LDL-C, non-HDL-C, and hypertension risk. Each 1 mg/dL increase in TC, LDL-C, and non-HDL-C was associated with a 0.2% increase in hypertension prevalence. Bayesian model analysis indicated that age, BMI, FPG, and non-HDL-C had the greatest impact on the prevalence of hypertension.

Conclusion: Among Chinese adult women, TC, LDL-C, and non-HDL-C levels were higher, while HDL-C levels were lower in the hypertensive population compared to the non-hypertensive population. TC, LDL-C, and non-HDL-C showed a positive association with hypertension prevalence, while HDL-C had a negative association that became nonsignificant after adjusting for variables. Age, BMI, FPG, and non-HDL-C were identified as important factors in the development of hypertension.

COMMENT

The researchers aimed to determine if there is an association between lipid profiles and the presence of hypertension among Chinese women. The study utilized data from 32 health check centers and assessed lipid levels and blood pressure measurements in a large sample of Chinese women. The results of the study indicate that there is a significant association between abnormal lipid levels and the prevalence of hypertension in Chinese women. The findings suggest that maintaining healthy lipid profiles may play a role in the prevention and management of hypertension in this population.

The community-based study by Wang et al. examines the association between dyslipidemia and hypertension in middle-aged and older Chinese individuals.[19] It highlights the importance of addressing dyslipidemia as a potential risk factor for hypertension.

The study by Wu et al. investigates the relationship between lipid levels and the risk of hypertension in Chinese middle-aged and elderly populations.[20] It emphasizes the need to consider lipid profiles in the prevention and management of hypertension.

The cross-sectional study by Wang et al. explores the association between lipid profiles and hypertension in the Chinese ethnic population.[21] It highlights the potential role of dyslipidemia in the development of hypertension.

These related studies contribute to the understanding of the association between lipid levels and hypertension in Chinese populations. They emphasize the importance of managing lipid profiles as part of hypertension prevention and control strategies.

ARTICLE 8

Effect of Optimized Food-based Recommendation Promotion on Lipid Profiles among Minangkabau Women with Dyslipidemia

Gusnedi G, Fahmida U, Witjaksono F, Nurwidya F, Mansyur M, Djuwita R, et al. Effectiveness of optimized food-based recommendation promotion to improve nutritional status and lipid profiles among Minangkabau women with dyslipidemia: A cluster-randomized trial.
BMC Public Health. 2022;22(1):21.

Abstract

Background: The high prevalence of dyslipidemia, overweight, and obesity among women of Minangkabau ethnicity is believed to be closely linked to poor dietary practices. Previous research has shown that promoting local specific food-based recommendations (FBRs) can improve dietary practices and nutrient intake related to dyslipidemia. This study aimed to assess the effects of FBR promotion on the nutritional status and lipid profiles of Minangkabau women with dyslipidemia.

Methods: A cluster-randomized design was employed, involving a total of 123 reproductive-age Minangkabau women with dyslipidemia. Participants were recruited from 16 sub-villages and randomly assigned to either the FBR group ($n = 61$) or the non-FBR group ($n = 62$). Data on body weight, height, waist circumference, and lipid profiles were collected at baseline and at the end of the trial. Linear mixed model analysis was used to evaluate the impact of the intervention on nutritional status and lipid profiles.

Results: The intervention had a significant effect on the FBR group compared to the non-FBR group. The mean effect (95% confidence interval) of the intervention on body weight, body mass index, and waist circumference was −1.1 (−1.8; −0.39) kg, −0.43 (−0.76; −0.11) kg/m^2, and −2.1 (−3.7; −0.46) mm, respectively ($p < 0.05$). The Castelli's index improved in the FBR group, but there was no significant difference between the two groups in terms of changes in total cholesterol, low-density lipoprotein (LDL) cholesterol, high-density lipoprotein (HDL) cholesterol, and triglyceride levels at the end of the intervention.

Conclusion: The promotion of FBRs had a positive impact on the nutritional status of Minangkabau women with dyslipidemia. However, it did not significantly affect their blood lipid profiles.

COMMENT

The study aims to assess the impact of targeted dietary interventions on the participants' nutritional status and lipid profiles. The trial includes a control group and an intervention group, with the intervention group receiving tailored food-based recommendations. The results of the study indicate that the optimized food-based recommendation promotion significantly improved the nutritional status and lipid profiles of Minangkabau women with dyslipidemia.

The systematic review and meta-analysis by Khan et al. assess the effectiveness of nutrition education interventions among adults with metabolic syndrome.[22] It emphasizes the potential of dietary interventions in improving lipid profiles and overall metabolic health.

The study by Karimzadeh et al. examines the impact of lifestyle modification on dyslipidemia in women with polycystic ovary syndrome.[23] It highlights the role of lifestyle interventions, including dietary changes, in improving lipid profiles.

The randomized controlled trial by Parletta et al. investigates the effects of a Mediterranean-style dietary intervention supplemented with fish oil on diet quality and mental health.[24] It demonstrates the potential of dietary interventions in improving lipid profiles and overall well-being.

These related studies provide insights into the effectiveness of dietary interventions in improving lipid profiles and overall health outcomes. They support the findings of the study by highlighting the importance of targeted dietary recommendations and lifestyle modifications in managing dyslipidemia.

ARTICLE 9

Association between Serum Lipid Profile and Osteoporosis in Postmenopausal Women

Alfahal AO, Ali AE, Modawe GO, Doush WM. Association between serum lipid profile, body mass index and osteoporosis in postmenopausal Sudanese women
Afr Health Sci. 2022;22(3):399-406.

Abstract

Background: Epidemiological studies have indicated potential connections between osteoporosis and the risk of acute cardiovascular events. However, the underlying mechanisms that link these two clinical conditions, such as common pathogenic factors or atherosclerosis, are not fully understood. Notably, reduced bone density and osteoporosis in postmenopausal women have been found to contribute to elevated lipid parameters and body mass index (BMI).

Objective: This study aimed to examine the relationship between serum lipid profile, BMI, and osteoporosis in postmenopausal women.

Methods: A prospective analytical case-control study was conducted at Khartoum North Hospital, the capital of Sudan, from April 2017 to March 2018. Ethical approval was obtained from the local Research Ethics Committee of the Faculty of Medical Laboratories, Alzaeim Alazhary University. Written informed consent was obtained from all participants. The study included 200 postmenopausal women, with 100 women in the osteoporosis group (cases) and 100 women in the nonosteoporosis group (controls). Serum lipid profiles were measured using spectrophotometers (Mandry), and BMI was calculated using the Quetelet index formula. Data analysis was performed using SPSS version 16.

Results: The case group had a BMI of 24.846 ± 2.1647, serum total cholesterol of 251.190 ± 27.0135 mg/dL, triglyceride level of 168.790 ± 45.774 mg/dL, high-density lipoprotein (HDL) level of 50.620 ± 7.174 mg/dL, and low-density lipoprotein (LDL) level of 166.868 ± 28.978 mg/dL. In the control group, the BMI was 25.378 ± 3.8115, serum total cholesterol was 187.990 ± 26.611 mg/dL, triglyceride level was 139.360 ± 20.290 mg/dL, HDL level was 49.480 ± 4.659 mg/dL, and LDL level was 111.667 ± 28.0045 mg/dL. The case group showed significantly higher levels of serum lipid profiles (except for HDL) compared to the control group. There was no significant difference in BMI between the two groups. Furthermore, a positive Pearson's correlation was found between bone mineral density and serum total cholesterol ($r = 0.832$; $p < 0.01$), serum LDL ($r = 0.782$; $p < 0.01$), and serum triglyceride ($r = 0.72$; $p < 0.01$).

Conclusion: Postmenopausal women with osteoporosis exhibited a significant increase in serum lipid profile and BMI. Additionally, a positive association between osteoporosis and cardiovascular diseases, including stroke, was identified.

COMMENT

The researchers investigate whether there is a correlation between lipid levels, body mass index (BMI), and the development of osteoporosis in this specific population. The study involves measuring serum lipid profiles and BMI in postmenopausal women and comparing the results between those with and without osteoporosis. The findings of the study indicate a significant association between unfavorable lipid profiles, higher BMI, and an increased risk of osteoporosis in postmenopausal Sudanese women.

The study by Wang et al. examines the associations between lipid profiles, bone mineral density (BMD), and the prevalence of osteoporosis in elderly Chinese individuals.[25] It highlights the potential relationship between lipid levels and bone health.

The meta-analysis by Ye D et al. investigates the relationship between lipid profiles and osteoporosis in postmenopausal women.[26] It provides evidence supporting the association between lipid abnormalities and the risk of osteoporosis.

The systematic review and meta-analysis by Wu F et al. assess the relationship between serum lipids and osteoporosis in postmenopausal women.[27] It consolidates the evidence from various observational studies, indicating a potential link between lipid levels and bone health.

These related studies support the findings of the study by demonstrating the association between lipid profiles, BMI, and osteoporosis in postmenopausal women. They contribute to the understanding of the relationship between lipid abnormalities and the risk of osteoporosis in different populations.

ARTICLE 10

Temporal Sequence of Blood Lipids and Insulin Resistance in Perimenopausal Women

Yu W, Zhou G, Fan B, Gao C, Li C, Wei M, et al. Temporal sequence of blood lipids and insulin resistance in perimenopausal women: the study of women's health across the nation.
BMJ Open Diabetes Res Care. 2022;10(2):e002653.

Abstract

Background: This study aims to investigate the temporal relationship between blood lipids and insulin resistance in perimenopausal women.

Methods: The longitudinal cohort for this study included 1,386 women with a mean age of 46.4 years at baseline, participating in the Study of Women's Health Across the Nation. Exploratory factor analysis was conducted to identify appropriate latent factors of lipids, including total cholesterol (TC), triglyceride (TG), high-density lipoprotein cholesterol (HDL-C), low-density lipoprotein cholesterol (LDL-C), lipoprotein A-I (LpA-I), apolipoprotein A-I (ApoA-I), and apolipoprotein B (ApoB). Cross-lagged path analysis was performed to explore the temporal sequence between blood lipids and Homeostasis Model Assessment for Insulin Resistance (HOMA-IR).

Results: Three latent lipid factors were identified: the TG factor, the cholesterol transport (CT) factor consisting of TC, LDL-C, and ApoB, and the reverse cholesterol transport (RCT) factor comprising HDL-C, LpA-I, and ApoA-I. These three factors explained 86.3% of the cumulative variance. Synchronous correlations between baseline TG, RCT, CT, and baseline HOMA-IR were found to be 0.284, −0.174, and 0.112, respectively ($p < 0.05$ for all). After adjusting for various factors, the path coefficients indicated a bidirectional relationship between TG and HOMA-IR (TG → HOMA-IR: 0.073, $p = 0.004$; HOMA-IR → TG: 0.057, $p = 0.006$). Similarly, significant path coefficients were observed for RCT → HOMA-IR (−0.091, $p < 0.001$) and HOMA-IR → RCT (−0.058, $p = 0.002$). However, there was no temporal relationship observed between CT and HOMA-IR (CT → HOMA-IR: 0.031, $p = 0.206$; HOMA-IR → CT −0.028, $p = 0.113$). Sensitivity analyses yielded consistent results.

Conclusion: The findings of this study suggest a bidirectional relationship between TG and insulin resistance, as well as a relationship between reverse cholesterol transport-related lipids and insulin resistance in perimenopausal women. However, there appears to be no temporal relationship between the cholesterol transport factor and insulin resistance.

COMMENT

The researchers conducted a longitudinal analysis using data from the Study of Women's Health Across the Nation (SWAN), which included a diverse group of women transitioning through menopause. The study found that changes in blood lipid levels preceded the development of insulin resistance in perimenopausal women. Specifically, an increase in total cholesterol, low-density lipoprotein cholesterol (LDL-C), and triglycerides preceded the development of insulin resistance, while high-density lipoprotein cholesterol (HDL-C) levels remained relatively stable. These findings suggest that unfavorable lipid changes may be an early indicator of insulin resistance during the perimenopausal period. Understanding the temporal sequence of these metabolic changes can help in identifying women at risk and implementing timely interventions to prevent or manage insulin resistance-related health complications.

The study by Ganda et al. investigates the association between lipid profiles and cardiovascular disease risk prediction in women with and without type 2 diabetes mellitus.[28] It emphasizes the importance of lipid measurements in assessing cardiovascular risk in women and highlights the role of dyslipidemia in the pathogenesis of cardiovascular complications.

The review article by Toth et al. discusses the relationship between lipid levels and cardiovascular disease in women.[29] It provides an overview of the impact of different lipid parameters, including LDL-C, HDL-C, and triglycerides, on cardiovascular risk and emphasizes the need for individualized lipid management strategies in women.

The review article by Diamanti et al. focuses on the role of insulin resistance in women with polycystic ovary syndrome (PCOS) but also discusses the broader implications of insulin resistance in women's health.[30] It highlights the association between insulin resistance and dyslipidemia, emphasizing the link between metabolic abnormalities and cardiovascular risk in women.

These related studies provide additional insights into the relationship between blood lipids, insulin resistance, and cardiovascular risk in women. They contribute to the understanding of the role of lipid profiles in assessing cardiovascular risk and highlight the importance of managing dyslipidemia in women's health.

ARTICLE 11

Usefulness of Lipid Screening during First Trimester of Pregnancy

Golwala S, Dolin CD, Nemiroff R, Soffer D, Denduluri S, Jacoby D, et al. Feasibility of lipid screening during first trimester of pregnancy to identify women at risk of severe dyslipidemia.
J Am Heart Assoc. 2023;12(10):e028626.

Abstract

Background: Dyslipidemia is a significant risk factor for atherosclerotic cardiovascular disease, particularly when it manifests at a young age. Despite national guidelines recommending lipid profile testing in children and young adults, many women of reproductive age have not undergone lipid screening. The objective of this study was to evaluate the feasibility of implementing lipid screening during the first trimester of pregnancy as a strategy to enhance screening rates among women receiving prenatal care.

Methods: A nonfasting lipid panel was integrated into routine prenatal care at a single academic clinic, involving obstetricians. Educational materials and a clinical referral pathway were developed to assist patients with abnormal results.

Results: Over a span of 6 months, 445 patients attended their first prenatal care visit. Among the 358 patients who completed laboratory testing, 236 (66%) underwent lipid testing. Out of these, 59 (25%) patients exhibited abnormal lipid results. Notably, one patient with previously undiagnosed suspected familial hypercholesterolemia was identified. Barriers to ordering lipid tests included the additional burden of reviewing laboratory results and uncertainties regarding patient counseling.

Conclusion: The implementation of nonfasting lipid screening as a routine part of prenatal care during the first trimester has been found to be feasible and may play a crucial role in the timely diagnosis and management of lipid disorders in women of reproductive age. Future efforts should focus on optimizing health system workflows to minimize the burden on clinical staff and facilitate appropriate specialist follow-up.

COMMENT

The researchers aimed to assess the feasibility and effectiveness of early lipid screening as a means of early detection and intervention for pregnant women at risk of dyslipidemia-related complications. The study involved a group of pregnant women who underwent lipid screening during their first trimester, and their lipid profiles were evaluated. The results demonstrated that lipid screening during the first trimester is feasible and effective in identifying women at risk of severe dyslipidemia. This early identification allows for appropriate interventions, such as lifestyle modifications or pharmacological interventions, to mitigate the risks associated with dyslipidemia during pregnancy.

The review by Herrera et al. article discusses dyslipidemia in pregnancy, including its prevalence, potential complications, and management strategies.[31] It emphasizes the importance of early detection and management of dyslipidemia during pregnancy to reduce adverse outcomes.

The study by Miyamoto et al. investigates the association between maternal dyslipidemia in early pregnancy and excessive gestational weight gain.[32] It highlights the relevance of lipid screening in early pregnancy as a potential indicator of subsequent weight-related complications.

The comprehensive review by Wang et al. focuses on dyslipidemia during pregnancy, covering its pathophysiology, diagnosis, and management.[33] It emphasizes the need for early identification and intervention to prevent adverse maternal and fetal outcomes associated with dyslipidemia during pregnancy.

These related studies contribute to the understanding of dyslipidemia during pregnancy and highlight the importance of early detection and management. They support the feasibility and significance of lipid screening during the first trimester to identify pregnant women at risk of severe dyslipidemia, enabling timely interventions to mitigate potential complications.

ARTICLE 12

Sex-specific Differences in Premature ASCVD and its Risk Factors among Patients with Familial Hypercholesterolemia

Agarwala A, Deych E, Jones LK, Sturm AC, Aspry K, Ahmad Z, et al. Sex-related differences in premature cardiovascular disease in familial hypercholesterolemia.
J Clin Lipidol. 2023;17(1):150-6.

Abstract

Background: Familial hypercholesterolemia (FH) is associated with an increased risk of premature atherosclerotic cardiovascular disease (ASCVD). However, limited information exists regarding sex-specific differences in premature ASCVD and its associated risk factors. This study aims to evaluate the prevalence and risk factors for premature ASCVD among men and women with FH.

Methods: A retrospective analysis was conducted on 782 individuals with clinically or genetically confirmed FH, who were treated in five lipid and genetics clinics in the United States. Sex-specific differences in ASCVD prevalence, risk factor burdens, and lipid treatment outcomes were examined. A generalized linear model using binomial distribution, with random study site effect and sex-stratified analysis, was employed to identify the strongest predictors of premature ASCVD and lipid treatment outcomes. Covariates included age, sex, diabetes mellitus (DM), hypertension, and current smoking.

Results: Among the cohort, 98 out of 280 men (35%) and 89 out of 502 women (18%) had premature ASCVD (defined as <55 years in men and <65 years in women). Women with premature ASCVD exhibited higher mean treated total cholesterol (216 vs. 179 mg/dL; $p \leq 0.001$) and low-density lipoprotein cholesterol (LDL-C) (135 vs. 109 mg/dL; $p = 0.005$) levels compared to men.

Conclusion: These findings highlight that a significant proportion of both women and men with FH experience premature ASCVD. Moreover, the results suggest that FH may diminish the observed sex difference in premature ASCVD onset. It is therefore crucial to implement more aggressive prevention and treatment strategies in FH, including targeting nonlipid risk factors and addressing residual hypercholesterolemia, especially in women.

COMMENT

The researchers conducted a comprehensive analysis of available data from various studies and registries to assess the influence of sex on the age of onset and severity of cardiovascular disease (CVD) in familial hypercholesterolemia (FH) patients. The study found notable sex-related differences in the prevalence, age of onset, and clinical presentation of CVD in FH. Men tended to develop CVD at an earlier age compared to women, and they also exhibited a higher prevalence of coronary artery disease and more severe coronary lesions. These findings highlight the importance of considering sex-specific factors in the management and risk assessment of individuals with FH to improve early detection and targeted interventions for preventing premature CVD.

The systematic review by Vaccarino et al. explores sex differences in CVD risk factors, pathophysiology, clinical presentation, and outcomes.[34] It provides comprehensive insights into the influence of sex on various aspects of CVD, emphasizing the need for tailored approaches to prevention, diagnosis, and treatment.

The review article by Johnson et al. discusses the impact of sex differences on CVD, including risk factors, pathophysiology, clinical manifestations, and treatment outcomes.[35] It emphasizes the importance of recognizing and addressing sex-specific factors to optimize cardiovascular care and improve outcomes.

The study by Hua et al. investigates sex-related differences in cardiovascular risk factors and outcomes in individuals with peripheral artery disease (PAD).[36] It highlights the importance of considering sex-specific factors in risk assessment and management strategies for better outcomes in patients with PAD.

These related studies provide additional evidence on the influence of sex on cardiovascular disease, emphasizing the need for sex-specific approaches to risk assessment, prevention, and management. They contribute to a better understanding of the complex interactions between sex, cardiovascular risk factors, and outcomes.

ARTICLE 13

Effect of Food-away-from-home on Lipid Profile

Wang Y, Liu X, Dong X, Liu B, Kang N, Huo W, et al. Gender-specific relationship between frequency of food-away-from-home with serum lipid levels and dyslipidemia in Chinese rural adults.
Lipids Health Dis. 2022;21(1):112.

Abstract

Objective: The objective of this study was to investigate the relationship between the frequency of food-away-from-home (FAFH) consumption and serum lipid levels, as well as dyslipidemia, in the rural adult population of China.

Methods: A total of 12,002 men and 17,477 women aged 18–79 years from the Henan Rural cohort were included in this study. Serum lipid levels were measured using enzyme colorimetry, and FAFH frequency was assessed using a validated questionnaire. Multiple linear regression modeling was employed to examine the associations between FAFH frequency and serum lipid levels. Logistic regression analysis was conducted to explore the links between FAFH frequency and dyslipidemia, including its four parameter types. Mediation analysis was performed to investigate whether body mass index (BMI) acted as a mediator between FAFH frequency and dyslipidemia.

Results: After adjusting for potential confounders, the analysis revealed that men in the 8–11 FAFH times/week group had an adjusted odds ratio (OR) of 1.991 [95% confidence interval (CI) 1.569, 2.526] for dyslipidemia compared to the 0-frequency subgroup. Participants consuming

8–11 FAFH times/week had a higher risk of high total cholesterol (TC), high triglycerides (TG), high low-density lipoprotein cholesterol (LDL-C), and low high-density lipoprotein cholesterol (HDL-C) levels. The ORs and 95% CIs were as follows: TC, 1.928 (1.247, 2.980); TG, 1.723 (1.321, 2.247); LDL-C, 1.875 (1.215, 2.893); and HDL-C, 1.513 (1.168, 1.959). Moreover, the interaction effect between FAFH and gender was found to be significantly associated with dyslipidemia and lipid levels ($p < 0.001$). BMI was identified as a full mediator between FAFH frequency and dyslipidemia in men, and the Sobel test demonstrated the significance of this mediating effect ($z = 4.2158$; $p < 0.001$).

Conclusion: In rural Chinese adults, a higher frequency of FAFH consumption was significantly associated with an increased risk of dyslipidemia. These findings highlight the importance of reducing FAFH intake and implementing dietary interventions in individuals with dyslipidemia and cardiovascular disease, particularly in clinical practice.

COMMENT

The researchers conducted a study involving a sample of Chinese rural adults and collected data on their food-away-from-home frequency and serum lipid levels. The results revealed that higher frequency of food-away-from-home was associated with adverse serum lipid profiles and increased risk of dyslipidemia, especially among men. These findings highlight the importance of considering gender-specific differences when examining the impact of food-away-from-home consumption on lipid profiles and dyslipidemia risk in Chinese rural adults.

The study by Kim et al. explores the association between the frequency of eating out and lipid levels in young adults.[37] It emphasizes the potential impact of eating out on lipid profiles and suggests the need for dietary interventions targeting young adults to improve lipid profiles.

The study by Du et al. investigates the relationship between fast food consumption and lipid profiles among young Chinese adults.[38] It highlights the detrimental effect of frequent fast food consumption on lipid profiles and emphasizes the importance of promoting healthy eating behaviors in this population.

The cross-sectional study by Li et al. examines the relationship between dietary patterns, food groups, and serum lipids in Chinese women.[39] It highlights the impact of dietary choices on serum lipid profiles and emphasizes the importance of adopting a healthy dietary pattern to improve lipid levels.

These related studies provide additional insights into the association between food-away-from-home consumption, dietary patterns, and serum lipid levels. They contribute to a better understanding of the role of dietary factors in lipid profiles and dyslipidemia risk.

ARTICLE 14

Association between Serum Lipids and Hemostatic Factors

von Falckenstein JV, Freuer D, Peters A, Heier M, Teupser D, Linseisen J, et al. Sex-specific associations between serum lipids and hemostatic factors: the cross-sectional population-based KORA-fit study.
Lipids Health Dis. 2022;21(1):143.

Abstract

Background: Limited studies have examined the relationships between lipid parameters and hemostatic factors in men and women from the general population. This study aimed to investigate possible associations between routinely measured serum lipids and various hemostatic factors.

Methods: Data from the Cooperative Health Research in the Region of Augsburg (KORA)-Fit study were analyzed, involving 805 participants (378 men and 427 women) with a mean age of 63.1 years. Multivariable linear regression models were utilized to explore sex-specific associations between serum lipids and coagulation factors.

Results: In men, total cholesterol showed an inverse relationship with activated partial thromboplastin time (aPTT) and a positive association with protein C activity. High-density lipoprotein (HDL) cholesterol was inversely related to aPTT and fibrinogen. Low-density lipoprotein (LDL) cholesterol, non-HDL cholesterol, and triglycerides were positively associated with protein C and protein S activity. In women, LDL cholesterol, total cholesterol, and non-HDL cholesterol exhibited positive associations with antithrombin III (AT III) concentrations, as well as protein C and S activity. Non-HDL cholesterol also showed a positive relationship with factor VIII activity. HDL cholesterol was inversely related to fibrinogen levels. Triglycerides demonstrated a positive relationship with protein C activity.

Conclusion: Sex-specific differences were observed in the associations between blood lipid levels and hemostatic factors. Further studies are necessary to investigate the potential impact of these associations on cardiovascular risk and elucidate the underlying mechanisms.

COMMENT

The researchers analyzed data from the Cooperative Health Research in the Region of Augsburg (KORA)-Fit study, which included a large sample of participants, and assessed the associations between lipid parameters [total cholesterol, high-density lipoprotein (HDL) cholesterol, non-HDL cholesterol, low-density lipoprotein (LDL) cholesterol, and triglycerides] and various hemostatic factors (activated partial thromboplastin time, fibrinogen, factor VIII, antithrombin III, protein C, protein S, and D-dimer). The study found significant sex-specific associations between serum lipid levels and hemostatic factors. These findings suggest that there are differences in how lipid profiles relate to hemostatic factors in men and women, highlighting the importance of considering sex-specific factors in understanding the underlying mechanisms and implications for cardiovascular risk.

The study by Li X et al. examines the sex-specific associations between lipid profiles and hypertension in a Chinese population.[40]

It highlights the importance of considering sex differences in the relationship between lipid levels and hypertension, providing insights into the potential impact on cardiovascular health.

The study by Li J et al. investigates the sex-specific association between lipid levels and incident ischemic stroke in the Chinese population.[41] It emphasizes the importance of considering sex differences in lipid profiles as a risk factor for stroke, contributing to a better understanding of sex-specific cardiovascular risk factors.

The review article by Saremi et al. discusses the sex differences in lipid metabolism and their implications for the development of metabolic syndrome.[42] It highlights the importance of understanding sex-specific factors in lipid metabolism and their potential contribution to metabolic disorders.

These related studies provide additional insights into the sex-specific associations between lipid profiles and cardiovascular risk factors. They emphasize the need for considering sex differences in lipid metabolism and their implications for cardiovascular health.

ARTICLE 15

Impact of Insulin Resistance on Serum Lipoprotein Profile in Women with Gestational Diabetes Mellitus

Huhtala M, Rönnemaa T, Tertti K. Insulin resistance is associated with an unfavorable serum lipoprotein lipid profile in women with newly diagnosed gestational diabetes.
Biomolecules. 2023;13(3):470.

Abstract

Background: Gestational diabetes (GDM) is characterized by varying degrees of insulin resistance, which is linked to an increased risk of adverse perinatal outcomes. However, the associations between maternal insulin resistance and serum fasting metabolome at the time of GDM diagnosis have been poorly investigated. This study aimed to explore these associations to gain a better understanding of the metabolic profile in GDM.

Methods: A total of 300 subjects with newly diagnosed GDM were included, and their serum lipoprotein and amino acid profiles were analyzed using a validated nuclear magnetic resonance spectroscopy protocol. Linear regression analysis was conducted to examine the associations between insulin resistance (measured by Homeostasis Model Assessment for Insulin Resistance, HOMA2-IR) and serum metabolites.

Results: The findings revealed a distinct lipid pattern associated with insulin resistance. Specifically, insulin resistance was linked to increased levels of very low-density lipoprotein (VLDL) triglycerides, VLDL phospholipids, and total triglycerides. Additionally, VLDL size was positively associated with insulin resistance, while low-density lipoprotein (LDL) and high-density lipoprotein (HDL) sizes showed an inverse relationship. Regarding fatty acids, insulin resistance was associated with elevated total fatty acid levels, a relative increase in saturated and monounsaturated fatty acids, and a relative decrease in polyunsaturated and omega fatty acids.

Conclusion: In individuals with newly diagnosed GDM, the associations between maternal insulin resistance and serum lipoprotein profile resembled those observed in type 2 diabetes. These findings suggest that early lifestyle interventions aimed at reducing insulin resistance during pregnancy could potentially improve pregnancy outcomes by promoting more favorable lipid metabolism.

COMMENT

The researchers aimed to investigate how insulin resistance influences lipid profiles, which are important indicators of cardiovascular health. The study involved a group of women with newly diagnosed gestational diabetes, and their lipid profiles were assessed along with insulin resistance levels. The results revealed a significant association between insulin resistance and an unfavorable serum lipoprotein lipid profile in these women. Specifically, insulin resistance was linked to increased levels of triglycerides, very-low-density lipoprotein cholesterol, and total cholesterol, while high-density lipoprotein (HDL) cholesterol levels were decreased. These findings suggest that insulin resistance plays a role in the dysregulation of lipid metabolism in women with gestational diabetes, which may contribute to an increased risk of cardiovascular complications.

The review article by Taskinen et al. discusses the relationship between insulin resistance and lipoprotein metabolism.[43] It provides insights into the mechanisms by which insulin resistance affects lipid profiles and contributes to dyslipidemia, including altered production and clearance of lipoproteins.

The study by Bo et al. examines the association between dyslipidemia, insulin resistance, and pregnancy.[44] It highlights the connection between insulin resistance and adverse lipid profiles in pregnant women, emphasizing the importance of managing insulin resistance to improve lipid metabolism during pregnancy.

The study by Wandji et al. investigates the relationship between insulin resistance and lipid abnormalities in African individuals with type 2 diabetes mellitus.[45] It sheds light on the impact of insulin resistance on lipid profiles and underscores the importance of addressing insulin resistance to manage dyslipidemia in diabetic patients.

These related studies contribute to the understanding of the relationship between insulin resistance and serum lipoprotein lipid profiles. They provide further evidence of the association between insulin resistance and dyslipidemia, emphasizing the need to manage insulin resistance for improved lipid metabolism and cardiovascular health.

ARTICLE 16

Correlation of Trends in Lipid Profiles from First to Second Trimester with Trends in Insulin Indices and Gestational Diabetes Mellitus

Shen L, Wang D, Huang Y, Ye L, Zhu C, Zhang S, et al. Longitudinal trends in lipid profiles during pregnancy: Association with gestational diabetes mellitus and longitudinal trends in insulin indices.
Front Endocrinol (Lausanne). 2023;13:1080633.

Abstract

Objective: The objective of this study was to examine the correlation between trends in lipid profiles from the first to second trimester and trends in insulin indices and gestational diabetes mellitus (GDM).

Methods: A secondary analysis was conducted on data from an ongoing prospective cohort study involving 1,234 pregnant women at a single center. Lipid profiles, glucose metabolism, and insulin indices were collected during the first and second trimesters. The trends in lipid profiles were categorized into four subgroups: low-to-low, high-to-high, high-to-low, and low-to-high. Insulin indices, including homeostasis model assessment for insulin resistance and quantitative insulin sensitivity check index, were calculated to evaluate insulin resistance (IR). The trends in insulin indices were described as follows: no IR, persistent IR, first-trimester IR alone, and second-trimester IR alone. Pearson correlation analysis and multivariate logistic regression were used to assess the associations between lipid profile subgroups, insulin indices, and GDM.

Results: Total cholesterol (TC), triglycerides (TG), and high-density lipoprotein cholesterol levels in the first and second trimesters were strongly correlated with insulin indices in both trimesters. Among the lipid profiles, only TG showed a sustained correlation with glucose metabolism indices. High-to-high low-density lipoprotein cholesterol (LDL-C) was identified as an independent risk factor for GDM. The high-to-high TG and high-to-low TG subgroups were independent risk factors for persistent IR. Additionally, the high-to-high TG and low-to-high TG subgroups were independent risk factors for second-trimester IR alone.

Conclusion: Triglyceride levels showed a sustained correlation with insulin indices and glucose metabolism indices throughout pregnancy. Persistently high TG levels were identified as independent risk factors for persistent IR and second trimester IR alone. Irrespective of the presence of first trimester IR, maintaining lower TG levels during early and middle pregnancy can help reduce the risk of persistent IR or subsequent development of IR. These findings emphasize the importance of lowering TG levels in early and middle pregnancy to prevent the development of insulin resistance.

COMMENT

The researchers conducted a longitudinal study involving pregnant women and measured their lipid profiles and insulin indices at different stages of pregnancy.

The results showed that lipid profiles, including total cholesterol, triglycerides, and low-density lipoprotein cholesterol, increased progressively during pregnancy. Additionally, women with gestational diabetes mellitus (GDM) had higher lipid levels compared to those without GDM. The study also examined the relationship between lipid profiles and insulin indices, highlighting the associations between lipid levels and insulin resistance. These findings suggest the importance of monitoring lipid profiles during pregnancy, particularly in women with GDM, to assess the risk of metabolic complications.

The systematic review by Zhang et al. and meta-analysis explore the association between maternal lipid profiles and adverse pregnancy outcomes.[46] It highlights the potential impact of lipid abnormalities on pregnancy complications and emphasizes the importance of monitoring lipid levels during pregnancy.

The retrospective cohort study by Zhang et al. investigates the changes in maternal lipid profiles during normal pregnancy and their association with infant's birthweight.[47] It emphasizes the role of lipid metabolism in pregnancy and its potential implications for fetal development.

The review article by Zhu et al. focuses on lipid metabolism in GDM.[48] It provides insights into the alterations in lipid profiles and lipid metabolism in women with GDM and discusses the potential mechanisms underlying these changes.

These related studies contribute to a better understanding of the association between lipid profiles, pregnancy outcomes, and GDM. They provide valuable insights into the metabolic changes that occur during pregnancy and highlight the importance of monitoring lipid levels for the management of gestational diabetes and the prevention of adverse pregnancy outcomes.

ARTICLE 17

Impact of Early Midlife Cardiovascular Health on Future HDL Metrics in Women

Nasr A, Matthews KA, Brooks MM, Barinas-Mitchell E, Orchard T, Billheimer J, et al. Early midlife cardiovascular health influences future HDL metrics in women: The SWAN HDL study.
J Am Heart Assoc. 2022;11(21):e026243.

Abstract

Background: The assessment of high-density lipoprotein cholesterol (HDL-C) alone may not adequately reflect the antiatherogenic properties of HDL in midlife women. It is important to explore novel metrics of HDL function, lipid contents, and subclasses to better understand the atheroprotective capacities of HDL. This study aimed to investigate the relationship between cardiovascular health, as measured by Life's Simple 7 (LS7) score, and various HDL metrics, as well as the impact of LS7 score on changes in HDL metrics over time in women.

Methods and results: A total of 529 women [baseline age: 46.4 (2.6) years, 57% White] from the Study of Women's Health Across the Nation HDL (SWAN HDL) study were included. Baseline

LS7 scores were assessed and repeated measurements of HDL metrics were obtained over time. Multivariable linear mixed models were utilized for analysis. Higher LS7 scores were associated with more favorable future HDL profiles, characterized by higher HDL-phospholipid levels, total HDL particle count (HDL-P), and large HDL-P, as well as lower HDL-triglyceride levels and larger overall HDL size. Maintaining an ideal body mass index was associated with higher HDL-cholesterol efflux capacity, HDL-phospholipid levels, and large HDL-P, while exhibiting lower HDL-triglyceride levels and small HDL-P, along with a larger overall HDL size. Engaging in ideal physical activity was linked to higher HDL-phospholipid levels, as well as increased total, large, and medium HDL-P. Ideal smoking status was associated with lower levels of HDL-triglycerides. Diet, however, did not show a significant association with HDL metrics. Higher LS7 scores and ideal body mass index were also related to slower progression of HDL size over time.

Conclusion: Novel HDL metrics provide additional insight into the clinical utility of HDL in midlife women. Adopting a healthier lifestyle, particularly maintaining an ideal body mass index, is associated with improved future HDL phenotype. These findings underscore the importance of cardiovascular health in shaping HDL functionality and highlight the potential of lifestyle interventions in optimizing HDL-related cardiovascular protection.

COMMENT

The study aimed to determine the associations between cardiovascular health factors, such as blood pressure, cholesterol levels, and smoking status, in early midlife and subsequent high-density lipoprotein (HDL) metrics. The results revealed that better cardiovascular health in early midlife was associated with favorable HDL metrics later in life. Specifically, women with healthier blood pressure, lipid profiles, and non-smoking status in early midlife had higher levels of HDL cholesterol (HDL-C) and improved HDL function in the future. These findings highlight the importance of maintaining cardiovascular health early in life to promote favorable HDL metrics and potentially reduce the risk of cardiovascular diseases in women.

The prospective cohort study by Wilson et al. examines the lifetime risk factors associated with reduced HDL-C levels.[49] It provides insights into the long-term impact of various risk factors on HDL-C and highlights the importance of early prevention and management of these factors.

The longitudinal study by El K et al. investigates the changes in lipoprotein measurements during the menopausal transition and their association with the age at the final menstrual period.[50] It provides insights into the influence of menopause on lipid profiles, including HDL-C levels, and their potential impact on cardiovascular health in women.

The study by Stefanick et al. examines the effect of physical activity on lipid profiles in young women.[51] It highlights the role of exercise in improving HDL-C levels and overall lipid profiles, emphasizing the importance of lifestyle interventions for cardiovascular health.

These related studies provide additional insights into the factors influencing HDL metrics and their long-term impact on cardiovascular health in women. They contribute to the understanding of preventive strategies and interventions to maintain favorable HDL profiles and reduce the risk of cardiovascular diseases.

REFERENCES

1. Fulcher J, O'connell R, Voysey M, Emberson J, Blackwell L, Mihaylova B, et al. Efficacy and safety of LDL-lowering therapy among men and women: meta-analysis of individual data from 174,000 participants in 27 randomised trials. Lancet. 2015;385(9976):1397-405.
2. Nordestgaard BG, Chapman MJ, Humphries SE, Ginsberg HN, Masana L, Descamps OS, et al. Familial hypercholesterolaemia is underdiagnosed and undertreated in the general population: guidance for clinicians to prevent coronary heart disease: consensus statement of the European Atherosclerosis Society. Eur Heart J. 2013;34(45):3478-90a.
3. Schmidt N, Schmidt B, Dressel A, Gergei I, Klotsche J, Pieper L, et al. Familial hypercholesterolemia in primary care in Germany. Diabetes and cardiovascular risk evaluation: Targets and Essential Data for Commitment of Treatment (DETECT) study. Atherosclerosis. 2017;266:24-30.
4. Noda H, Iso H, Irie F, Sairenchi T, Ohtaka E, Ohta H. Gender difference of association between LDL cholesterol concentrations and mortality from coronary heart disease amongst Japanese: the Ibaraki Prefectural Health Study. J Intern Med. 2010;267(6):576-87.
5. Cho L, Davis M, Elgendy I, Epps K, Lindley KJ, Mehta PK, et al. Summary of Updated Recommendations for Primary Prevention of Cardiovascular Disease in Women: JACC State-of-the-Art Review. J Am Coll Cardiol, 2020;75:2602-18.
6. Puymirat E, Simon T, Steg PG, Schiele F, Guéret P, Blanchard D, et al. Association of changes in clinical characteristics and management with improvement in survival among patients with ST-elevation myocardial infarction. JAMA. 2012;308:998-1006.
7. Bihuniak JD, Ramos A, Huedo-Medina T, Hutchins-Wiese H, Kerstetter JE, Kenny AM. Adherence to a Mediterranean-style diet and its influence on cardiovascular risk factors in postmenopausal women. J Acad Nutr Diet. 2016;116(11):1767-75.
8. Hamza RZ, EL-Megharbel SM, Altalhi T, Gobouri AA, Alrogi AA. Hypolipidemic and hepatoprotective synergistic effects of selenium nanoparticles and vitamin E against acrylamide-induced hepatic alterations in male albino mice. Appl Organomet Chem. 2020;34(3):e5458.
9. Smethers AD, Rolls BJ. Dietary Management of Obesity: Cornerstones of Healthy Eating Patterns. Med Clin North Am. 2018;102(1):107-24.
10. Vadiveloo M, Parker H, Raynor H. Increasing low-energy-dense foods and decreasing high-energy-dense foods differently influence weight loss trial outcomes. Int J Obes (Lond). 2018;42(3):479-86.
11. Schoenfeld BJ, Aragon AA, Krieger JW. Effects of meal frequency on weight loss and body composition: a meta-analysis. Nutr Rev. 2015;73(2):69-72.
12. Kim BY, Choi DH, Jung CH, Kang SK, Mok JO, Kim CH. Obesity and Physical Activity. J Obes Metab Syndr. 2017;26:15-22.
13. Thompson PD, Crouse SF, Goodpaster BH, Kelley DE, Moyna NM, Pescatello LS. The effects of exercise on high-density lipoprotein cholesterol levels and particle size: A meta-analysis. Metabolism. 2001;50(10):1253-8.
14. Laughlin MH, Newcomer SC, Bender SB. Exercise training improves size and oxygenation of coronary arteries and increases coronary flow capacity in sedentary humans. J Appl Physiol (1985). 2008;105(5):1664-70.
15. Kelley GA, Kelley KS. Effect of aerobic exercise on high-density lipoprotein cholesterol: A meta-analysis of randomized controlled trials. Eur J Cardiovasc Prev Rehabil. 2008;15(6):659-66.
16. Duntas LH, Brenta G. Subclinical hypothyroidism and dyslipidemia: A systematic review and meta-analysis. Thyroid. 2018;28(5):634-42.
17. Xu L, Sun L, Xu X, et al. Effect of levothyroxine supplementation on lipid profile in patients with subclinical hypothyroidism: A systematic review and meta-analysis. Endocrine. 2019;64(3):546-55.
18. Valentina L, Laura MM, Paolo R, et al. The effect of thyroid function on lipid profile in the population-based Carolina Atherosclerosis Study. Eur J Intern Med. 2018;50:e20-2.
19. Wang Y, Wang QJ. Association of dyslipidemia with hypertension in middle-aged and older Chinese: a community-based study. PLoS One. 2014;9(12):e115251.
20. Wu J, Zhu Y, Li Y, et al. Lipid levels and the risk of hypertension in Chinese middle-aged and elderly populations. PLoS One. 2017;12(11):e0187946.
21. Wang J, Zhang L, Wang F, et al. Association between lipid profiles and hypertension in Chinese ethnic population: a cross-sectional study. Lipids Health Dis. 2018;17(1):209.
22. Khan NI, Nazir N, Siddiqui AA, et al. Effectiveness of nutrition education interventions among adults with metabolic syndrome: A systematic review and meta-analysis. PLoS One. 2019;14(4):e0215123.
23. Karimzadeh M, Javedani M, Almasi-Hashiani A, et al. Impact of lifestyle modification on dyslipidemia in women with polycystic ovary syndrome. Clin Exp Reprod Med. 2020;47(2):148-55.
24. Parletta N, Zarnowiecki D, Cho J, Wilson A, Bogomolova S, Villani A, et al. A Mediterranean-style dietary intervention supplemented with fish

oil improves diet quality and mental health in people with depression: A randomized controlled trial (HELFIMED). Nutr Neurosci. 2019;22(7):474-87.
25. Wang L, Tian Y, Ou Y, et al. Associations of lipid profile with bone mineral density and prevalence of osteoporosis in elderly Chinese individuals. Clin Interv Aging. 2019;14:963-72.
26. Ye D, Zhang L, Li H, et al. Relationship between lipid profiles and osteoporosis in postmenopausal women: a meta-analysis. Clin Interv Aging. 2019;14: 9-18.
27. Wu F, Koenig W, Hou L, et al. Serum lipids and osteoporosis in postmenopausal women: a systematic review and meta-analysis of observational studies. Horm Metab Res. 2014;46(3):173-80.
28. Ganda OP, Bhatt DL, Mason RP, Miller M, Boden WE. Lipid profiles and cardiovascular disease risk prediction in women with and without type 2 diabetes. Circulation. 2019;139(22):2670-2.
29. Toth PP, Potter D, Ming EE. The relationship between lipid levels and cardiovascular disease in women. J Clin Lipidol. 2013;7(5):447-62.
30. Diamanti-Kandarakis E, Dunaif A. The role of insulin resistance in women with polycystic ovary syndrome. Endocrinol Metab Clin North Am. 1999;28(2):341-63.
31. Herrera E, Ortega-Senovilla H. Dyslipidemia in pregnancy. Reprod Biol Endocrinol. 2018;16(1):1.
32. Miyamoto S, Nagai Y, Oba M, Asai-Sato M, Sakuta R, Suzuki S. Maternal dyslipidemia in early pregnancy predicts excessive gestational weight gain in a cohort of Japanese women. J Obstet Gynaecol Res. 2019;45(9):1871-79.
33. Wang C, Zhu W, Wei Y, Su R, Feng H, Lin L. Dyslipidemia during pregnancy: implications for maternal health. J Biomed Res. 2017;31(1):1-12.
34. Vaccarino V, Badimon L, Bremner JD, Cenko E, Cubedo J, Dorobantu M, et al. Sex differences in cardiovascular disease risk and outcomes: A systematic review. J Am Coll Cardiol. 2017;70(3): 321-35.
35. Johnson JL, Greaves L, Repta R. Sex differences in cardiovascular disease: Impact on care and outcomes. Front Neuroendocrinol. 2019;52:1-8.
36. Hua P, Vemulapalli S, Lopes RD, Anand I, Diaz R, Fox KAA, et al. Sex-specific differences in cardiovascular risk factors and outcomes in peripheral artery disease: Insights from the EUCLID trial. J Am Heart Assoc. 2019;8(15):e012159.
37. Kim S, Haines PS, Siega-Riz AM, Popkin BM. Association between frequency of eating out and lipid levels in young adults. Nutr J. 2004;3:13.
38. Du SF, Neiman A, Batis C, Wang HJ, Zhang B. Fast food consumption and lipid profiles among young Chinese adults. J Acad Nutr Diet. 2019;119(6): 957-66.
39. Li J, Wang F, Yang X, Yang Y, Zhang L, Gao X, et al. Dietary patterns, food groups, and serum lipids in Chinese women: a cross-sectional study. Lipids Health Dis. 2018;17(1):223.
40. Li X, Wang X, Zhang S, Xu M, Ding Y, Ji X, et al. Sex differences in the association between lipid profiles and hypertension in a Chinese population. Medicine (Baltimore). 2016;95(40):e5022.
41. Li J, Wang Y, Li D, Chen Y, Wang Y, Zhao X, et al. Sex-specific association between lipid levels and incident ischemic stroke in the middle-aged and elderly Chinese population. Sci Rep. 2016;6:34273.
42. Saremi A, Asghari M, Ghorbani A. Sex differences in lipid metabolism and metabolic syndrome: From bench to bedside. Lipids Health Dis. 2014;13:186.
43. Taskinen MR, Borén J. Insulin resistance and lipoprotein metabolism. Curr Opin Lipidol. 2016; 27(3):257-61.
44. Bo S, Valpreda S, Menato G, Bardelli C, Botto C, Gambino R, et al. Dyslipidemia and insulin resistance in pregnancy. Atherosclerosis. 2006;189(1):201-7.
45. Wandji CN, Sobngwi E, Djouogo CF, Ngassam E, Gautier JF. Association between insulin resistance and lipids abnormalities in African type 2 diabetic patients. Lipids Health Dis. 2010;9:118.
46. Zhang J, Zhang Y, Wang X, Zhao Y, Li R, Zhang L, et al. Association between maternal lipid profile and adverse pregnancy outcomes: a systematic review and meta-analysis. J Matern Fetal Neonatal Med. 2020;33(4):614-23.
47. Zhang C, Liu S, Solomon CG, Hu FB. Maternal lipid profile changes during normal pregnancy and its association with infant's birthweight: a retrospective cohort study. PLoS Med. 2016;13(9): e1002091.
48. Zhu L, Hou X, Xu Y, Li Z, Li X, Chen X, et al. Lipid metabolism in gestational diabetes mellitus. Adv Clin Chem. 2019;91:209-39.
49. Wilson PW, Abbott RD, Castelli WP. Lifetime risk factors for reduced high-density lipoprotein cholesterol: the Framingham Offspring Study. Am J Clin Nutr. 1988;48(4):707-17.
50. El Khoudary SR, Wildman RP, Matthews KJ, Thurston RC, Bromberger JT, Sutton-Tyrrell K. Longitudinal changes in lipoprotein measurements during the menopausal transition and association with age at the final menstrual period. J Clin Endocrinol Metab. 2010;95(8):3844-52.
51. Stefanick ML, Mackey S, Sheehan M, Ellsworth N, Haskell WL, Wood PD. Effect of physical activity on lipid profiles in young women. Med Sci Sports Exerc. 1998;30(6):892-98.

SECTION 4

Diabetes Mellitus and CVD in Women

Section Editor: J Cecily Mary Majella

Associate Editors: Vatchala Sree Varadharajan, K Meenakshi, T Neelambujan, Aarathy Kannan, Rohith Velusamy, J Nandhini, Sundar C, S Arulrhaj, Manikandan, Nikhil Govind, Arun Ranganathan, P Deepa

ARTICLE 1

Cardiovascular Risk and Lifetime Benefit from Preventive Treatment in Type 2 Diabetes Mellitus: A Post Hoc Analysis of the CAPTURE Study

Østergaard HB, Humphreys V, Hengeveld EM, Honoré JB, Mach F, Visseren FLJ, et al. Cardiovascular risk and lifetime benefit from preventive treatment in type 2 diabetes: A post hoc analysis of the CAPTURE study. *Diabetes Obes Metab.* 2023;25(2):435-43.

Abstract

Objective: The objective of this study is to evaluate the likely number of life-years accomplished without (recurrent) cardiovascular disease (CVD) episodes with maximum cardiovascular risk management (CVRM) and initiation of glucose-lowering agents with established cardiovascular benefit in cohort with type 2 diabetes Mellitus (T2DM)

Materials and methods: The CAPTURE study population (n = 9,416) were taken for assessment. CAPTURE is a multinational cross-sectional study that involved 13 countries and 5 continents, that looked at the prevalence of CVD in T2DM patients. The individual 10-year and lifetime CVD risk in T2DM cohort was calculated using the diabetes lifetime-perspective prediction model. An estimate of the usage of preventive medications was assessed in line with expected CVD risk and laminated for history of CVD. The total sole gain from continuing preventive treatment including best CVRM and the inclusion of glucagon-like peptide-1 receptor agonists (GLP-1 RAs) and sodium-glucose cotransporter-2 inhibitors (SGLT-2is) was computed by amalgamating the treatment sequel from prevailing evidence.

Results: There was not much diversity in the usage of GLP-1 RA or SGLT-2i in T2DM with or without CVD. However, T2DM patients with CVD were taking more antihypertensives, statins, and aspirin when compared to T2DM patients without CVD. Mean [standard deviation (SD)] life-time benefit from best CVRM was 3.9 (3.0) for T2DM patients with proven CVD and 1.3 (1.9) for T2DM patients without CVD. T2DM patients with established CVD gained an extra 1.2 (0.6) years when treated with GLP-1 RA and SGLT-2i, this benefit was not extended to T2DM patients without CVD.

Conclusion: The CVD status of an individual is detrimental in gleaning benefit from best CVRM and treatment with GLP-1 RA or a SGLT-2i in terms of life-years gained without recurrent CVD.

COMMENT

What was Known Prior to this Study?

Type 2 diabetes mellitus (T2DM) is a common clinical entity with a global prevalence of 9% which is expected to increase by 25% in 2030 and by 51% by 2045. The incidence worldwide is growing expeditiously.[1] T2DM patients are at two-fold excess risk of developing cardiovascular disease (CVD). T2DM confers an independent risk to develop CVD irrespective of other conventional risk factors.[2] CVD contributes for increased mortality and morbidity in T2DM patients in addition to associated poor quality of life and increasing the healthcare cost.

Glucagon-like peptide-1 receptor agonist (GLP-1 RA) and sodium-glucose cotransporter-2 inhibitors (SGLT-2is), the newer glucose-lowering oral agents have established cardiovascular (CV) benefits by significantly reducing the mortality and morbidity in T2DM patients with CVD. The benefit obtained by these agents is irrespective of their effect on the glycemic control. Hence, latest guidelines recommend their use in high-risk T2DM patients with CVD. However, the use of these agents in real world scenario is limited despite being advocated by guidelines. The use of statins, antihypertensives, and aspirin for secondary prevention and smoking cessation are also proved to reduce the mortality and morbidity due to CVD in T2DM patients in addition to good glycemic control by guidelines recommend treatment strategy.[3]

The benefit gleaned through best CVRM by strategies like achieving optimal glycemic control through GLP-1 RA and SGLT-2is, blood pressure lowering, lipid lowering, smoking cessation, and usage of aspirin is not normally distributed rather widely distributed. This is influenced by the risk factor burden, baseline risk, and duration of treatment. The DIAbetes Lifetime-perspective prediction (DIAL) model, forecasts the CVD risk in patients with T2DM while atoning for non-CVD mortality as a combative risk. Additionally, the tool lets incarnation of treatment aftermath [hazard ratio (HR) or meta-analyses] to calculate the number of life-years accomplished without a (recurrent) CVD event with commencement of preventive medication strategies. This allows the clinicians to educate individual patient regarding their possible CVD risk and the advantages of starting them on preventive treatment options thereby providing a tailored treatment protocol for that individual patient. This facilitates a shared decision-making between the patient and the clinician.[4]

What this Study Adds? Older men with longer duration of T2DM had CVD more often compared to T2DM patients who did not have CVD. In addition, patients with CVD and T2DM were taking CV preventive medicines regularly compared to those who did not develop CVD. 96% of the T2DM patients with prior CVD had a 10% chance of having a 10-year risk of recurrent event and 80% of cohort had a lifetime risk of recurrent event of >50%. However, in T2DM patients without CVD, only 0.4% had a lifetime risk of a first CV event of > 50%. 14% had a 10-year risk of a first CV event of >10%.

Information regarding the usage of CV preventive medications in T2DM patients with or without CVD has revealed several important data. Generally, the usage of antihypertensives, statins, and aspirin are higher in T2DM patients with CVD compared to those without CVD. In T2DM patients with CVD and a high predicted risk of further CVD, the usage of BP-lowering medications was high, but the usage of statins and aspirin were low. There was not much difference in the usage of glucose-lowering agents particularly GLP-1 RA and SGLT-2i in T2DM patients with or without CVD. Generally, GLP-1 RA was used less compared to SGLT-2i. About 10% of T2DM patients with CVD received GLP-1 RA and 11% of T2DM patient without CVD received the same. Likewise, SGLT-2i was used in 18% of T2DM patients with CVD and in 16% of T2DM patients without CVD. Furthermore, the usage of GLP-1 RA and SGLT-2i was low in T2DM patients with CVD and higher predicted risk for future CVD.

The overall mean [standard deviation (SD)] lifetime benefit gained through best CVRM in T2DM patients with CVD was 3.9 (3.0) years. The overall mean (SD) lifetime benefit gained through best CVRM in T2DM patients without CVD was much lower at 1.3 (1.9) years. T2DM patients with CVD gained a mean (SD) 0.9 (0.5) years and 0.6 (0.4) years without recurrent CVD when treated with GLP-1 RA and SGLT-2i, respectively. T2DM patients with CVD and higher predicted CVD risk gained maximum with optimum CVRM through greater lifetime benefit. Furthermore, when glucose-lowering agents like GLP-1 RA and SGLT-2i were added to CVRM in T2DM patients with CVD, they gained an overall mean (SD) of 1.2 (0.6) life-years free of recurrent CVD event. The gain thus obtained was higher when treatment was initiated at a younger age. The addition of GLP-1 RA and SGLT-2i in T2DM patients with no CVD, but with higher predicted risk for CVD gained maximum.

Major strengths of the study: This study allows the patients to gain an insight on the individual lifetime CVD risk and life-years free of CVD with and without a particular treatment. This facilitates the patient to take an informed decision about their health after discussion with the clinician. Patients with T2DM more often play a crucial role in deciding their treatment pathway and such conversation between the patient and treating clinician may foster a greater adherence to treatment or lifestyle changes as long as the primary physician tailors the information to the individual. The DIAL model chosen in this study is a well validated tool currently in use to evaluate the absolute risk reduction and gain in life-years without CVD with preventive treatment. The model itself is obtained through clearly endorsed large studies involving current T2DM-based cohort from various regions. Hence, the tool is applicable to all T2DM patients regardless of their geographical distribution in routine clinical settings making it suitable worldwide.

Major limitations of the study: The DIAL model only accommodates CVD risk prediction as the outcome; hence no assessment could be made on the risk of chronic kidney disease and heart failure hospitalization which are equally relevant outcome in T2DM treatment. Also, it is not devisable to authenticate the DIAL model beyond 10-year life span prediction. As the DIAL model is applied to CAPTURE study, which is a cross-sectional study and no follow up data is available, it is not possible to recalibrate the model to current cohort. The usage of glucose-lowering medications like GLP-1 RA and SGLT-2i in the CAPTURE study was significantly found to be lower than expected. Also, there was no difference in the percentage of patients with or without CVD who used these medications although guidelines explicitly advocate their use in T2DM patients with high risk for CVD. The study did not evaluate the reason behind this lower usage in terms of lack of reimbursement from healthcare providers or contraindication in high-risk patients.

Type 2 diabetes mellitus and cardiovascular disease in women: In females, CVDs tend to occur at a later age compared to male. However, in female patients with T2DM this age-related discrepancy is diluted. Therefore, women with T2DM develop myocardial infarction as the same age like male. The incidence of CV complications is five to four times higher in diabetic women and three to two times higher in diabetic males. Latest medical guidelines lack clarity on sex-specific or gender-sensitive prevention strategies and management. Hence more research is needed in this area

Conclusion: This study explains the trend in T2DM management and the usage of various guidelines recommended treatment options including glucose-lowering medicines, BP-lowering medications, lipid-lowering medications, and aspirin. Generally, the usage of guideline recommended glucose-lowering medications like GLP-1 RA and SGLT-2i is lower than expected. T2DM patients with CVD gained an extra 1.2 (0.6) years of lifetime free of recurrent CVD events, and such difference was not noted in T2DM patients without CVD.

ARTICLE 2

Association of Gestational Diabetes Mellitus with Overall and Type Specific Cardiovascular and Cerebrovascular Diseases: Systematic Review and Meta-analysis

Xie W, Wang Y, Xiao S, Qiu L, Yu Y, Zhang Z. Association of gestational diabetes mellitus with overall and type specific cardiovascular and cerebrovascular diseases: Systematic review and meta-analysis.
BMJ. 2022;378:e070244.

Abstract

Introduction: Gestational diabetes mellitus (GDM), defined as first-onset glucose intolerance in pregnancy, has a prevalence from 1 to >30%. Women who had GDM experience a 10-fold higher risk of developing type 2 diabetes mellitus (T2DM) and a two-fold higher risk of overall subsequent cardiovascular (CV) disease than women without GDM.[5] However, there is very little evidence on the associations between GDM and type-specific CV diseases.

Methodology: The aim of the meta-analysis was to assess the risk of overall and type-specific CV, cerebrovascular, and venous thromboembolism in women with a history of GDM. This meta-analysis of 15 studies involved more than eight million women, with data was obtained from PubMed, Embase, and the Cochrane Library from inception to 1st November 2021. Studies included were observational studies with a retrospective or prospective cohort or case–control studies. Cross-sectional studies, studies without eligible control group, reviews, and editorials were excluded. The study was reported in accordance with the Preferred Reporting Items for Systematic Reviews and Meta-Analysis (PRISMA) guidelines.[6] The primary outcome was the association of GDM with overall and type-specific CV and cerebrovascular diseases. Secondary outcomes were the association of GDM with type-specific CV and cerebrovascular diseases and venous thromboembolism including deep vein thrombosis and pulmonary embolism. Extracted data were analysed with Stata Statistical Software version 13.0 and R statistical language version R 3.6.0. The p values of <0.05 were considered significant. Additional subanalyses was performed to determine whether the association of GDM with CV and cerebrovascular disease were influenced by factors including race, smoking, body mass index, socioeconomic status, level of education, parity, comorbidities, and pregnancy complications.

Results: Women with a history of GDM showed a 45% increased risk of developing overall CV and cerebrovascular diseases compared to women without GDM. Increased risks of subsequent coronary artery disease (CAD), myocardial infarction, heart failure, angina pectoris, and CV procedures was seen in women with a history of GDM when compared to non-GDM group even after accounting for ethnicity, sociodemographic characteristics, education level, conventional CV risk factors, and future T2DM. The risk for overall stroke, ischemic stroke, hemorrhagic stroke, and venous thromboembolism was also increased in the GDM group over the non-GDM group. The test for subgroup differences in GDM patients showed a statistically significant subgroup effect for smoking ($p = 0.03$), body mass index ($p = 0.01$), and socioeconomic status ($p = 0.006$), and for comorbidities ($p = 0.05$), suggesting that these factors might statistically significantly modify the association between GDM and CV and cerebrovascular diseases.

Conclusion: The meta-analysis showed that women with a history GDM are subject to a higher risk of future CV and cerebrovascular diseases which cannot be solely due to conventional CV risk factors. The results highlight the need for further studies and continuous follow-up of women with GDM.

COMMENT

Although gestational diabetes mellitus (GDM) usually resolves after child birth, there is growing evidence that it imparts a lifelong cardiovascular (CV) and cerebrovascular disease risk in the mother. GDM can promote CV diseases in many ways, viz., (1) By increasing risk of type 2 diabetes mellitus (T2DM), metabolic syndrome, and hypertension.[6] (2) The chronic β-cell dysfunction and insulin resistance in GDM could increase levels of low-density lipoprotein (LDL) cholesterol, blood pressure, and adiposity and decrease high-density lipoprotein (HDL) cholesterol.[7] (3) Abnormal expression of CV diseases associated microRNAs and inflammatory markers including tumor necrosis factor-alpha, C-reactive protein (CRP), and adiponectin in patients with GDM may also contribute to endothelial dysfunction.[7] (4) Even a short-period hyperglycemia could cause reduction of cardiac function in GDM women.[7] (5) These patients also had a two-fold higher prevalence of coronary artery calcification, which was independent of traditional CV risk factors.[7] Barker's hypothesis states that epigenetic factors may predispose to CV risk abnormalities in GDM offspring also.[7]

Data from the 2007–2014 NHANES showed that except for a lower HDL cholesterol, GDM mothers did not significantly have other abnormalities. This indicates that HDL cholesterol may be the contributing factor for the future development of CV diseases in GDM. A meta-analysis of 32 studies had reported that the risk from CV diseases was reduced by 23% with each 1 mmol/L increment in HDL cholesterol by its high cholesterol efflux capacity and antioxidant and anti-inflammatory effects.[7] However, HDL subspecies could exert diverse effects on the development of CV disease.[7] Atheroprotective effects were observed with of HDL containing APOE or APOC-I and APOC-III-containing HDL was associated with higher carotid intima-media thickness and HDL subspecies containing haptoglobin, complement C3, α-2 macroglobulin, or plasminogen were also associated with higher risk of coronary heart disease (CHD).[7]

There are several studies for and against the observations that women who had experienced GDM are at a higher risk of CV disease independent of other CV risk factors.

Insulin and metformin are recommended for the treatment of GDM if glycemic levels are not controlled with diet alone.[7] Two meta-analyses have reported that metformin treatment in GDM could reduce the further risk of CV diseases.[7] In the DPP/DPPOS trial (the longest and largest trial of metformin treatment for diabetes prevention) with a 21-year median follow-up, neither indicated that metformin nor lifestyle interventions reduced the risks of myocardial infarction and stroke. Although there are no high quality nutritional studies, nutritional interventions could significantly reduce the risk of postpartum diabetes.[7]

Conclusion: Gestational diabetes mellitus had stronger associations with CAD and heart failure than cerebrovascular disease, and the excess risks cannot be solely attributed to conventional CV risk factors, which are partially mediated by the onset of T2DM. The American Heart Association recommends that GDM be considered as a gender-specific risk factor for identifying women at increased risks of type-specific CV diseases. Continuous monitoring of women with a history of GDM is mandatory. There is also need for further studies on the associations between GDM and levels of HDL subspecies. Long-term studies are needed to study effects of diet modification and antidiabetics on risks of CV diseases among women with a history of GDM.

ARTICLE 3

Cardiovascular Outcomes in Type 1 and Type 2 Diabetes Mellitus

Rosengren A, Dikaiou P. Cardiovascular outcomes in type 1 and type 2 diabetes. *Diabetologia. 2023;66(3):425-37.*

Abstract

The incidence and prevalence of type 1 diabetes mellitus (T1DM) and type 2 diabetes mellitus (T2DM) are on the rise worldwide. The global burden of diabetes is around 536.6 million and is set to increase to 783.2 million by 2045. Even though T1DM and T2DM are two different phenotypes, overlap between these two types occurs. The risk for cardiovascular disease in diabetes is contributed by conventional risk factors and also by vasculogenic risk factors like arterial stiffness and coronary flow reserve. Intensive glycemic control reduces coronary events but all-cause mortality did not benefit. Increased glycemic variability is also an independent cardiovascular risk factor.

Type 1 diabetes mellitus patient being younger in age will have a lower short-term absolute cardiovascular risk but will have a longer exposure to dysglycemia. T2DM being older will have a higher absolute risk. Young-onset T2DM is the most serious health challenge today. Increase in childhood obesity is another factor which will have adverse impact on the cardiovascular outcome. The difference in risk between younger and older people in terms of absolute versus lifetime risk of T2DM complication should promote different strategies to improve the cardiovascular disease.

COMMENT

Introduction

There is a worldwide increase in the incidence and prevalence of type 1 diabetes mellitus (T1DM) and type 2 diabetes mellitus (T2DM). The global burden of diabetes is estimated to be around 536.6 million with 10.5% of adults in the age group of 20–79 years being affected. The incidence of diabetes is also set to increase to 783.2 million by 2045 mainly due to lifestyle changes.

The largest increase in T2DM is seen in low- and middle-income countries. India has more than 101 million people living with diabetes compared to 70 million in 2019 according to ICMR study. While 11.4% of India's population is in diabetics and another 15.3% is prediabetic, one-third of people with prediabetes will develop diabetes and another one-third remains as prediabetic in the follow-up. This sets the stage for further increase in diabetes and cardiovascular problems in the next two decades. The reason for this increasing trend is due to changes in physical activity and the diet pattern leading to obesity. While 28.6% Indians have generalized obesity and 39.5% have abdominal obesity. The incidence of T1DM is also on the rise even though there is no adequate data when compared to T2DM.

Overlap between Type 1 and Type 2 Diabetes Mellitus

People with T1DM and T2DM are two different phenotypes with regard to age of onset, diabetes duration, and lifetime glycemic load. However, there occurs overlap between these two types of diabetes leading to misdiagnosis and wrong estimation of cardiovascular risk.

Even though the mean age of onset of T1DM and T2DM differs by decades, both types can occur at any age. LADA (latent autoimmune diabetes in adults) is considered as an intermediate of T1DM and T2DM. This group is associated with overweight, insulin resistance, and underlying autoimmunity. They show a faster progression to insulin therapy than the usual T2DM.

Late-onset T1DM can be misdiagnosed as T2DM. Conversely, onset of T1DM in younger people who are obese can be misdiagnosed as T2DM. These caveats have to be taken into consideration when assessing the cardiovascular outcomes in T1DM and T2DM.

Gender Differences in Diabetes Mellitus

One's sex is a fundamental biological factor, which plays a key role in regulation of homeostasis in health and causes vulnerability to cardiometabolic risk factors, as well as manifestation, clinical picture, and management of T2DM. Severity of injury differs in a sex-specific way regarding various diabetes-related comorbidities, especially cardiovascular and renal disease. Psychosocial factors also impact development and progression of diabetes and coping in a gender-dimorphic way. Reproductive factors and sexual function have to be considered. The care of diabetic pregnancy demands special attention, because this vulnerable phase programs health of offspring even in a sex-specific way. Otherwise hyperglycemic parents beget diabetic offspring, further contributing to pandemic increase of T2DM. Biomedical basic and clinical research in endocrinology should benefit both women and men in a balanced manner. Modern personalized treatment has to consider differences in biological factors, such as genetic predisposition, sex hormones, neurohumoral pathways, and behavioral and environmental differences between men and women.

For example, males with diabetes have a higher risk for microvascular complications, such as retinopathy and nephropathy, whereas several studies report a higher relative risk for cardiovascular diseases (CVDs) in females with diabetes compared to their male counterparts.

Women with T2DM have earlier risk of major cardiovascular events by 20–30 years and males by 15–20 years compared to the people without diabetes. The overall incidence of myocardial infarction, stroke, and heart failure is about two-fold in T2DM compared to the people without diabetes. The diabetes-related excess risk of myocardial infarction is much higher for women than for men, while for the other CVDs, people with T2DM of the two sexes have a similar excess risk. In light of finding possible mechanisms to explain the partial loss of advantage for myocardial infarction and not for the other two types of events, we foresee a second study to investigate the determinants of CVD events only in population with T2DM using information about prescribed drug and on other areas of care such as tests and lifestyle factors and diabetes duration.

Cardiovascular Risk Factors in Diabetes

The additional risk for CVD in diabetes is due to the presence of multiple factors. The conventional risk factors, such as elevated low-density lipoprotein (LDL)-cholesterol, hypertension, smoking, advanced age, and sex have a role to play irrespective of the type of diabetes. Factors specific to diabetes like HbA1c levels, micro- and macroalbuminuria contributes significantly for cardiovascular risk.

Various studies have emphasized the importance of having the blood glucose levels under control in both T1DM and T2DM. The Diabetes Control and Complications Trial (DCCT) compared individuals with T1DM assigned to intensive versus standard therapy for a mean period of 6.5 years. During 30 years of follow-up, those assigned to intensive therapy had a one-third reduced incidence of any CVD and major adverse cardiovascular events (MACEs). Similarly, in T2DM intensive glycemic control had reduced coronary events when compared to standard glycemic control from the data analysis of landmark trials, such as UKPDS, ADVANCE, ACCORD, and VADT. However, all-cause mortality did not benefit with the degree of glycemic control. The beneficial effect of intensive glycemic control can be explained by the impact of legacy effect.

In T1DM, certain vasculogenic risk factors play a significant role for CVD. Arterial stiffness in the small resistance arteries have been associated with all-cause mortality

In an Australian study, 470 individuals with T1DM and 354 individuals with T2DM in the age group of 15–30 years with mean duration of diabetes of 14.7 and 11.6 years respectively were enrolled. During long-term follow-up, it was found that despite similar metabolic control and shorter duration of diabetes, T2DM had more albuminuria and marked excess of macrovascular disease compared with T1DM (ischemic heart disease 12.6% vs. 2.5%; stroke 4.3% vs. 0.7%) and higher death rates [11% vs. 6.8%; HR 2.0; 95% CI 1.2, 3.2]. Among the middle-aged individuals with T1DM and T2DM there was no difference with regard to cardiovascular mortality and long-term outcomes as shown by a Finnish study with 173 participants with T1DM and 834 participants with T2DM aged 45–64 years.[8]

Another factor which influences a higher cardiovascular risk in T2DM is obesity. Overweight individuals with T2DM were 15 times more likely to develop a cardiovascular event when compared with individuals with T1DM. No statistical differences were noted between normal weight T2DM and T1DM group.

Trends in Cardiovascular Outcomes in Type 1 and Type 2 Diabetes Mellitus

With expanding knowledge about the cardiovascular risk factors operating in type 1 and T2DM there should be a decline in the occurrence of CVD globally. With adequate control of various cardiovascular risk factors using lifestyle modifications and usage of drugs like statins, there should be a favorable outcome. Last decade had witnessed a marked decline in coronary mortality in high-income countries. The CVD rates in the low- and middle-income countries are on the rise.

In a US noninstitutionalized population study, major CVD mortality had declined in the last two decades in adults with diabetes mainly in men. There had been reduction in mortality from ischemic heart disease and stroke. Heart failure and arrhythmia related deaths did not change. Vascular diseases accounted for almost half of deaths in people with diabetes which is seen to be reducing in the last decade. Studies have also shows greater reduction in cardiovascular outcomes in type 1 diabetes than T2DM.

Cardiovascular Outcomes in Type 1 and Type 2 Diabetes Mellitus in Our Population

Type 1 diabetes mellitus is conventionally considered as a disease of younger age and T2DM is considered as a disease of middle and older age. However, there are overlaps between the two phenotypes of diabetes with regard to age of presentation. In our population with increasing incidence of diabetes, we come across T2DM diagnosed at an younger age group. There is also increase in the incidence of childhood obesity which puts us on peril. The combination of younger age of onset of diabetes and obesity will have adverse impact on the cardiovascular outcome.

In the young diabetic study from Chennai, the mean age of T1DM participants were 17.1 ± 4.2 years and type 2 diabetes were 21.6 ± 3.6 years. The incidence of microvascular and macrovascular complications was 2.11 times (95% CI 1.27–3.51) higher among the type 2 diabetes when compared to T1DM.

Being a genetically predisposed race of Southeast Asians and higher incidence of metabolic syndrome, the impact of younger age of diabetes onset on the cardiovascular outcome needs a large-scale study for our Indian population.[9,10]

In a meta-analysis by Natalie Nanayakkara et al.,[11] it was shown that each 1 year increase in age of diabetes diagnosis was associated with a 4%, 3%, and 5% decreased risk of all-cause mortality, macrovascular disease, and microvascular disease, respectively.

and cardiovascular mortality in T1DM. The simple clinical parameter of pulse pressure, which is a surrogate of arterial stiffness has been found to be increased in patients with T1DM. Coronary flow reserve is also found to be reduced in young individuals with T1DM.

Increased glycemic variability has been found to be an independent cardiovascular risk factor both in type 1 and type 2 diabetic patients. An association between glycemic variability and coronary artery calcium scores has been reported in T1DM study. Nonenzymatic glycation, oxidative stress, activation of inflammatory pathways, and endothelial dysfunction are considered to be the proposed mechanisms. Symptomatic and asymptomatic hypoglycemia can trigger cardiac arrhythmias and increase mortality in diabetic patients, especially in patient with CVD or those with increased cardiovascular risk.

Cardiovascular Outcomes in Type 1 and Type 2 Diabetes Mellitus

Majority of data for cardiovascular outcomes in diabetes is related to T2DM. In a meta-analysis of 102 prospective studies with 698,782 people without initial vascular disease, adjusted hazard ratios (HRs) for diabetes versus no diabetes were 2.00 [95% confidence interval (CI) 1.83, 2.9] for coronary heart disease (CHD), 2.27 (95% CI 1.95, 2.65) for ischemic stroke, 1.84 (95% CI 1.59, 2.13) for unclassified stroke, and 1.73 (95% CI 1.51, 1.98) for other vascular deaths. HRs for CHD were also noted to be higher in woman than in men, in younger than in older patients.

In another meta-analysis of 10 observational studies involving 166,027 patients with T1DM and matched control from general population, the overall relative risk for CHD was 9.38 (95% CI 5.56, 15.82). The relative risk was extremely high in individuals with T1DM with onset at an age of 10 years and younger. The relative risks were also lower among those with onset after 20 years of age. The EURODIAB IDDM complications study which included 3,250 T1DM patients, CVD prevalence increase with diabetes duration and age from 6% in the age group of 15–29 years to 25% in the age group of 45–59 years.

Comparison of Cardiovascular Outcomes between Type 1 and Type 2 Diabetes Mellitus

Comparison of cardiovascular outcomes between T1DM and T2DM is fraught with difficulty because of differences in the phenotype and also difference in the absolute risk between T1DM and T2DM. The mean age, age at onset, and diabetes duration vary between these groups. In one study involving 36,869 individuals with T1DM and 457,473 individuals with type 2 diabetes, the mean age at entry was 35.3 years for T1DM and 65.2 years for T2DM, a difference of 30 years. The mean duration of diabetes was also longer for T1DM (20 years) when compared to T2DM (5.7 years). The mean HbA1c levels were also higher in T1DM (HbA1c 8.2%) when compared to T2DM (HbA1c 7.1%). The difference in population characteristics lead to difficulties in comparing the outcomes in T1DM and T2DM. T1DM patients being younger in age will have a lower short-term absolute cardiovascular risk but will have longer exposure to dysglycemia. On the other hand, T2DM patients being older will have a higher absolute risk. As the baseline factors are opposite, the comparison also becomes an unbalanced one.

With altered lifestyle, more and more individuals develop T2DM at a young age. These young individuals with T2DM may be at higher risk of cardiovascular complications when compared to T1DM. Young-onset T2DM is termed as the most serious health challenges today. Earlier onset of T2DM represents an aggressive phenotype with more rapid deterioration of β-cell function.

Older people with diabetes have the highest short-term absolute risk while diabetes at younger age puts them at a longer lifetime risk of developing significant complication. This difference in risk between younger and older people in terms of absolute versus lifetime risks of T2DM complication should promote increased screening programs in older people with T2DM and a greater emphasis on preventive measures for younger people with T2DM. Risk stratification methods using age at diagnosis may provide a method of identifying those at greatest risk of complication who would be targeted for individualized treatment regimens for reaping the most benefit.

Younger people with T2DM underestimate the risk of complications and have lower adherence to therapy with poor glycemic control when compared to older people. Research and clinical guidelines should address the younger people with T2DM and ensure that they receive optimal medical attention with good glycemic control to improve the cardiovascular outcome among the diabetes in our population.

ARTICLE 4

Cardiovascular Risk Factors in Diabetic Patients with Metabolic Syndrome

Bazmandegan G, Abbasifard M, Nadimi AE, Alinejad H, Kamiab Z. Cardiovascular risk factors in diabetic patients with and without metabolic syndrome: a study based on the Rafsanjan cohort study.
Sci Rep. 2023;13(1):559.

Abstract

Background: Cardiovascular disease (CVD) is the leading cause of death and disability in people with diabetes mellitus (DM), because finding a correlation between DM and cardiovascular risk factors can be effective prevent patient morbidity and mortality.

Objective: The purpose of this study was to find out prevalence of cardiovascular risk factors in women with and without metabolic syndrome (MetS).

Methods: This cross-sectional study in women aged 35–70 years without MetS in DM. Indicators of CVD risk factors, including age, blood pressure, dyslipidemia, fasting blood sugar, creatinine, blood urea, waist circumference, body mass index, family history, physical inactivity, and fruit and vegetable consumption were collected. Data were analyzed using SPSS software version 22. Overweight from the MetS, participants were estimated to be 80% (95% confidence interval 78.1–81.8%). In logistic regression model, triglycerides were identified as factors associated with MetS while there was an association of smoking, alcohol consumption in men in Pioneering studies.

Results: Our results show that, based on our study, there is a prevalence risk factors for CVD were high in women. The suggested solutions in this field are control of hypertension and dyslipidemia.

COMMENT

Cardiovascular disease (CVD) is the leading determinant of mortality and disability among individuals with diabetes mellitus (DM), as correlating DM with cardiovascular risk factors can significantly reduce the risk of disease and mortality. DM is a persistent risk factor for CVD due to its ability to raise fasting plasma glucose levels before they reach a point where they can be diagnosed.[9] As a result, DM has been linked to a shortened life expectancy of up to 10 years, with over 50% of patients dying of a cardiovascular event. Women with DM are at a higher risk of developing CVD than those without diabetes, with a 10% increased risk of CVD, a 53% increased risk of multiple myelodysplastic syndromes [myocardial infarction (MI)], a 58% increase in stroke risk, and a 12% increased risk of heart failure compared to the general population. Therefore, DM is a significant contributor to the development of CVD and its associated risks.

Although premenopausal women are protected against CVD compared to males of the same age, the risk of CVD increases exponentially for women after menopause.

The risk of CVD in women with DM is subject to a gradual increase, and the extent of this increase is dependent on the combination of multiple risk factors. The majority of the additional risks associated with DM are related to the increased prevalence of risk factors, such as high blood pressure, obesity, and hypertension. Over the past decade, research has demonstrated the importance of treating known risk factors in patients with DM in order to reduce the risk of CVD. Poor control of cardiovascular risk factors is commonly observed in women with diabetes. However, it is not possible to solely attribute additional risks of CVD in DM patients to the prevalence of these risk factors, thus other risk factors may be relevant. DM is characterized by a set of interconnected risk factors including high blood pressure, high blood sugar, obesity, and diabetes. The disease is associated with an increase in cardiovascular events, diabetes, and mortality. In India, the prevalence of DM was estimated at 45.8 and 57.7%, respectively.

The prevalence of risk factors associated with CVD in women has been extensively studied in research, as the identification of a connection between DM risk factors and CVD can be beneficial in avoiding the occurrence of mortality and morbidity in patients.[12] Endocrinology and cardiology professionals recommend that further efforts be made to enhance risk factors for CVD in diabetic women, as they are more likely to develop heart attack and have a higher mortality rate.

Metabolic syndrome is associated with a range of risk factors including chronic mild inflammation biomarkers, such as CRP, increased oxidant stress, thrombophiliac disorders [such as plasminogen activator inhibitor-1 (PAI-1) and E-selectin] and a predisposition to atherosclerosis and cardiovascular events.[13] Consequently, metabolic syndrome is one of a number of risk factors associated with atherosclerosis and is strongly associated with DM. This type of diabetes is characterized by insulin resistance with secondary hyperinsulinemia, and is often associated with hypertension, dyslipidemia, CVD, and obesity, particularly central obesity.

Diabetes mellitus is characterized by high levels of low-density lipoprotein (LDL) and hypertension, which are the primary determinants of CVD. Additionally, women with low high-density lipoprotein (HDL) cholesterol levels, insulin resistance, high blood sugar levels, and inflammation had more cardiovascular complications.

Women with high risk of metabolic syndrome should be identified through primary health center screening and so that multifactorial interventions, such as management of hypertension, hyperlipidemia, and obesity can be done.

The article adds to the literature in the domain of obesity, diabetes, and metabolic syndrome in women and emphasizes the risk factors and highlights on the methods to decrease the risk of metabolic syndrome.

ARTICLE 5

14 Sex-specific Predictors of Coronary Microvascular Function in a Multiethnic Cohort of 455 Asymptomatic People with Type 2 Diabetes Mellitus

Yeo JL, Gulsin GS, Dattani A, Marsh AM, Brady EM, Xue H, et al. 14 Sex-specific predictors of coronary microvascular function in a multiethnic cohort of 455 asymptomatic people with type 2 diabetes. *Heart. 2023;109:A10-A11.*

Abstract

Introduction: Type 2 diabetes mellitus (T2DM) confers 10% higher relative risk of heart failure in women than men,[14] which may be linked to higher prevalence of coronary microvascular dysfunction. We aimed to determine the prevalence and sex-specific determinants of coronary microvascular dysfunction in asymptomatic people with diabetes mellitus.

Materials and methods: A multiethnic cohort of people with diabetes mellitus and no evidence of cardiovascular disease and sex- and ethnicity-matched nondiabetic controls underwent echocardiography and stress perfusion cardiac magnetic resonance imaging. Quantitative myocardial blood flow analysis was performed for measurement of myocardial perfusion reserve (MPR), an index of microvascular function. Multivariable linear regression was undertaken to identify the independent clinical and imaging predictors of MPR in people with diabetes mellitus.

Results: Excluding silent myocardial infarction ($n = 7$), 455 participants with diabetes mellitus [42% women, age 57 ± 11 years, body mass index (BMI) 32 ± 6 kg/m^2] and 88 nondiabetic controls (43% women, age: 52 ± 12 years, BMI: 25 ± 4 kg/m^2) were included in study. Women and men with diabetes mellitus had increased left ventricular (LV) concentricity, systolic, and diastolic dysfunction. MPR was significantly lower in diabetes mellitus than controls (2.9 ± 0.9 vs. 3.5 ± 1.1, $p < 0.001$) and lower in diabetic women than men (2.7 ± 0.9 vs. 3.0 ± 0.9, $p < 0.001$). A greater proportion of women with diabetes mellitus had MPR of <2.5 (45% vs. 28%, $p < 0.001$). In a regression model adjusting for clinical risk factors, only age ($\beta = -0.184$, $p = 0.004$), female sex ($\beta = -0.210$, $p < 0.001$) and systolic blood pressure (SBP) ($\beta = -0.119$, $p = 0.021$) were independently associated with MPR in diabetes mellitus. Sex-stratified analysis showed independent associations with MPR: age ($\beta = -0.221$, $p = 0.022$), SBP ($\beta = -0.122$, $p = 0.131$), and BMI ($\beta = -0.188$, $p = 0.026$) in women, and age ($\beta = -0.150$, $p = 0.085$) and SBP ($\beta = -0.155$, $p = 0.027$) in men. Diffuse fibrosis did not independently predict MPR in T2DM.

> **Conclusion:** Age and SBP are independent predictors of MPR in people with diffuse fibrosis did not independently predict MPR in diabetes mellitus. BMI is an additional independent risk factor for MPR in women but not men.

COMMENT

How does study contribute? In adults without cardiovascular disease, women who developed diabetes mellitus had a greater reduction in MPR compared to men without subclinical cardiac remodeling. Early interventions focused on blood pressure reduction and weight loss may prevent coronary microvascular dysfunction. Chest pain in the absence of obstructive coronary artery disease (CAD) (≥50% stenosis in ≥1 major coronary artery) is common in women,[14] and associated with debilitating symptoms. It leads to repeated evaluations and at times false reassurance. Diagnosis of normal coronary arteries is five times more common in women as compared to men during evaluation of CAD. Coronary microvascular dysfunction is a problem of the small arteries of the heart with reduced blood flow without any accompanying large vessel obstructive disease. Endothelial function is an independent predictor of cardiovascular events.

Cardiovascular medicine is less evidence based in women than in men due in part to underrepresentation in clinical trials and the misperception that women are "protected" against cardiovascular disease. In the entity of microvascular angina, syndrome X, or microvascular coronary dysfunction studies like this have been invaluable.

Changes in heart failure: Microvascular dysfunction is an important mechanism in the development of heart failure with preserved ejection fraction (HFpEF). HFpEF is characterized by severe exercise intolerance and is associated with adverse clinical outcomes. Myocardial perfusion reserve is reduced compared with that of age- and sex-matched controls in many cross-sectional studies. Reduced myocardial perfusion reserve (analogous to microvascular dysfunction) is present in the absence of CAD and it corresponds with impaired exercise tolerance test. Early impairment in peak oxygen consumption is one of the first signs of heart failure. Microvascular dysfunction may be present in asymptomatic individuals who are at risk of HFpEF in the future. Abnormalities of resting and stress blood flow suggestive of microvascular dysfunction have been reported in individuals with metabolic syndrome and obesity. Microvascular dysfunction is an independent predictor of HFpEF development and associated with worse LV diastolic function (E/e′).[15]

In diabetic women: Coronary endothelial function is impaired in hypertensive, hyperlipidemic, smoking, and diabetic women.[16] Coronary endothelial dysfunction (CED) in the coronary microcirculation is said to be the trigger for pathogenesis of ischemic heart disease (IHD). CED leads to unfavorable functional consequences such as inadequate tissue perfusion during stress, contributing to myocardial ischemia. CED could trigger an imprecise augmentation of the response to all vasoconstrictor stimuli. Inability to release endothelium-dependent NO changes a net dilator response to a net constrictor response with sympathetic stimulation. Myocardial ischemia may occur with impaired endothelium-dependent coronary flow reserve.

Coronary microvascular tone due to cardiac autonomic nervous system imbalance has been implicated in microvascular dysfunction. Gulli and colleagues[17] found that among almost two-thirds of syndrome X patients, symptoms could be related to the attenuated parasympathetic tone, rather than to an enhanced sympathetic activity.

Angina in microvascular dysfunction may be either typical or atypical and may occur with exertion or at rest. It is sometimes difficult to differentiate microvascular dysfunction from obstructive CAD. Some clinical features provide clues such as episodes of chest pain lasting longer and poor response to sublingual nitrates.

Box 1 summarizes different invasive and noninvasive techniques used to assess functional abnormalities in coronary microvasculature **(Box 1)**.

Treatment of Microvascular Coronary Dysfunction

Treatment of microvascular dysfunction is often unsuccessful. The goals of treatment are to control debilitating symptoms and improve quality of life, to reduce incidence of hospitalization/repeated invasive testing, and to improve event-free survival. Antiatherosclerotic and anti-ischemic treatment strategies include nitrates, β-blockers/α-β blockers, ranolazine, calcium channel blockers, angiotensin-converting enzyme inhibitors (ACE-Is), hydroxymethylglutaryl coenzyme A (HMG-CoA) reductase inhibitors (statins), L-arginine supplementation, aerobic exercise, and cognitive behavioral therapy.

BOX 1 Investigations.

Assessment of myocardial ischemia:
- Stress ECG test
- Positron emission tomography (metabolic tracers)
- Magnetic resonance spectroscopy
- Transmyocardial metabolic studies

Myocardial perfusion techniques:
- Myocardial scintigraphy
- Positron emission tomography (blood flow tracers)
- Magnetic resonance imaging
- Contrast echocardiography
- Angiographic myocardial blush

Coronary blood flow techniques:
- Coronary sinus thermodilution
- Intracoronary Doppler FloWire
- Angiographic frame count
- Doppler echocardiography

ARTICLE 6

Pregestational Diabetes Mellitus and Congenital Heart Defects

Maduro C, Castro LF, Moleiro ML, Guedes-Martins L. Pregestational diabetes and congenital heart defects. *Rev Bras Ginecol Obstet.* 2022;44(10):953-61.

Abstract

The adverse effects of maternal diabetes on the fetus during the gestational period have been well documented. Pregestational diabetes is a risk factor for offspring born with congenital heart disease. Retrospective cohort studies have indicated a four-fold increase in cardiovascular malformation, in particular congenital heart defects, in offspring born to mothers with preexisting diabetes compared with nondiabetic mothers. The effect of pregestational diabetes on congenital heart anomalies is profound.

COMMENT

Introduction

Diabetes is a chronic metabolic disorder caused due to insulin resistance and/or insufficient insulin production. Pregestational diabetes mellitus, higher maternal glycated hemoglobin (HbA1c) levels, and poor maternal glycemic control in the first trimester are associated with increased risk of the fetus developing congenital heart disease. The adverse effects of maternal diabetes on the fetus during the gestational period have been well documented. Pregestational diabetes is a risk factor for offspring born with congenital heart disease. Retrospective cohort studies have indicated a four-fold increase in cardiovascular malformation, in particular congenital heart defects, in offspring born to mothers with preexisting diabetes compared with nondiabetic mothers. The effect of pregestational diabetes on congenital heart anomalies is profound.

Maternal Hyperglycemia and Fetal Cardiac Development

The teratogenic effect of pregestational hyperglycemia on the development, structure, and function of fetal heart is profound. Research has proven that prenatal diabetes mellitus affects the structure and function of fetal heart and fetal-placental circulation.[18] The extent of fetal heart damage is determined by the duration and degree of hyperglycemia, hyperketonemia, and HbA1c levels during the first 6 weeks, the period of organogenesis. Hyperglycemia during early gestation, particularly the first and second trimesters in mothers, with pregestational diabetes is found to induce diabetic embryopathy, pathological heart rates, fetal cardiomyopathy, congenital cardiac malformations, alterations in the left-right patterning. Hypertrophy of insulin-sensitive tissues including the heart is induced by chronic fetal hyperinsulinemia which in turn is induced by chronic intrauterine (environmental) hyperglycemia. Diabetic fetopathy is observed during the second and third trimesters leading to fetal hyperglycemia, insulinemia, and macrosomia.[19]

The phenotypes of cardiovascular malformations observed in the fetus of prediabetic mothers include heterotaxia, conotruncal defects, atrioventricular septal defect, anomalous pulmonary venous return, left ventricular outflow tract obstruction, right ventricular outflow tract obstruction, atrial septal defect, ventricular septal defect, complex defect, and valve defect.[20] **Table 1** includes the subtypes of the fetal cardiac abnormalities and their subtypes.

Heart conditions, such as persistent foramen ovale, ventricular hypertrophy, and pulmonary valve stenosis were observed in neonatal infants. Congenital malformations are associated with 50% perinatal mortality rate in infants of mothers with diabetes.[21]

TABLE 1: Subtypes of the fetal cardiac abnormalities and their subtypes.	
Fetal heart malformation	**Subtypes**
Conotruncal defect	• Truncus arteriosus • Transposition of the great arteries • Tetralogy of Fallot • Double-outlet right ventricle
Ventricular outflow tract obstruction	• Coarctation of the aorta • Valvular aortic stenosis
Right ventricular outflow tract obstruction	Valvular pulmonary stenosis

Around two-thirds of congenital anomalies found in infants with diabetic mothers are associated with either the cardiovascular or the nervous system.

Risk of Congenital Heart Defects in Offspring of Pregestational Diabetic Mothers

Clinical trials have revealed a four-fold increase in the development of congenital heart defects in the fetus of mothers with pregestational diabetes when compared with mothers without diabetes.[22] The risk is more pronounced in mothers with pregestational diabetes than mothers with gestational diabetes. This clearly proves that pregestational diabetes is a risk factor which can be modified to mitigate the congenital heart defects in fetus and neonates. Maternal hyperglycemia may have a detrimental effect on the fetal cardiogenesis which occurs between the third and seventh weeks of gestation. It has also been found that maternal hyperglycemia is associated with fetal myocardial hyperplasia and hypertrophy.

Tests for the Evaluation of Mothers and Fetus

Testing of A1c before conception is advised in mothers who are at high risk of developing diabetes.

Ultrasound and Growth Monitoring

Ultrasound is the gold standard for monitoring the fetus and the state of pregnancy. Fetal viability is monitored during the first trimester and structural integrity is observed in the second trimester. Fetal health and growth are observed during the third trimester. Fetal abnormality is diagnosed at around or before 20 weeks of gestation.[23]

Other Tests

Fetal echocardiogram can detect fetal heart sounds and cardiac abnormalities. Fetal magnetic resonance imaging (MRI) is recommended only under certain conditions such as suspicion of congenital abnormalities. Fetal α-protein is measured between 16 and 18 weeks for detecting neural tube defects.[24] Fetal lung assessment is performed at 32 weeks of gestation. Nonstress tests are performed twice a week after the completion of 32 weeks of gestation and contraction stress test is warranted in case of a failed nonstress test.

Treatment/Management

Women belonging to high-risk group should be screened for diabetes mellitus and counseled prior to conception as organogenesis occurs during the first few weeks of conception.[25] Tight glycemic control and supplementary diets play a key role in the prevention and management of diabetes. Maintaining the HbA1c level below 6.1% and body mass index (BMI) below 25 is imperative during the preconception period. Nutritional/dietary interventional, lifestyle modification with light exercise, and maintaining normal blood sugar levels should be the main goal. It has been proven that exercise can reduce postprandial hyperglycemia and decrease insulin resistance.[25] A diet with low carbohydrates and increased fiber and less calories is recommended for maintaining optimal blood sugar levels and preventing maternal hyperglycemia. Vitamin D plays a key role in increasing the insulin sensitivity and insulin secretion.[26] Supplements such as inositol and fish oil are found to be beneficial for gestational diabetes. Drug therapy using insulin and metformin should be recommended only when the dietary interventions fail to bring about the optimal control of hyperglycemia. Diabetic mothers should be managed by a team of healthcare professionals which include gynecologists, obstetricians, maternal-fetal specialists, pediatricians, geneticists, pharmacists, and radiologists.[27] Neonatologists help manage child with complicated medical problems, such as congenital heart defects, neural defects, and other structural and functional abnormalities.

Conclusion

The negative outcome of pregestational diabetes on fetal heart development is undisputed. This clearly necessitates the importance of continued research on the association between pregestational diabetes and fetal cardiac defects which would result in early intervention and prenatal detection for preventing adverse cardiac outcomes. Studies have proved that adequate glycemic control in mothers with pregestational diabetes does not mitigate the risk of congenital heart defects in offspring. Research must be carried out to find additional safe and accessible interventions which support current treatment regimen.

ARTICLE 7

Rising Prediabetes, Undiagnosed Diabetes, and Risk Factors in Young Women

Yoshida Y, Wang J, Zu Y, Fonseca VA, Mauvais-Jarvis F. Rising prediabetes, undiagnosed diabetes, and risk factors in young women.
Am J Prev Med. 2023;64(3):423-7.

Abstract

Introduction: Women of reproductive age tend to be at a lower risk of developing cardiovascular disease compared to men. However, this benefit is outweighed by the risk associated with diabetes mellitus. The prevalence of preexisting cardiovascular risk factors and their associated changes in prevalence in women prior to menopause have not been clearly elucidated.

Methods: This study looked at the age-related prevalence of obesity, dyslipidemia, prediabetes, and diabetes in women before and after menopause. It used logistic regression to look at cardiovascular risk factors related to young diabetes, such as obesity (central obesity), hypercholesterolemia, hypertension, associated with young, diagnosed, or undetected diabetes mellitus. The size of the association was compared with age-matched men.

Results: Young women were more likely to have preexisting diabetes mellitus and diabetes mellitus that had not been diagnosed. Obesity risk among young women is comparable to that of age-matched men, and is higher than that of postmenopausal women with diabetes mellitus. Hypercholesterolemia and hypertension associated with undetected diabetes mellitus were more pronounced in men and women of the same age.

Conclusion: Over the past two decades, young women have been associated with an elevated level of prediabetes mellitus and undiagnosed diabetes mellitus. As a result, they are exposed to a significant cardiovascular risk associated with prediabetes and diabetes mellitus. Therefore, it is essential to improve cardiometabolic risk screening and patient education in the younger and early middle age groups.

COMMENT

Women of childbearing age are less likely to develop cardiovascular disease (CVD) than men, partly due to the cardiac protection of estrogen. Diabetes mellitus (DM), however, negates this female advantage. Women may develop CVD with lower glucose levels than men, and may have a higher risk of prediabetes-related CVD.[28] Undiagnosed diabetes (UDD) mellitus is more common in women than in men, due to inequitable access to healthcare and screening, as well as a lack of awareness of disease risk. Untreated DM is associated with higher mortality risk and CVD-related hospitalization compared to diagnosed/controlled DM. Young women with DM or prediabetes may already have more publicly known cardiovascular risk factors than men at the same age, which has yet to be confirmed.[29] The relationship between diabetes and prediabetes mellitus in young women has not been fully elucidated.[30,31] This research examined the patterns of premenopausal, diagnosed, undetected DM, as well as the cardiovascular risk factors associated with premenopausal and postmenopausal women, compared to those observed in age-matched males and females.

This study enrolled 3,366 male and female participants aged <49 years, with data on diagnostic dimensions (DM), menopause status, and other relevant covariates. For the purpose of regression analysis, those with a prior history of CVD were excluded.

In this study, young women were defined as age group of <49 years, irrespective of their menopausal status, young women can be premenopausal or postmenopausal. Premenopausal women were defined as those who had not had menstrual cycles in the preceding 12 months, and postmenopausal women were those who had not experienced menstrual cycles in the past 12 months as a result of menopause (e.g., pregnancy, breastfeeding, medical conditions, or treatments such as contraceptive use). Diagnosis of diabetes (DM) was based on fasting glucose (FG) levels of 100–126 mg/dL, elevated blood glucose levels [heart failure (HF)], oral glucose tolerance test, outcome variables included obesity [body mass index (BMI)] < 30; waist circumference >102 cm in men and >88 cm in women; hypercholesterolemia (total cholesterol >240 mg/dL); and systolic (high) and diastolic (high) blood pressure.

This study quantified the prevalence of young women (premenopausal and postmenopausal), age-matched men, who had premenopausal disease (DM), diagnosed DM, or DM undiagnosed. Additionally, multivariable logistic regression was employed to evaluate the relationship between cardiometabolic risk factors, premenopausal and postmenopausal DM, diagnosed DM, or undiagnosed DM.

The prevalence of diagnosed DM also increased in young women. Compared to those with normoglycemia, those with premenopausal DM were associated with a nearly three-fold risk of obesity [odds ratio (OR) 2.8; 95% confidence interval (CI) 3.1] and a more than fourfold risk of central obesity (OR 4; 95% CI). The association was less pronounced in age-matched males or postmenopausal women.

Young women were the only group of individuals to experience an association between young disease (DM) and hypertension; however, the relationship between premenopausal disease (PMD) and hypertension was only statistically significant in male age-matched patients. Additionally, premenopausal women were associated with a risk of hypertension in all age-matched groups, with the risk being highest in premenopausal men (OR 3.1; 95% CI 1.4). Postmenopausal women, however, were not affected by the risk of hypertension.

The study revealed an increase in the prevalence of UDD mellitus and pre-diabetes mellitus (PDD) in young female adults. The decrease in the prevalence of UDD in all adults was associated with alterations in diabetes diagnosis and screening procedures. The increasing prevalence of UDD and PDD in young females suggests a deficiency in screening and a lack of awareness of the risk of UDD in this demographic compared to men of similar age and elderly women. Furthermore, the rise in PDD and PDD among young women coincided with the rise in the overall prevalence of UDD.

The study quantified the relationship between premenopausal and postmenopausal women with cardiovascular risk factors. The risk profiles of premenopausal women and those with premenopausal diabetes (DM) were comparable to, or worse than, those of men in their same age and postmenopausal age. This highlights the potential cardiovascular consequences of not adequately controlling for these risk factors, and suggests that the decline in cardiovascular health in women may begin in young adulthood. These findings may partially explain the women's disadvantage in diabetic CVD during middle and late adulthood.

This work adds to the literature in the domain of young diabetic CVD and emphasizes the importance of screening young women for diabetic CVD.

ARTICLE 8

Can Artificial Intelligence Predict Heart Disease in Diabetic and Prediabetic Women: Hype or Hope?

Wang M, Francis F, Kunz H, Zhang X, Wan C, Liu Y, et al. Artificial intelligence models for predicting cardiovascular diseases in people with type 2 diabetes: A systematic review.
Intell-Based Med. 2022;6:100072.

Abstract

Cardiovascular disease (CVD) is the leading cause of mortality in both men and women, particularly patients with diabetes. CVD usually presents later in life in women. However, this age-related difference is reduced in women with diabetes, who would have their first myocardial infarction (MI) at about the same age as men with diabetes. Diabetes mellitus could increase the risk of CVD by three to four times in women and two to three times in men, after adjusting for other risk factors. Artificial intelligence (AI) is a field in computer science that incorporates the use of computational algorithms which simulate and perform tasks that traditionally require human intelligence such as problem-solving and learning. Although medicine is plausibly the last to apply AI in its daily routine, cardiology is at the forefront of the AI revolution in the field of medicine. The evolution of AI methods for precise prediction of CVD outcomes, noninvasive diagnosis of CVD, detection of arrhythmia via wearables, diagnostics, management strategies, and prediction of outcomes for heart failure (HF) patients, reveals the potential of AI in future cardiology. With the recent advancements in AI, the Internet of Things (IoT), and the promotion of precision medicine, the cardiology future would be based on these innovative digital technologies. Furthermore, this article highlights the importance of sex-specific analyses in clinical research to improve our knowledge of CVD in women in general and in women with diabetes and prediabetes in particular.

COMMENT

Cardiovascular disease (CVD), despite a lot of significant advances in the diagnosis and treatments, still constitutes the leading cause of morbidity and mortality worldwide. Prediabetes is characterized by impaired fasting glucose or impaired glucose tolerance.[32] According to the American Diabetes Association (ADA) guideline, fasting plasma glucose concentration of 100–125 mg/dL or glycated hemoglobin (HbA1c) concentration of 5.7–6.4% indicates prediabetes. Recent studies have emphasized that people with prediabetes resulted in long-term complications of diabetes such as microvascular and macrovascular diseases. The macrovascular disorders associated with prediabetes include stroke, CVD, and peripheral vascular disease. Epidemiologic studies including DECODE and Funagata Diabetes Study[33] have reported that prediabetes is a strong predictor of CVD. The prediabetic prevalence is more than 400 million and expecting more than 470 million people with prediabetes by 2030 worldwide.

Diabetes is the most common and rapidly growing disease that affects more than 380 million people worldwide and is the well-established risk factor for CVD with distinctive effects on women compared to men. The International Diabetes Federation has forecasted that the number of people with diabetes in the world will increase from 387 million in 2014 to 592 million by 2035. The predominant cause of morbidity and mortality among people with diabetes is CVD. The incidence of CVD resulted in 17.6 million deaths in 2016, an increased prevalence of 14.5% from 2006 to 2016. In developing regions, the mortality and morbidity rates of CVD are increasing year by year, particularly in low- and middle-income countries.

Burden of Disease: Increasing Prediabetic and Diabetic Population in Women

Gender analysis from the INTERHEART study revealed that various risk factors such as hypertension, diabetes, high alcohol intake, and low physical activity were stronger among women than in men and were more strongly associated with MI in women below the age of 60 years compared with older women.

Artificial Intelligence

Artificial intelligence is a modern digital tool wherein machines are programmed to think like humans and mimic their actions. It performs tasks using algorithms, heuristics, pattern matching, rules, deep learning, and cognitive computing.

The objective of this article is to understand the recent advances in research modalities such as AI in CVDs in diabetes and especially prediabetes among women.

The Era of Artificial Intelligence, Machine Learning, Internet of Things

The recent advancement of AI has increasingly attracted clinicians in improving novel integrated, effective, and competitive strategies in delivering quality healthcare approaches.

The subdomains in AI (as given in **Fig. 1**) are:
- Machine learning (ML)
- Deep learning (DL)

Machine learning is a subset of AI that teaches computers with the help of complicated computation and statistical algorithms to analyze several datasets quickly, precisely, accurately, and effectively.[34] ML can be classified into three groups (as depicted in **Fig. 2**):
1. Supervised learning (e.g., logistic regression, support vector machine, and neural networks)
2. Unsupervised learning (e.g., cluster analysis)

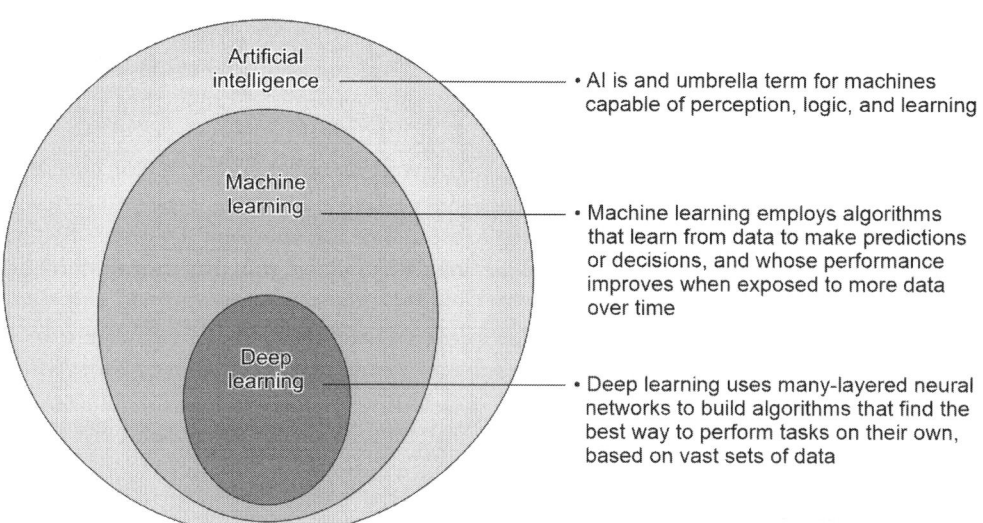

FIG. 1: Definitions of artificial intelligence (AI) terms.

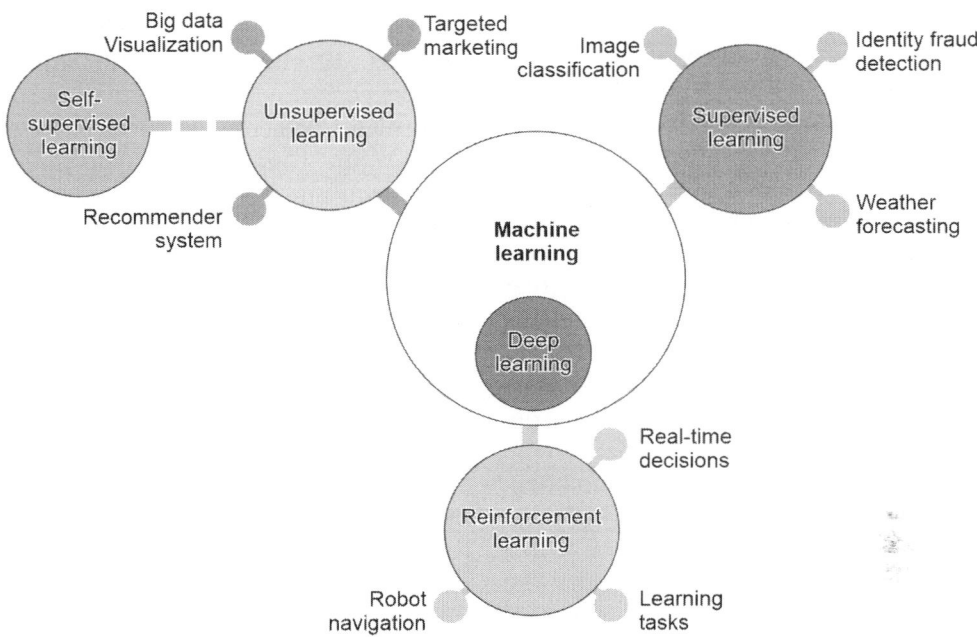

FIG. 2: Overview of various components of artificial intelligence.

3. *Reinforcement learning/semi-supervised learning*: Reward-driven learning (usually deployed in games and robotic apps)

Machine learning helps in promoting decision-making and forecasting the robust volume of knowledge provided by the healthcare industry.[35]

Deep learning is a supervised approach to ML that incorporates neural networks which can be explained by artificial algorithm processes in capturing meaningful patterns of data collection.[34] It emulates the complex human brain, being suitable for learning from information with complex hierarchical representations which have multiple abstraction layers. Based on their history, expertise, and training, doctors diagnose them. At this phase, DL may be very effective, which expands and improves medical knowledge, particularly for nonexpert doctors.

Importance and Advantage of using AI in the Evaluation of Prediabetes, Diabetes, and Cardiovascular Diseases

Blood Glucometers

Continuous glucose monitoring (CGM) sensors are compact medical equipment, which measure interstitial glucose concentrations in subcutaneous tissue almost continuously every 1–5 minutes for several consecutive days or weeks,[35] used in daily management of diabetes mellitus. In contrast to self-monitoring blood glucose (SMBG), CGM sensors allow tracking glucose dynamics and ensure prompt detection of even asymptomatic glycemic variability, difficult to capture using SMBG.

Continuous glucose monitoring sensors can be classified into two main types:
1. Professional CGM sensors
2. Real-time CGM sensors

Professional CGM sensors are unique in one way that the readings could be accessed by the healthcare professional only and patients are not aware of the readings. Based on the readings, drug modifications are done.

Real-time glycemic variability alerts have been recently introduced in flash glucose monitoring (FGM) systems. Real-time CGM (rt-CGM) sensors are different in the way that the readings could be accessed by the patients also and they could understand their food pattern and can even adjust medications as per doctor's advise. Real-time CGM sensors consist of an electrode which is placed in the subcutaneous tissue of the arm or abdomen. It reads the interstitial glucose and transmits the signal to a portable receiver from which the readings can be obtained in real time. The electrode needs to be replaced once in 7–14 days. Going one step further, in the western world, advanced implantable real-time CGM sensors have come where the electrode is placed by means of a minimal surgical intervention.

Yet another CGM called flash CGMs are available where the readings are made by just scanning the device.

The advantage of rt-CGM sensors is that these provide not only the glucose concentration in real time but also the details about the glucose trend, which can be used for making more efficient therapeutic decisions such as insulin dosing. Also, rt-CGM devices provide vibratory or auditory alerts when hypoglycemic or hyperglycemic events are detected. Nowadays, smartphone apps are available which have become easy to install and data can be retrieved anytime.

Artificial Intelligence in Cardiovascular Disease Intervention

Artificial intelligence techniques such as ML, DL, and cognitive computing, especially in cardiovascular imaging, will influence the practice of cardiology and cardiovascular medicine in a serene manner.

Artificial Intelligence Stethoscope

Artificial intelligence stethoscope is a mobile, economical device for early cardiac abnormality detection. It is a special wireless stethoscope that has been designed for monitoring the actual cardiac signals and transferring them to our smartphone app for simultaneous cloud assessment. Heart sounds are preprocessed to identify heart diseases by using algorithms such as audio slicing and segmentation, which can then be transformed into top-notch spectrograms, categorized by our pretrained cloud based on convolutional neural network (CNN).

Artificial Intelligence ECG

An electrocardiography (ECG) sensor system with an ECG-sensing-enabled front-end device is connected to the patient's chest portion involving low energy consumption analog front-end circuit, with an integrated commercial energy management (IC) circuit and a commercial Bluetooth module. The single-lead wearable ECG tracking device could use up to 24 hours of daily use.

Artificial Intelligence and Imaging Modalities

Cardiac imaging analysis has revealed tremendous growth opportunities in recent years, with the evolution of DL.[34] DL will discuss coronary angiography and ECG and echocardiography. The predominant interventions in CVD in developing countries in recent times are procedures such as coronary angiography and percutaneous coronary intervention (PCI), especially for coronary heart disease (CHD) and acute coronary syndrome (ACS). AI will be able to identify coronary atherosclerotic plaques more efficiently than physicians in the near future, using DL.[36]

Artificial Intelligence ECHO

With the help of AI, a large amount of preformed data are stored in large data bases.

By using advance echocardiography such as 3D and speckle tracking,[37] where echo images are obtained within a short period, analysis can be done and reproduced in the same pattern whenever needed. This is especially useful in complex congenital heart disease, valvular heart disease, and various cardiomyopathies. Software algorithms such as heart model have advanced software systems which enable to analyze faster and come to a conclusion faster than human minds. AI echo has the ability to estimate chamber volumes such as left atrium, left ventricle, right atrium, and right ventricle. Similarly, ejection fraction estimation and flow velocity calculations are made very easy.

Artificial Intelligence Computed Tomography Coronary Angiogram

In the risk assessment and treatment of coronary artery disease (CAD) and atherosclerosis, methodologies for ML image processing in cardiac CT are coronary artery calcium scoring and fractional flow estimation.[37] Coronary computed tomographic angiography (CCTA) is a noninvasive way of diagnosing CAD where the stenosis estimation is exaggerated when compared to invasive coronary angiogram. In order to overcome this difficulty, noninvasive fractional flow reserve (FFR) is incorporated. When FFR is incorporated, the stenosis calculations are better correlated with invasive coronary angiogram. With the advancement in software tools, it has become easy to make early analysis in a swift manner. SMARTTOOL techniques are new endeavors which work very smartly and are more reliable without human error.

Artificial Intelligence MRI

In cardiac MRI, ventricular segmentation has more potential for the implementation of ML models.[34] It enables volumetry to be quantified and diagnostic monitoring accuracy and increased reproducibility. DL algorithms (i.e., CNNs and stacked autoencoders) by cardiac MRI datasets are defined for the automated classification and extraction of the right ventricular (RV) chamber. In addition, multiple artificial neural networks were successfully introduced for left ventricular segmentation, especially in cardiac cine MRIs. Subacute or chronic myocardial scar recognition is another utilization of ML in cardiac MRI.

Remote Application

Device (hardware) – interface (software) – cloud storage – rapid analysis and feedback – early diagnosis – early treatment

Application of Artificial Intelligence in Cardiovascular Disease

Precision Medicine

Artificial intelligence would be implemented from the patient's point of view to capture voice information such as patient history, remote follow-ups, drug alerts, real-time therapy, and earlier indication warnings. Simultaneously, it would be helpful to link clinicians' electronic medical record systems and reduce clinicians' workload. Cognitive systems (ML devices or DL algorithms that can solve challenges without any human assistance) assist doctors to make accurate decisions and also predict health performance. People accept that doctors would not be replaced by AI. Physicians, on the other hand, must learn about using AI technologies and attain proficiency in the clinical practice in implementing AI in improving the evaluation and management of CVD by using data processing, thus assisting to evolve to the age of precision medicine.

Intelligent Robots

With the recent advances in surgical robotics, the amalgamation of AI and minimally invasive surgical systems, along with the da

Vinci surgical robot, would make robotic surgery more realistic, improve surgical protection, minimize patient trauma, and shorten hospital stays.[34] AI could perform cardiac interventional procedures on patients such as PCI procedures and atrial fibrillation catheter ablation, which can use automatic subtraction angiography to reduce the radiation exposure of clinicians. By using augmented learning, the incorporation of AI would be much superior to that of a human being. The AI could be able to practice more easily than human doctors in performing complicated procedures. In short, the simultaneous utilization of AI and surgical robotics would make the conventional medicine revolution simpler.

Conclusion

Diabetes is a strong risk factor for cardiovascular complications and in women, diabetes reduces the routine advantage in preventing atherosclerosis. Recent research in diabetes mellitus is implementing considerable effort in support systems for patient use, which automatically analyze the patient's data collected by CGM sensors and other portable devices, and also providing personalized guidelines about therapy adjustments to patients. Due to the large amount of data collected by patients with DM and their variety, AI techniques are increasingly being adopted in these decision support systems.

Artificial intelligence is the next advanced step in the practice of cardiovascular medicine. The integration of AI and cardiovascular medicine requires not only professional skills and advanced technologies but also a considerable investment.

In our fast-paced world, time is limited and precious. AI will be a part of every cardiologist's daily routine to provide the opportunity for an effective clinical history of patients and the design of predictive models for different diseases. AI will accelerate the use of noninvasive diagnostics and decrease the need for costly and complicated invasive tests to diagnose CAD. Future cardiologists will be able to give clues to an asymptomatic patient, whether they will develop an arrhythmia or an MI in the future, and preventive measures can be taken to avoid this. However, there is a need to take into consideration the ethical dilemmas generated in areas where AI is replacing human decisions and aim to integrate their knowledge and AI-derived suggestions, for mature and accurate decision-making in every step in the decision process. AI in the field of cardiology brings wide feasibility in providing personalized care.

REFERENCES

1. Saeedi P, Petersohn I, Salpea P, Malanda B, Karuranga S, Unwin N, et al. Global and regional diabetes prevalence estimates for 2019 and projections for 2030 and 2045: Results from the International Diabetes Federation Diabetes Atlas, 9th edition. Diabetes Res Clin Pract. 2019;157:107843.
2. Emerging Risk Factors Collaboration; Sarwar N, Gao P, Seshasai SR, Gobin R, Kaptoge S, et al. Diabetes mellitus, fasting blood glucose concentration, and risk of vascular disease: a collaborative meta-analysis of 102 prospective studies. Lancet. 2010;375(9733):2215-22.
3. Sattar N, McMurray JJ, Cheng AY. Cardiorenal risk reduction guidance in diabetes: can we reach consensus? Lancet Diabetes Endocrinol. 2020;8(5):357-60.
4. Østergaard HB, Hageman SHJ, Read SH, Taylor O, Pennells L, Kaptoge S, et al. Estimating individual lifetime risk of incident cardiovascular events in adults with Type 2 diabetes: an update and geographical calibration of the DIAbetes Lifetime

perspective model (DIAL2). Eur J Prev Cardiol. 2023;30(1):61-9.
5. Vounzoulaki E, Khunti K, Abner SC, Tan BK, Davies MJ, Gillies CL. Progression to type 2 diabetes in women with a known history of gestational diabetes: systematic review and meta-analysis. BMJ. 2020;369:m1361.
6. Page MJ, McKenzie JE, Bossuyt PM, Boutron I, Hoffmann TC, Mulrow CD, et al. The PRISMA 2020 statement: an updated guideline for reporting systematic reviews. BMJ. 2021;372:n71.
7. Mao Y, Hu W, Xia B, Liu L, Han X, Liu Q. Association Between Gestational Diabetes Mellitus and the Risks of Type-Specific Cardiovascular Diseases. Front Public Health. 2022;10:940335.
8. Colom C, Rull A, Sanchez-Quesada JL, Pérez A. Cardiovascular Disease in Type 1 Diabetes Mellitus: Epidemiology and Management of Cardiovascular Risk. J Clin Med. 2021;10(8):1798.
9. Patel N, Chen O, Donahue C, Wang B, Fang Y, Donnino R, et al. Impact of diabetes on heart failure incidence in adults with ischemic heart disease. J Diabetes Complications. 2017;31(11):1597-1601.
10. Amutha A, Anjana RM, Venkatesan U, Ranjani H, Unnikrishnan R, Narayan KMV, et al. Incidence of complications in young-onset diabetes: Comparing type 2 with type 1 (the young diab study). Diabetes Res Clin Pract. 2017;123:1-8.
11. Nanayakkara N, Curtis AJ, Heritier S, Gadowski AM, Pavkov ME, Kenealy T, et al. Impact of age at type 2 diabetes mellitus diagnosis on mortality and vascular complications: systematic review and meta-analyses. Diabetologia. 2021;64(2):275-87.
12. Bonora E. The metabolic syndrome and cardio-vascular disease. Ann Med. 2006;38(1):64-80.
13. Hajar R. Risk Factors for Coronary Artery Disease: Historical Perspectives. Heart Views. 2017;18(3):109-14.
14. Maruhashi T, Soga J, Fujimura N, Idei N, Mikami S, Iwamoto Y, et al. Relationship between flow-mediated vasodilation and cardiovascular risk factors in a large community-based study. Heart. 2013;99(24):1837-42.
15. Bottcher M, Botker HE, Sonne H, Nielsen TT, Czernin J. Endothelium-dependent and -independent perfusion reserve and the effect of L-arginine on myocardial perfusion in patients with syndrome X. Circulation. 1999;99(14):1795-1801
16. Roman MJ, Naqvi TZ, Gardin JM, Gerhard-Herman M, Jaff M, Mohler E, et al. Clinical application of noninvasive vascular ultrasound in cardiovascular risk stratification: a report from the American Society of Echocardiography and the Society of Vascular Medicine and Biology. J Am Soc Echocardiogr. 2006;19(8):943-54.
17. Gulli G, Cemin R, Pancera P, Menegatti G, Vassanelli C, Cevese A. Evidence of parasympathetic impairment in some patients with cardiac syndrome X. Cardiovasc Res. 2001;52(2):208-16.
18. Al-Biltagi M, El Razaky O, El Amrousy D. Cardiac changes in infants of diabetic mothers. World J Diabetes. 2021;12(8):1233-47.
19. Bhandari J, Thada PK, Khattar D. Diabetic Embryopathy. StatPearls [Internet]. Treasure Island (FL): StatPearls Publishing; 2023.
20. Chen ZY, Mao SF, Guo LH, Qin J, Yang LX, Liu Y. Effect of maternal pregestational diabetes mellitus on congenital heart diseases. World J Pediatr. 2023;19:303-14.
21. Correa A. Pregestational Diabetes Mellitus and Congenital Heart Defects. Circulation. 2016;133(23):2219-21.
22. Hunter LE, Sharland GK. Maternal Gestational Diabetes and Fetal Congenital Heart Disease: An Observational Study. J Preg Child Health. 2015;2:132.
23. Lemaitre M, Bourdon G, Bruandet A, Lenne X, Subtil D, Rakza T, et al. Pre-gestational diabetes and the risk of congenital heart defects in the offspring: A French nationwide study. Diabetes Metab. 2023;49(4):101446.
24. Øyen N, Diaz LJ, Leirgul E, Boyd HA, Priest J, Mathiesen ER, et al. Prepregnancy Diabetes and Offspring Risk of Congenital Heart Disease: A Nationwide Cohort Study. Circulation. 2016;133(23):2243-53.
25. Riskin A. (2023). Infants of mothers with diabetes (IMD). [online] Available from https://www.uptodate.com/contents/infants-of-mothers-with-diabetes-imd [Last accessed October 2023].
26. Tinker SC, Gilboa SM, Moore CA, Waller DK, Simeone RM, Kim SY, et al. Specific birth defects in pregnancies of women with diabetes: National Birth Defects Prevention Study, 1997-2011. Am J Obstet Gynecol. 2020;222(2):176.e1-11.
27. Wren C, Birrell G, Hawthorne G. Cardiovascular malformations in infants of diabetic mothers. Heart. 2003;89(10):1217-20.
28. Mauvais-Jarvis F. Gender differences in glucose homeostasis and diabetes. Physiol Behav. 2018;187:20-3.
29. Hubbard D, Colantonio LD, Tanner RM, Carson AP, Sakhuja S, Jaeger BC, et al. Prediabetes and risk for cardiovascular disease by hypertension status in black adults: the Jackson Heart study. Diabetes Care. 2019;42(12):2322-9.

30. Ballantyne CM, Hoogeveen RC, McNeill AM, Heiss G, Schmidt MI, Duncan BB, et al. Metabolic syndrome risk for cardiovascular disease and diabetes in the ARIC study. Int J Obes (Lond). 2008;32 Suppl 2(Suppl 2):S21-4.
31. Wong ND, Zhao Y, Patel R, Patao C, Malik S, Bertoni AG, et al. Cardiovascular risk factor targets and cardiovascular disease event risk in diabetes: a pooling project of the atherosclerosis risk in communities study, multi-ethnic study of atherosclerosis, and Jackson Heart study. Diabetes Care. 2016;39(5):668-76.
32. DeFronzo RA, Abdul-Ghani M. Assessment treatment of cardiovascular risk in prediabetes: impaired glucose tolerance impaired fasting glucose. Am J Cardiol. 2011;108:3B-24B.
33. The DECODE Study Group. Consequence of the new diagnostic criteria for diabetes in older men and women. Diabetes Care. 1999;22:1667-71.
34. Romiti S, Vinciguerra M, Saade W, AnsoCortajarena I, Greco E. Artificial intelligence (AI) and cardiovascular diseases: An unexpected Alliance. Cardiol Res Pract. 2020:2020:4972346.
35. Klonoff DC, Ahn D, Drincic A. Continuous glucose monitoring: A review of the technology and clinical use. Diabetes Res Clin Pract. 2017;133: 178-92.
36. Lin YJ, Chuang CW, Yen CY, Huang SH, Huang PW, Chen JY. Artificial Intelligence of things wearable system for cardiac disease detection. In: 2019 IEEE International Conference on Artificial Intelligence Circuits and Systems (AICAS); 2019. pp. 67-70.
37. Desai U, Martis RJ, Acharya UR, Nayak CG, Seshikala G, Ranjan SK. Diagnosis of multiclass tachycardia beats using recurrence quantification analysis and ensemble classifiers. J Mech Med Biol. 2016;16(01): 1640005.

SECTION 5

Metabolic Syndrome and CVD in Women

Section Editor: Hetan C Shah

Associate Editors: Tamagna Ghosh, Bhavik Shah, Chandrakant Chavan, Malav Jhala

ARTICLE 1

Assessment of Cardiovascular Risk in Women: Progress So Far and Progress to Come

Tschiderer L, Seekircher L, Willeit P, Peters SAE. Assessment of cardiovascular risk in women: Progress so far and progress to come.
Int J Womens Health. 2023;5:191-212.

Abstract

The leading cause of death in women worldwide is cardiovascular disease. The prediction, diagnosis, and treatment of cardiovascular disease in women are not without uncertainty, though. The use of risk scores is a pillar in the prediction of cardiovascular disease. Numerous reproductive and pregnancy-related factors have been linked to a lower or higher risk of cardiovascular disease. Therefore, the question of whether these female-specific factors also contribute to the prediction of cardiovascular risk has been raised. In this review, the article gives a general overview of the literature on the relationship between female-specific risk factors and cardiovascular risk and the sex differences in the association of known cardiovascular risk factors with cardiovascular disease. In addition, the author conducted a thorough literature search for studies that evaluated the added value of female-specific factors over and above already known cardiovascular risk factors. There has not been much, if any, improvement in the prediction of cardiovascular events as a result of including female-specific factors in models with established cardiovascular risk factors. However, analyses mainly used information from women who were below 40 years of age. In order to support effective risk factor treatment and improve cardiovascular disease prevention in women, future studies are required to quantify whether pregnancy-related factors improve cardiovascular risk prediction in young women.

COMMENT

Cardiovascular diseases remain the leading cause of death among women worldwide. Nonetheless, there exist several uncertainties pertaining to their risk stratification when it comes to women. A variety of gender-specific factors such as pregnancy and menopause have been associated with a higher risk of cardiovascular risk prediction. In this review, the authors provide an overview of the existing literature on sex differences in the association of established cardiovascular risk factors with cardiovascular diseases.[1]

The main modifiable risk factors related to the high risk of cardiovascular mortality remain obesity, high blood pressure, diabetes, smoking, and lipid abnormalities. To address them, cardiovascular risk scores have been developed. However, they have been criticized in the past, especially in cardiovascular risk prediction in women. For instance, it has been shown that the Framingham risk score underestimates cardiovascular risk factors and do not take into account female-specific risk factors.[2]

Sex differences in risk factors associated with cardiovascular events have been identified and included in risk prediction tools as they are usually developed separately for women and men. Adding female-specific factors to models containing established cardiovascular risk factors in younger women.[3,4]

Consequently, future investigations are needed to quantify whether pregnancy-related factors improve cardiovascular risk prediction in young women in order to support adequate treatment of risk factors and enhance prevention of cardiovascular diseases in women.

ARTICLE 2

Cardiometabolic Biomarkers in Women with Polycystic Ovary Syndrome

van der Ham K, Louwers YV, Laven JSE. Cardiometabolic biomarkers in women with polycystic ovary syndrome. *Fertil Steril. 2022;117(5):887-96.*

Abstract

The most prevalent endocrine condition affecting women of reproductive age is polycystic ovary syndrome (PCOS). PCOS affects adolescents, postmenopausal women, and their offspring as well as other first-degree relatives. In addition to reproductive issues, PCOS is also linked to metabolic disturbances. Teenagers with PCOS exhibit unfavorable cardiometabolic biomarkers, such as overweight/obesity and hyperandrogenism, more frequently than controls. Studies also point to an unfavorable lipid profile. Women with PCOS who are of reproductive age develop additional cardiometabolic biomarkers, such as metabolic syndrome, hypertension, and insulin resistance. Inflammatory cytokines play a significant role in these women's cardiovascular health, according to mounting evidence. Some PCOS traits improve as the menopausal transition occurs, while other biomarkers such as body mass index, insulin resistance, type 2 diabetes mellitus, and hypertension rise. Children of PCOS-afflicted mothers have lower birth weights and later in life have higher body mass indices than controls. In addition, unfavorable cardiometabolic biomarkers are present in the parents, mothers, and siblings of women with PCOS. Therefore, it is crucial to screen for cardiovascular disease and monitor PCOS-affected women, their children, and siblings.

COMMENT

This study, after examining all available evidence about cardiometabolic biomarkers in women with polycystic ovary syndrome (PCOS), found that these women exhibit unfavorable cardiometabolic biomarkers during their whole life span. Apart from the more established biomarkers such as body mass index (BMI), visceral fat, insulin resistance (IR), and dyslipidemia, which increase the prevalence of metabolic syndrome, the presence of raised inflammatory markers is high risk for future cardiovascular (CV) events. Characteristics such as hyperandrogenism decrease with age, but other cardiometabolic factors increase exponentially. In fact, all these biomarkers are related to each other in a complex network of interactions. Assessing some of these biomarkers is relevant as it will help in early intervention and preventing CV events. Tumor necrosis factor-alpha, interleukin-6 (IL-6), monocyte chemoattractant protein-1 (MCP-1), and advanced glycation end products (AGEs) could have the potential to be used in clinical care, but further research is needed to determine reference values. Follow-up studies on women with PCOS until very old age will eventually provide definitive answers on that risk and the involved mechanisms.

Sisters and female offspring of women with PCOS should be screened for PCOS and cardiometabolic disturbances, including measurements of BMI, blood pressure, lipid profile, and insulin and glucose levels, directly after diagnosis of their sister and if they are >3 years after menarche because reliable information about menstrual cycle can then be obtained.

Brothers and male offspring should be screened on cardiometabolic parameters, including measurements of blood pressure, lipid profile, and insulin and glucose levels, around the age of 20 years because differences in dyslipidemia and blood pressure were already observed during the age of 30 years and it is important to screen and create awareness for that time.

The study of cardiometabolic biomarkers in women with PCOS is important since it determines a huge burden of preventable CV events if screened early and intervened. Equally important is screening of first-degree relatives including both sexes as there are enough data to support affection on them. Inflammatory markers and their estimation are the future area of research into cardiometabolic biomarkers beyond the traditional markers of metabolic syndrome which may aid in detecting population at risk of imminent CV events.

ARTICLE 3

Cardiovascular Health in the Menopause Transition: A Longitudinal Study of up to 3,892 Women with up to Four Repeated Measures of Risk Factors

Clayton GL, Soares AG, Kilpi F, Fraser A, Welsh P, Sattar N, et al. Cardiovascular health in the menopause transition: A longitudinal study of up to 3892 women with up to four repeated measures of risk factors.
BMC Med. 2022;20(1):299.

Abstract

Background: Women's cardiovascular health deteriorates in middle age; whether the menopausal transition affects these changes is hotly contested. This study's objective was to examine relationships between chronological and reproductive ages [time since last menstrual period or final menstrual period (FMP)], changes in carotid intima media thickness (CIMT), and cardiovascular risk factors.

Methods: The article used information from 1,702 UK women who underwent a natural menopause and had up to four repeat cardiovascular health measurements between the ages of 51 [standard deviation (SD) = 4.0] and 56 (SD = 3.6) years. In order to account for the effects of confounding variables (socioeconomic factors, body mass index, smoking, alcohol, parity, and age at menarche) as well as the inherent effects of chronological age, multilevel models were used to analyze the relationship between cardiovascular measures and time since FMP (reproductive age). In addition, using data from women who had and had not gone through menopause (n = 3,892), we examined the relationship between cardiovascular measures by chronological age according to menopausal stages (premenopause, perimenopause, and postmenopause).

Results: Contrary to the strong positive association of chronological age [7.6 μm/year; 95% confidence interval (CI) 6.3, 8.9] with CIMT, there was no strong evidence that reproductive age was associated with CIMT [difference in mean 0.8 m/year, 95% CI −0.4, 2.1]. Consistent with this, we found weaker linear associations of reproductive compared with chronological age for atherosclerotic risk factors, such as with systolic blood pressure (SBP) (−0.1 mm Hg/year, 95% CI −0.3, 0.1 and 0.4 mm Hg/year, 95% CI 0.2, 0.5, respectively) and non-high-density-lipoprotein (HDL) cholesterol (0.02 mmol/L/year, 95% CI 0.005, 0.03, and 0.06, 95% CI 0.04, 0.07, respectively). Contrarily, associations with C-reactive protein and fat mass (0.01, 95% CI 0.001, 0.02, and 0.01, 95% CI −0.001, 0.02 natural logged mg/L/year, respectively) were stronger for reproductive age than for chronological age (0.06 kg/m^2/year, 95% CI 0.03, 0.10, and 0 kg/m^2/year, 95% CI 0.04, respectively). Glucose was (weakly) positively correlated with both chronological age and reproductive age (0.002, 95% CI 0.0001, 0.003, and 0.002, 95% CI 0.0001, 0.003, respectively).

Conclusion: Our findings imply that beyond the effects of aging, the menopausal transition does not further increase women's risk of atherosclerosis (measured by CIMT). Along with aging, menopausal transition may slightly raise blood sugar levels and adiposity, possibly increasing the risk of developing diabetes.

COMMENT

Cardiovascular disease (CVD) is the leading cause of death in women, who have a notable increase in the risk for this disease after menopause and typically develop coronary heart disease several years later than men. This observation led to the hypothesis that the menopause transition (MT) leads to increase CVD events in a female. Until now, longitudinal studies of women traversing menopause have shown a relationship between the MT and CVD risk. Following up women over this period, researchers have been able to disentangle chronological and ovarian aging with respect to CVD risk. Studies have documented distinct patterns of sex hormone changes, as well as adverse alterations in body composition, lipids and lipoproteins, and measures of vascular health over the MT, which can increase in developing CVD postmenopausally. The reported findings underline the significance of the MT as a time of accelerating CVD risk, thereby emphasizing the importance of monitoring women's health during midlife which enables early intervention strategies to reduce CVD risk. The 2011 American Heart Association guidelines for CVD prevention in women did not include information now available about the contribution of the MT to increased CVD in women. Therefore, there is an unmet need to discuss the contemporary literature on menopause and CVD risk in order to increase awareness of the significant adverse cardiometabolic health–related changes accompanying midlife and the MT. This scientific statement provides an up-to-date synthesis of the existing data on the MT and how it relates to CVD.

This study suggests that reproductive age (reflecting the menopausal transition) does not independently influence change in subclinical atherosclerosis (CIMT) or risk factors [e.g., systolic blood pressure (SBP), non-HDL-cholesterol, and triglycerides] strongly associated with atherosclerosis, as shown in randomized trials and/or Mendelian randomization studies to causally influence coronary heart disease.[5-7] Reproductive age group has shown to increase the risk of diabetes mellitus and adiposity modestly which is supported strongly by linear association with reproductive age than chronological age. Hormone replacement therapy (HRT) may not identically reflect endogenous hormonal and other changes associated with a natural menopause. However, this study has shown findings consistent with randomized controlled trials (RCTs) of HRT which have shown no protection or some increased risk of coronary artery disease (CAD) but decrease in the risk of developing diabetes mellitus.[8]

The strength of this study is that it is the largest prospective study to date with two repeat CIMT measures and up to four repeated cardiovascular risk factor measures that span the late reproductive period, from menopausal transition into postmenopause. The average 5-year follow-up period with up to four repeat measures in women of different baseline ages allowed the description of associations from 4 years before to 16 years after the menopause, a longer postmenopausal period than described in previous studies.

The limitations of this study are that reproductive age is a self-reported measure and measured with more error than chronological age. It may be that this causes some bias toward the null for reproductive age and correspondingly away from the null for chronological age. The outcomes and confounders were similar between women included and excluded from the main analysis. This study is also predominantly of white European origin women, and previous studies have shown ethnic differences in cardiovascular risk factors,[9] so our findings cannot be extrapolated to women of other race/ethnic groups. As our study recruited women during an index pregnancy and only followed those with a live birth from that pregnancy, all participants had at least one live birth and we cannot assume that our findings would generalize to women with no previous pregnancies or live births. As we know that the risk of cardiovascular disease increases with an increase in live births,[10] the association between reproductive age and cardiovascular health may differ in studies that also include nulliparous women.

This study adds importantly to the limited research in this area and, taken together with the small number of previous, generally smaller studies, suggests that reproductive age, defined as time since FMP (independent of chronological age), is unlikely to have a major impact on subclinical atherosclerosis but may increase adiposity and risk of type 2 diabetes mellitus modestly. Women can be reassured that transitioning through the menopause does not appear to increase atherosclerosis, contrary to the previous studies and belief. The increase in fat mass and fasting glucose with advancing reproductive and chronological age, as well as increase in CIMT and its risk factors with chronological age in midlife, highlights the importance of cardiovascular monitoring in women and support to maintain healthy behaviors and early intervention to decrease CVD events in an elderly female during menopausal transition.

ARTICLE 4

Cumulative Burden of Metabolic Syndrome and Its Components on the Risk of Atrial Fibrillation: A Nationwide Population-based Study

Ahn HJ, Han KD, Choi EK, Jung JH, Kwon S, Lee SR, et al. Cumulative burden of metabolic syndrome and its components on the risk of atrial fibrillation: A nationwide population-based study. *Cardiovasc Diabetol. 2021;20(1):20.*

Abstract

Background: Atrial fibrillation (AF) development is linked to the metabolic syndrome (MetS) and its elements. The effect of MetS's time burden on the risk of AF is unknown, though. We looked into how MetS's cumulative longitudinal burden affected the onset of AF.

Methods: From the database of the Korean National Health Insurance service, the study included 2,885,189 people without AF who underwent four annual health examinations between 2009 and 2013. The following three criteria were used to assess metabolic burdens: (1) cumulative MetS diagnoses at each health examination (0–4), (2) cumulative MetS diagnoses for each MetS component at each health examination (0–4), and (3) cumulative total MetS components at each health examination (0 to a maximum of 20). Using Cox proportional-hazards models, the risk of AF was estimated in relation to the metabolic burden.

Results: About 62.4%, 14.8%, 8.7%, 6.5%, and 7.6% of all people met the MetS diagnostic criteria zero, once, twice, three times, and four times, respectively. The cumulative number of MetS diagnosed over four health examinations was positively correlated with the risk of AF over a mean follow-up of 5.3 years: Adjusted hazard ratios (HRs) with 95% confidence intervals (CIs) were 1.18 (1.13–1.24), 1.31 (1.25–1.39), 1.46 (1.38–1.55), and 1.72 (1.63–1.82), respectively; p for trend 0.001. When MetS was repeatedly diagnosed, each of the five components was independently linked to a higher risk of AF, with an adjusted HR (95% CI) ranging from 1.22 (1.15–1.29) for impaired fasting glucose to 1.96 (1.87–2.07) for elevated blood pressure. The risk of AF gradually increased from 0 to 20 counts of metabolic components, reaching a maximum of 3.1-fold (adjusted HR 3.11, 95% CI 2.52–3.83 in those with 20 cumulative components of MetS). Recovery from MetS was associated with a lower risk of AF, though.

Conclusion: The greatest effort should be made to identify and correct metabolic derangements even before MetS development in order to prevent AF and related cardiovascular diseases, given the positive correlations between the cumulative metabolic burdens and the risk of incident AF.

COMMENT

It is a well-known fact that the metabolic syndrome and its components are associated with the development of atrial fibrillation. However, its impact on the population at large is rather unknown. Hence, the authors published this study to investigate the cumulative burden of metabolic syndrome and its many components on the risk of atrial fibrillation. They searched for the Korean National Health Insurance database looking for patients with metabolic syndrome.

The authors concluded that the participants who presented with the same cumulative numbers of metabolic syndrome components were having an increased risk of developing atrial fibrillation. Given that recovery from metabolic syndrome is known to be significantly decreased risk of major adverse cardiovascular events, the risk of developing atrial fibrillation was also decreasing.[11] However, the limitation of the study included the fact that the majority of population included in the study had diabetes and hypertension which are known risk factors for atrial fibrillation. Besides, the metabolic syndrome status may change from time to time on active follow-up. Plus, the causality and underlying mechanism between metabolic syndrome and atrial fibrillation are poorly defined.[12]

Despite these limitations, we cannot overlook the fact that this study underlined the cumulative burden of metabolic syndrome diagnostic criteria and its components over time which have a positive correlation with the risk of incident atrial fibrillation which has also been proven by other studies. Given the close association between the cumulative number of total metabolic syndrome components and the risk of atrial fibrillation, maximal effort to detect and correct metabolic derangements even before the development of metabolic syndrome may be important in order to prevent atrial fibrillation and related cardiovascular morbidities.[13]

Since the South Asian population is at a higher risk of developing metabolic syndrome, the issue of preventing it should be highlighted as an immediate task at hand. Atrial fibrillation, once developed, has many adverse outcomes including heart failure with preserved ejection fraction (HFpEF). The risk factors for atrial fibrillation in a young age with metabolic syndrome should be thoroughly investigated and addressed accordingly.

ARTICLE 5

Fitness Attenuates Long-term Cardiovascular Outcomes in Women with Ischemic Heart Disease and Metabolic Syndrome

Quesada O, Lauzon M, Buttle R, Wei J, Suppogu N, Cook-Wiens G, et al. Fitness attenuates long-term cardiovascular outcomes in women with ischemic heart disease and metabolic syndrome.
Am J Prevent Cardiol. 2023;14:100498.

Abstract

Background: While fitness levels remain comparatively low, the prevalence of metabolic syndrome is steadily rising. It is still unclear how fitness affects mortality and longer-term cardiovascular outcomes in people with cardiovascular disease and metabolic syndrome.

Design: Women's Ischemia Syndrome Evaluation (WISE), a prospective cohort of women undergoing invasive coronary angiography with ischemic heart disease symptoms (enrolled 1996–2001).

Methods: The article examined the relationships between metabolic syndrome (ATPIII criteria) and dysmetabolism (ATPIII criteria and/or treated diabetes), as well as fitness, defined as >7 metabolic equivalents (METs) measured by self-reported Duke Activity Status Index (DASI), with long-term cardiovascular outcomes and the risk of all-cause mortality.

Results: Of the 492 women who were monitored for a median of 8.6 years (ranging from 0 to 11 years), 19.5% had a fit, healthy metabolism (reference), 14.4% had metabolic syndrome, 29.9% had a healthy metabolism but was unfit, and 36.2% had metabolic syndrome. Major adverse cardiovascular event (MACE) risk was 1.52 times higher in women with a fit metabolic syndrome [hazard ratio (HR) 1.52, 95% confidence interval (CI) 1.03–2.26] and 2.42 times higher in women with an unfit metabolic syndrome (HR 2.42; 95% CI 1.30–4.48) compared to the reference group. Fit women with dysmetabolism had a mortality risk that was 1.96 times higher than that of unfit women with dysmetabolism (HR 3.0; 95% CI 1.66–5.43) compared to the reference group.

Conclusion: Compared to fit-metabolically healthy women, women who were unfit and metabolically unhealthy were at a higher risk of long-term MACE and mortality in a high-risk cohort of women with signs and symptoms of ischemic heart disease. Women who were unfit and metabolically unhealthy were also at the highest risk. Our study shows that metabolic health and fitness are crucial for long-term outcomes, which calls for more research.

COMMENT

The prevalence of metabolic syndrome among women is increasing day-in and day-out, more so in developing countries. However, the focus on maintaining fitness has remained low despite its contribution on long-term cardiovascular outcomes, and mortality is rather mysterious. The authors here described a study where they proved that fitness attenuated long-term cardiovascular outcomes among women diagnosed with ischemic heart disease and metabolic syndrome.

Apparently, every fourth woman has a higher risk of metabolic syndrome compared to man.[14] In this study, Women's Ischemia Syndrome Evaluation (WISE) prospective cohort was utilized where the data of women undergoing coronary angiography with signs and symptoms of ischemic heart disease were included. While investigating the association of fitness, it was defined as >7 metabolic equivalents (METs) measured by self-reported Duke Activity Status Index (DASI). Among 492 women followed up for a median of 8.6 years, 19.5% were fit-metabolic syndrome, 29.9% unfit-metabolically healthy, and 36.2% categorized as unfit-metabolic syndrome.

Apparently, mortality was three-fold higher in unfit-dysmetabolism women. In a high-risk cohort of women with signs and symptoms of ischemic heart disease, metabolically unhealthy women were at the highest risk. According to the authors, this was the first study to evaluate the association of fitness and metabolic syndrome without and with diabetes with long-term cardiovascular outcomes.

Subclinical systemic inflammation has been found to be associated with metabolic syndrome and its components, physical inactivity, and cardiovascular disease (CVD).[15,16] The public health burden associated with metabolic syndrome and diabetes is substantial, yet it remains a tip of the iceberg. The concern needs to be addressed more so in developing countries where majority of the concerned population is overlooked. The women's cardiovascular health remains a thoroughly underestimated topic and it is high time to address them.

ARTICLE 6

Gender Differences and Cardiometabolic Risk: The Importance of the Risk Factors

Meloni A, Cadeddu C, Cugusi L, Donataccio MP, Deidda M, Sciomer S, et al. Gender differences and cardiometabolic risk: The importance of the risk factors.
Int J Mol Sci. 2023;24(2):1588.

Abstract

Proatherogenic dyslipidemia, increased blood pressure, dysglycemia, and abdominal obesity are the main risk factors for type 2 diabetes mellitus and cardiovascular disease (CVD) that make up the clinical condition known as metabolic syndrome (MetS). Each risk factor acts independently, but when combined, they have a synergistic effect that increases mortality from all causes by 1.5 times and doubles the risk of CVD. In this article, we will focus on how the epidemiology, etiology, pathophysiology, and clinical manifestation of the aforementioned MetS components differ depending on gender. We will also talk about gender differences in the new biochemical indicators of cardiovascular risk and the metabolic syndrome.

COMMENT

Metabolic syndrome is a complex disorder which is more prevalent in urbanized living conditions associated with sedentary lifestyle and high caloric food intake. It is defined as a cluster of causally interconnected metabolic and cardiovascular risk factors such as atherogenic dyslipidemia, arterial hypertension, dysregulated glucose homeostasis, and abdominal obesity.[17] Recently, the abnormalities like chronic inflammatory markers such as C-reactive protein, sleep apnea, and nonalcoholic fatty liver disease (NAFLD).

The authors described the current evidence of the syndrome in women and gender differences associated with cardiometabolic risk factors. The differences are due to different etiopathogeneses, clinical expressions, and management of metabolic syndrome and its various components. Atherogenic dyslipidemia has a direct correlation with cardiovascular disease. Abdominal fat accumulation, particularly visceral fat mass, contributes to worsening dyslipidemia and hypertensive profile detected in women with impaired glucose tolerance.[18]

As regards for the therapeutic strategies, the benefits of statins, ezetimibe, and proprotein convertase subtilisin/kexin type 9 (PCSK9) inhibitor therapy have been demonstrated to be comparable between men and women at similar levels. Besides, biochemical markers like uric acid in obesity are more associated among females compared to males. Moreover, factors such as pregnancy, gestational diabetes mellitus, preeclampsia, polycystic ovary disease, and menopause are associated with adverse cardiovascular outcomes among females since they are gender-specific.[19,20]

To conclude, metabolic syndrome is a heterogeneous entity with variations in age and gender. Sex-specific hormones influence gender differences, and they have a large impact on the expression and outcomes of cardiovascular diseases. As cardiologists, we need to consider the importance of a multimodality approach while addressing gender-specific metabolic syndrome involving other specialties such as general physicians, gynecologists, and endocrinologists for better outcomes.

ARTICLE 7

Menstrual Cycle Regularity and Length Across the Reproductive Lifespan and Risk of Cardiovascular Disease

Wang YX, Arvizu M, Rich-Edwards JW, Stuart JJ, Manson JE, Missmer SA, et al. Menstrual Cycle Regularity and Length Across the Reproductive Lifespan and Risk of Cardiovascular Disease.
JAMA Netw Open. 2022;5(10):e2238513.

Abstract

Importance: The risk of cardiovascular disease (CVD) may be raised by menstrual cycle characteristics. The few studies that have examined the mediating role of known CVD risk factors are few in number and are currently available.

Objective: The goal of this study was to determine whether and to what extent hypercholesterolemia, chronic hypertension, and type 2 diabetes mellitus were responsible for the associations between menstrual cycle characteristics and the risk of CVD across the reproductive life span.

Design, setting, and participants: Those who reported menstrual cycle regularity and length for ages 14–17 and 18–22 years at enrolment in 1989 and updated current cycle characteristics in 1993 (at ages 29–46 years) were included in this cohort study, which prospectively followed them from 1993 to 2017. The data analysis started in October 1, 2019, to January 1, 2022.

Exposures: The frequency and duration of menstruation throughout the reproductive life cycle.

Main outcomes and measures: Interest-worthy incident CVD events include stroke and coronary heart disease (CHD); myocardial infarction (MI) or coronary revascularization, both of which can be fatal.

Results: 80,630 Nurses' Health Study II participants in total, with a baseline body mass index of 25.1 (5.6) kg/m^2 and a mean (SD) age of 37.7 (4.6) years, were included in the analysis. During the potential follow-up period of 24 years, 1,816 women experienced their first CVD event. Compared to women reporting very regular cycles at the same ages, multivariable Cox proportional hazards models revealed that women who had irregular cycles or no periods at ages 14–17, 18–22, or 29–46 years had hazard ratios for CVD of 1.15 [95% confidence interval (CI), 0.99–1.34), 1.36 (95% CI, 1.06–1.75), and 1.40 (95% CI, 1.14–1.71), respectively. Women reporting a cycle length of 40 days or more, or a cycle that is too irregular to estimate, had hazard ratios for CVD of 1.44 (95% CI, 1.13–1.84) and 1.30 (95% CI, 1.09–1.57), respectively, compared to women reporting a cycle length of 26–31 days. Only 5.4–13.5% of the observed associations could be explained by type 2 diabetes mellitus, chronic hypertension, or hypercholesterolemia, according to mediation analyses.

Conclusion and relevance: In this cohort study, irregular and prolonged menstrual cycles were both linked to higher rates of CVD, and this association persisted even after taking into account later-identified CVD risk factors.

COMMENT

The menstrual cycle characteristics across the reproductive life span associated with the risk of cardiovascular disease and to what extent are these associations mediated by hypercholesterolemia, chronic hypertension, and diabetes. To explore the association of menstrual cycle characteristics across the reproductive life span with the risk of cardiovascular disease and to what extent these associations were mediated by other risk factors.[21]

The authors assessed the effect of menstrual cycle regularity and length across the reproductive life span and their risk of cardiovascular diseases. Incident cardiovascular events of interest included fatal and nonfatal coronary heart disease and stroke, which were identified based on a questionnaire. Consistent with prior literature, the association between cycle regularity and cardiovascular disease appeared to be primarily driven by an increased rate of cardiovascular events rather than stroke.[22]

They observed an increased rate of cardiovascular disease among women reporting oral contraceptive use only at ages 14-17 years which might represent confounding by indications for oral contraceptive use. Cycle dysfunction can also be indicative of endometriosis, depleted ovarian reserve, or disrupted hormonal environment, which are also associated with adverse cardiometabolic health.[23,24]

In this prospective cohort study, to conclude, irregular and long menstrual cycle lengths across the reproductive life span were associated with an increased risk of cardiovascular disease later in life. Furthermore, only a small proportion of the relation between cycle characteristics and cardiovascular disease risk was driven by hypercholesterolemia, chronic hypertension, and type 2 diabetes mellitus. These results suggest that menstrual cycle dysfunction may be a useful marker for identifying women who are more likely to develop cardiovascular events later in life.

ARTICLE 8

Metabolic Disorders in Menopause

Jeong HG, Park H. Metabolic disorders in menopause. *Metabolites.* 2022;12(10):954.

Abstract

An important stage of aging that lasts for one-third of a woman's lifetime is called menopause. Cardiometabolic diseases such as obesity, type 2 diabetes mellitus, cardiovascular illnesses, non-alcoholic fatty liver disease (NAFLD)/metabolic associated fatty liver disease (MFFLD), and metabolic syndrome (MetS) are all significantly more common in women after menopause. Many symptoms that women experience during the perimenopausal stage are distressing for most women. Controlling these factors may be a tactic to enhance the health of postmenopausal women. Many factors make a woman's menopausal experience worse. This study examined the pathophysiology, definition, prevalence, diagnosis, treatment, and prevention of metabolic diseases (especially MetS) and menopause.

COMMENT

Life expectancy differs between the genders, as it has been shown that females live longer than the males. Differences in life expectancy between the sexes are a result of the high incidence of cardiovascular diseases in men due to differences in cholesterol–lipoprotein profiles and other cardiovascular factors caused by sex hormones.[25] Generally, menopause is clinically diagnosed when a woman has not menstruated for 12 months, which usually occurs around the age of 45–55 years. The authors investigated the metabolic disorders that could occur in menopausal women and confirmed their causes, diagnoses, and treatment.

It is well known that abrupt cessation of menstruation affects bones, heart, and blood vessels. Body weight, metabolic, and cardiovascular changes are progressive and chronic that take place beyond menopause. They are important precursors for developing metabolic syndrome as well as cardiovascular diseases.[26]

In menopausal women, higher visceral fat is accumulated due to changes in metabolism and body composition, and adipose tissue is more lipolytic after estrogen reduction. Excessive hepatic steatosis accelerates non-alcoholic fatty liver disease progression by causing hepatic insulin resistance, oxidative stress, and inflammation. Hormone-replacement therapy provided the selected progestin and it does not antagonize estrogen action and may improve fat mass and distribution.[27]

To conclude, the importance of metabolic syndrome and non-alcoholic fatty liver disease is further emphasized because they increase the overall risk associated with cardiovascular morbidity and mortality. Recently, new facts regarding the relationship between diseases of skeletal muscle metabolism, such as sarcopenia, and metabolic syndrome have been revealed. It is hoped that strategies will be established to detect and prevent metabolic syndrome early and accurately before and after menopause.

ARTICLE 9

Cardiovascular Disease in Women: Clinical Perspectives

Garcia M, Mulvagh SL, Merz CNB, Buring JE, Manson JE. Cardiovascular disease in women: Clinical perspectives. *Circ Res.* 2016;118(8):1273-93.

Abstract

Cardiovascular disease (CVD) continues to be the leading cause of death among women in the United States, accounting for ≈1 of every 3 female deaths. Sex-specific data focused on

CVD have been increasing steadily, yet are not routinely collected nor translated into practice. This comprehensive review focuses on novel and unique aspects of cardiovascular health in women and sex differences as they relate to clinical practice in the prevention, diagnosis, and treatment of CVD. This review also provides current approaches to the evaluation and treatment of acute coronary syndromes that are more prevalent in women, including myocardial infarction associated with nonobstructive coronary arteries, spontaneous coronary artery dissection, and stress-induced cardiomyopathy (Takotsubo syndrome). Other CVD entities with higher prevalence or unique considerations in women, such as heart failure with preserved ejection fraction, peripheral arterial disease, and abdominal aortic aneurysms, are also briefly reviewed. Finally, recommendations for cardiac rehabilitation are addressed.

COMMENT

As it has been documented in recent years, awareness of cardiovascular disease (CVD) as the primary cause of mortality in women has been slowly increasing. Women are less likely to receive preventive treatment or guidance, such as lipid-lowering therapy, aspirin, and lifestyle changes, than are men at a similar atherosclerotic cardiovascular disease (ASCVD) risk.[28-30] Traditional ASCVD risk factors, particularly for women, include diabetes, obesity and overweight, physical inactivity, hypertension, and dyslipidemia. On the other hand, the emerging, nontraditional ASCVD risk factors include preterm delivery, hypertensive disorders of pregnancy, gestational diabetes, autoimmune disease, breast cancer treatment, and depression. The average lifetime risk of developing CVD in women at 50 years of age is nearly 40%, and this percentage rises as the number of risk factors increases.

Premenopausal women are relatively protected against CVD, compared with age-matched men. This long-standing observation led to a hypothesis that ovarian steroid hormones were rather cardioprotective. KEEPS (Kronos Early Estrogen Prevention Study) and ELITE (Early versus Late Intervention Trial with Estradiol) trials concluded that at the lowest effective dose, menopausal hormone therapy (MHT) remains an appropriate treatment for menopausal symptoms in early menopause, in the absence of contraindications, but should never be prescribed for the express purpose of preventing CVD. Further research into the mechanisms responsible for the observed sex differences in traditional risk factor effects would not only improve our understanding of the pathogenesis, but could also inform health policy makers and clinical guideline committees in tailoring gender-specific interventions for the treatment management of these risk factors.

For many decades, CVD research has focused primarily on men, thus leading to an underappreciation of sex differences from an etiologic, diagnostic, and therapeutic perspective. We encourage a new era in research where cardiovascular studies are designed with adequate power for sex-specific analysis to understand the underlying mechanisms and develop optimal treatment for CVDs in both genders.

ARTICLE 10

Metabolic, Behavioral, and Psychosocial Risk Factors and Cardiovascular Disease in Women Compared with Men in 21 High-income, Middle-income, and Low-income Countries: An Analysis of the PURE Study

Walli-Attaei M, Rosengren A, Rangarajan S, Breet Y, Abdul-Razak S, Al Sharief W, et al., on behalf of the PURE investigators. Metabolic, behavioural, and psychosocial risk factors and cardiovascular disease in women compared with men in 21 high-income, middle-income, and low-income countries: An analysis of the PURE study.
The Lancet. 2022;400(10355):P811-21.

Abstract

Background: Particularly from low- and middle-income countries, there is a dearth of information on the prevalence of risk factors and their associations with incident cardiovascular disease in women compared to men.

Methods: The study recruited participants from the general population in 21 high-, middle-, and low-income countries for the Prospective Urban Rural Epidemiological (PURE) study and followed them for roughly 10 years. The metabolic, behavioral, and psychosocial risk factors of the participants were noted. Participants with at least one follow-up visit and a baseline age between 35 and 70 years old were included in this analysis. The main result was a composite of major cardiovascular events, including heart failure, myocardial infarction, stroke, and deaths from cardiovascular disease. Each risk factor's prevalence in both men and women, along with its hazard ratio (HR) and population-attributable fraction (PAF), for a major cardiovascular disease was listed. ClinicalTrials.gov has the PURE study listed under NCT03225586.

Findings: In this analysis, we included 155,724 participants with a median follow-up of 10.1 years [interquartile range (IQR) 8.5–12.0], including 64,790 men and 90,934 women, who were enrolled and followed up between January 5, 2005, and September 13, 2021. Women were 49.8 years old on average at the start of the study, while men were 50.8 years old on average [standard deviation (SD) 9.8]. At the data cutoff date of September 13, 2021, there had been 4,911 major cardiovascular disease events in men and 4,280 major cardiovascular disease events in women [age-standardized incidence rate: 5.0 events (95% CI 4.9–5.2) per 1,000 person-years]. Women showed a better cardiovascular risk profile than men, especially when they were younger. Except for non-high-density-lipoprotein (non-HDL) cholesterol, which was associated with a hazard ratio (HR) for major cardiovascular disease of 111 (95% CI 101–121) in women and 128 (119–139) in men, the HRs for metabolic risk factors were similar in men and women. There was a consistent pattern of higher risk in men than in women for other lipid markers. Depression symptoms had an HR of 109 (098–211) for women and 142 (125–160) for men. Contrarily, women [117 (108–126)] than men [1.07 (0.99–1.15)] were more strongly linked to major cardiovascular disease by eating a diet with a PURE score of 4 or lower (score ranges from 0 to 8). Men (15.7%) had more PAFs overall associated with behavioral and psychosocial risk factors than women (8.4%), primarily because smoking contributed more to PAFs in men [i.e., 13% (95% CI 05–21) in women vs. 107% (88–126) in men].

Interpretation: While diet is more strongly associated with the risk of cardiovascular disease in women than in men, lipid markers and depression are more strongly associated with the risk in men. The similarities in other risk factor associations with cardiovascular disease in men and women highlight the significance of a similar strategy for cardiovascular disease prevention in both sexes.

COMMENT

Previous work has reported that diabetes, smoking, and hypertension are more strongly associated with cardiovascular disease in women than in men. *The Lancet*, Marjan Walli-Attaei and colleagues argue that studies on sex differences in cardiovascular risk factors are mainly from high-income countries and add to the literature by reporting their community-based study conducted in 21 high-income, middle-income, and low-income countries. In their analysis, Walli-Attaei and colleagues included 155,724 adults [90,934 (58.4%) women and 64,790 (41.5%) men] aged 35-70 years without a history of cardiovascular disease from the Prospective Urban Rural Epidemiological (PURE) study, who had a median follow-up of 10.1 years [interquartile range (IQR) 8.5–12.0], and assessed the primary composite outcome of major cardiovascular events (cardiovascular disease deaths, myocardial infarction, stroke, and heart failure).

The hazard ratios (HRs) for the composite outcome of major cardiovascular disease associated with metabolic risk factors were *similar in women and in men, except for high non-high-density-lipoprotein (non-HDL) cholesterol, for which larger HRs were found in men [1.11 (95% CI 1.01–1.21) in women vs. 1.28 (1.19–1.39) in men].* Larger HRs were observed in men compared to women with respect to depression.

Lipid markers and depression are more strongly associated with the risk of cardiovascular disease in men than in women, whereas diet is more strongly associated with the risk of cardiovascular disease in women than in men. The similar associations of other risk factors with cardiovascular disease in women and men emphasize the importance of a similar strategy for the prevention of cardiovascular disease in men and women.

High carbohydrate diet is associated with a higher risk of mortality, whereas total fat and individual type of fat were related to lower mortality. Saturated fat had an inverse relationship with stroke, and global dietary guidelines need to be rethought in light of the above findings.

This study stresses the sex difference in major adverse cardiovascular events (MACE) looking into various risk factors. There are no specific atherosclerotic cardiovascular disease (ASCVD) risk-prevention guidelines for female and we need to study the role of various risk factors which have shown higher HR in female like diet and household air pollution. We need to rule out the confounding effect of other risk factors when we attribute higher HRs to a certain risk factor. Moreover, it is the interaction between various risk factors which leads to a MACE; hence, tackling risk factors as a comprehensive screening and intervention effort is required to decrease future events.

ARTICLE 11

Modifiable Cardiovascular Risk Factors in Adults Less than 40 Years of Age

Laghari ZA, Attar N, Sadiq N, Baloch FG. Modifiable cardiovascular risk factors in adults less than 40 years of age. J Bahria Univ Med Dent Coll. 2022;13(01):24-8.

Abstract

Objectives: The main goal is to find out how common modifiable cardiovascular risk factors are in adults under the age of 40 years.

Study design and setting: At University of Sindh, Jamshoro, a cross-sectional study was conducted between 2018 and 2019.

Methodology: Using a convenient sampling technique, 263 participants were added to the study after receiving ethical review board approval. Subjects over the age of 40 years, those with a history of CVD, those taking medications, expectant mothers, smokers, and drug addicts were disqualified from the study. Data was gathered in conjunction with the administration of a structured questionnaire. Blood pressure and anthropometric measurements were taken. Blood was drawn, and total cholesterol, low-density lipoprotein (LDL), triglycerides (TG), high-density lipoprotein (HDL), and blood sugar levels were all measured. The percentages indicating the presence of modifiable risk factors and the gender difference were evaluated using the chi-square test.

Results: About 76% of the subjects as a whole had at least one risk factor. For both men and women, the risk of obesity was 29% and 30%, respectively. Compared to men (35%), females (61%) had a higher rate of central obesity. Males were more likely than females to have risk factors such as hypertension, high total triglycerides, and unfavorable HDL (p-value 0.0001). When compared to men, women had higher levels of risk factors such as total cholesterol and an inactive lifestyle (p-values of 0.012 and 0.0007, respectively).

Conclusion: Females were found to have higher rates of three risk factors (obesity, central obesity, and total cholesterol), whereas males had higher rates of four risk factors (hypertension, increased TG, raised LDL, and hyperglycemia).

COMMENT

Nearly 20 million people worldwide die of cardiovascular diseases every year, which remains the leading cause of noncommunicable mortality even in the 21st century. The South Asian population is rather at a higher risk which is a hugely unaddressed issue. Recently, in the post-COVID era, a large number of young people are being diagnosed with occult cardiovascular morbidity and mortality which is becoming rather not so uncommon. The premature coronary artery disease is one of the major concerns among Indian population with more incidence of young sudden cardiac deaths. Hence, it requires important health concerns to prevent such a malignant event.

From an early age, preventive measures should be taken to reduce the risk of cardiovascular diseases. As it has been rightly said, prevention is better than cure. Adults under the age of 60 years account for nearly a third of cardiovascular cases. Preventing future cardiovascular disease by gaining better knowledge of cardiovascular risk factors and their causes in young adults is only one benefit of a rather more comprehensive understanding of these variable parameters.[31]

In this study, the authors included 263 participants who were under 40 years of age. Variables pertaining to cardiovascular risk factors were recorded and analyzed. The authors concluded that the risk of obesity was 30% for women. Central obesity was higher in women. Risk factors such as total cholesterol and inactive lifestyle were more common in females compared to males.

The authors concluded that mainly three risk factors, namely obesity, central obesity, and total cholesterol, were found to be higher in females, while the rest of the conventional risk factors were found to be predominant in male population. Hayes et al. compared the activity levels of South Asians to those of Europeans and found that South Asians were not able to get enough time for exercise.[32] Less active than men, women may consider to increase their daily physical activity to at least two- to three-fold with a view to decreasing the conventional cardiovascular risk factors.[33]

Since there is an ongoing trend of increasing cardiovascular mortality among young South Asians, it is a need of the hour that these modifiable risk factors be controlled sooner rather than later as preventive strategy decreases the burden not only at a personal level but at a population level as well.

ARTICLE 12

Scoring Systems of Metabolic Syndrome and Prediction of Cardiovascular Events: A Population-based Cohort Study

Motamed N, Ajdarkosh H, Niya MHK, Panahi M, Farahani B, Rezaie N, et al. Scoring systems of metabolic syndrome and prediction of cardiovascular events: A population based cohort study.
Clin Cardiol. 2022;45(6):641-9.

Abstract

History and objectives: In contrast to conventional dichotomous approaches, continuous scoring systems were developed to define metabolic syndrome (MetS). The goal of the current study was to assess scoring systems' capacity to forecast both fatal and nonfatal cardiovascular events.

Resources and procedures: A population-based cohort study yielded data on 5,147 people who were at least 18 years old, and those data were examined. The associated outcome was defined as the development of atherosclerotic cardiovascular disease (ASCVD) over the course of a 7-year follow-up. As traditional definitions of the metabolic syndrome (MetS), the Joint Interim

Statement (JIS) definition and two MetS scoring systems based on standard regression weights from structural equation modeling (SEM) and the simple method for quantifying the metabolic syndrome (siMS) were taken into consideration as potential predictors.

Results: In multiple Cox proportional hazard regression analyses, it was found that the scoring systems, specifically those based on structural equation modeling (SEM), had a significant association with composite cardiovascular events [hazard ratio (HR) 1.388 (95% CI 1.153–1.670), p 0.001 in men and HR 1.307 (0.95% CI 1.120–1.526) in women], whereas the traditional definition of MetS did not. While both scoring systems [MetS score based on SEM: area of under curve (AUC) = 0.7438 (95% CI = 0.6195–0.7903) and simple method for quantifying the metabolic syndrome (siMS) AUC = 0.7207 (95% CI 0.6676–0.7738)] demonstrated acceptable predictive abilities for cardiovascular events in women, the two systems were not acceptable for identifying risk in men.

Conclusion: The scoring systems revealed an independent association with cardiovascular events, in contrast to the dichotomous definition of MetS. In particular, SEM-based scoring systems may be useful for the prediction of cardiovascular events in women.

COMMENT

Despite a large decrease in the burden of cardiovascular diseases worldwide compared to three decades back, the huge disparities in the total burden of cardiovascular diseases in different regions of the world can be attributed to the differences in exposure to some or the other modifiable risk factors. As the prevalence of chronic diseases rise globally, it is important to identify individuals at greater risks of disease progression by evaluating their metabolic syndrome status.[34] Scoring systems in metabolic syndrome can be considered as a "red flag" sign in early diagnosis of the same. They can be used for precise planning and should be user-friendly for early identification.

The authors evaluated different scoring systems of metabolic syndrome and their prediction of cardiovascular outcomes. The occurrence of atherosclerotic cardiovascular disease (ASCVD) in the period of 7 years follow-up was considered as the associated outcome. The scoring systems were observed to have a significant association with composite cardiovascular events. When the authors incorporated age into the model, an acceptable ability for the prediction of cardiovascular events was obtained. Hence, age may play a role in predicting the development of cardiovascular events using these scores.[35]

The limitations of this study include lack of ECG data in the initial phase of cohort. The authors detected 21 cases of ECG changes that were not included as outcomes in the present study. Besides, a scenario analysis including the outcomes of these participants did not show any significant and reportable changes.

Despite these limitations of this study, we can conclude that the early prediction of cardiovascular disease plays an important role in decreasing its incidence and developing effective target population-based strategies; the scoring system of metabolic syndrome can prove to be valuable in this instance.[36,37]

ARTICLE 13

Sex Differences in Adiposity and Cardiovascular Diseases

Li H, Konja D, Wang L, Wang Y. Sex differences in adiposity and cardiovascular diseases.
Int J Mol Sci. 2022;23(16):9338.

Abstract

Independent of total adiposity, the distribution of body fat is a well-established predictor of unfavorable medical outcomes. The analysis of body fat distribution sheds light on the origins of obesity and offers important knowledge regarding the emergence of various comorbidities. Body fat distribution is more closely linked to the risk of cardiovascular diseases than total adiposity. The current review focuses specifically on the genetic characteristics that are distinct from general obesity, the biological hints, and the sexual dimorphism in body fat distribution. The prevention and treatment of cardiovascular diseases (CVD) will be improved with a better understanding of the effects of gender on body fat distribution and adiposity.

COMMENT

Morbidity can be predicted by body fat distribution and is associated with adverse medical outcomes, independent of overall adiposity. Various causes of obesity can be diagnosed and predicted by studying body fat distribution and provides valuable information about the development of various comorbidities. Body fat distribution is more closely associated with the risks of cardiovascular diseases. Sex dimorphism refers to the characteristic differences between males and females. Dimorphism, which refers to the characteristic differences between males and females in a species, helps clinicians and researchers classify, treat, and offer the prognosis of a species differently. Men and women are both susceptible to obesity but differ in the health consequences, due largely to the different body fat distribution. Obesity is an important risk factor for cardiovascular diseases. Heterogeneity in the regional deposition of fat is more deleterious than total body adiposity. Many studies show associations between cardiovascular risk factors and directly measured visceral adipose tissue which are stronger than those observed with typical anthropometric measures. Men and women have different patterns of body fat distribution. While the former is associated with increased cardiovascular risk, the latter, on the other hand, has more subcutaneous adipose tissue and brown adipose tissue. The female pattern of fat distribution is associated with improved cardiovascular risk at a similar body mass index (BMI). However, ectopic fat deposition within the abdomen, pericardium, and neck is more strongly associated with women's adverse cardiovascular risk than men. Female fat distribution and expression regulation may be more genetically affected than males by environmental factors. The molecular mechanism of this sex dimorphism may be beyond the modulation of sex hormones. Understanding the sex determinations on body fat distribution and adiposity will aid in the improvement of the prevention and treatment of cardiovascular diseases (CVD).

ARTICLE 14

Subclinical Cardiovascular Disease and Polycystic Ovary Syndrome

Gomez JMD, VanHise K, Stachenfeld N, Chan JL, Merz NB, Shufelt C. Subclinical cardiovascular disease and polycystic ovary syndrome.
Fertil Steril. 2022;117(5):912-23.

Abstract

Around 6–10% of women worldwide are affected by polycystic ovary syndrome (PCOS), which is characterized by hyperandrogenism, irregular menstruation, infertility, and ovaries that appear polycystic on ultrasound. The risk for subclinical cardiovascular disease (CVD), which is the presence of altered vascular endothelium without overt CVD, is also increased by the association of PCOS with a number of endocrine and metabolic disorders, such as obesity, insulin resistance, diabetes mellitus, hypertension, dyslipidemia, and metabolic syndrome. Using markers such as flow-mediated dilation, arterial stiffness, coronary artery calcium scores, carotid intima-media thickness, and visceral and epicardial fat, the study reviewed the most recent research on subclinical CVD in women with PCOS.

COMMENT

Polycystic ovary syndrome (PCOS) is one of the most common endocrine disorders affecting women; its etiology is not entirely understood. Clinical symptoms of PCOS include acne, amenorrhea or oligomenorrhea, hirsutism, infertility, and mood disorders, which tend to be the primary focus of clinical management. However, the impact of PCOS on future cardiovascular disease (CVD) risk is unknown, and opportunities to implement CVD-prevention strategies in these women should be given high priority. The pathogenesis of PCOS commonly involves insulin resistance which leads to several cardiometabolic abnormalities (e.g., dyslipidemia, hypertension, glucose intolerance, diabetes, and metabolic syndrome), thereby putting women at an increased risk for CVD. Prior studies have found that subclinical CVD markers such as coronary artery calcium scores, C-reactive protein, carotid intima-media thickness (CIMT), and endothelial dysfunction are more likely to be increased in women with PCOS.

This review of the data indicates that women with PCOS have subclinical CVD, as measured by alterations in flow-mediated dilation (FMD), arterial stiffness, coronary artery calcium (CAC) scores, CIMT, and novel markers such as visceral fat thickness (VFT) and epicardial fat thickness (EFT). The contribution of these factors to the increased risk of future overt cardiovascular events and mortality is largely unknown. Confounding factors, such as age and metabolic syndrome components, such as obesity, dyslipidemia, and glucose intolerance, can make the data more difficult to interpret, as they are not consistently controlled for in current cross-sectional studies. Larger population studies have demonstrated lower cardiovascular event-free survival and increased risks of incident myocardial infarction, angina, and stroke in women with PCOS. Future longitudinal studies with extended follow-up periods are needed to better understand the role of subclinical CVD markers in the future risk of major cardiovascular events in women with PCOS. These studies support current guideline recommendations for early screening in this patient population, with early glucose and lipid screening, consideration of measurement of markers for subclinical CVD, and initiation of targeted interventions such as weight and blood pressure management and smoking cessation. An aging longitudinal PCOS cohort would afford the opportunity to observe fluctuations of androgens and potential metabolic disturbances in the menopausal transition. A well-characterized, phenotyped PCOS cohort with detailed data on race and ethnicity will be necessary to determine how these variables impact subclinical CVD and future cardiometabolic risk.

This study includes literature from January 2017 to December 2021 with all peer-reviewed articles in English being included irrespective of study design. There is evidence that women of reproductive age have elevated subclinical CVD, but whether this translates to CV risk after menopause is unknown. The article has investigated various parameters of CVD risk including FMD, arterial stiffness, carotid intimal thickness, and CAC which are directly related to increased CV risk.

The study is limited by the fact that it has included studies irrespective of study design and varied study population; hence, it is difficult to extrapolate the findings to other study population.

The study has large implications, and all high-risk elderly females with PCOS need to undergo early screening and management of specific risk factors to decrease CV events in future and in turn decrease morbidity and mortality and dependency.

An important area of research is the impact of subclinical CVD on children of women with PCOS. There is a need for head-to-head study of CV risk in different age groups and negate confounding factors such as age in PCOS-affected females. Also, these studies should be backed up with physiological studies with an eye on the mechanism of CVD.

ARTICLE 15

Women's Reproductive Milestones and Cardiovascular Disease Risk: A Review of Reports and Opportunities from the CARDIA Study

Kim C, Catov J, Schreiner PJ, Appiah D, Wellons MF, Siscovick D, et al. Women's reproductive milestones and cardiovascular disease risk: A review of reports and opportunities from the CARDIA study.
J Am Heart Assoc. 2023;12(5):e028132.

Abstract

The Coronary Artery Risk Development in Young Adults (CARDIA) study recruited 5,115 Black or White participants between the ages of 18 and 30 years, including 2,788 women, between the years of 1985 and 1986. The CARDIA study gathered extensive longitudinal data on women's reproductive milestones, spanning menarche to menopause, over the ensuing 35 years. More than 75 CARDIA study publications address relationships between reproductive factors and events with cardiovascular and metabolic risk factors, subclinical and clinical cardiovascular disease, and social determinants of health, even though the study was not initially intended to focus on the health of women. One of the earliest population-based studies to note Black–White differences in menarche age and associations with cardiovascular risk factors was the CARDIA study. Negative pregnancy outcomes, in particular gestational diabetes and preterm birth, as well as postpartum behaviors, such as lactation, have been assessed. Studies that have already been conducted have looked at the risk factors for unfavorable pregnancy and lactation outcomes as well as how these factors relate to future cardiovascular and metabolic risk factors, diagnoses, and subclinical atherosclerosis. Examining the reproductive health of a population-based cohort of young adult women has been made easier by ancillary studies looking at polycystic ovary syndrome components and ovarian biomarkers such as anti-Müllerian hormone. Examining the significance of premenopausal cardiovascular risk factors along with menopause has improved our understanding of shared mechanisms as the cohort underwent menopause. Women will start to experience a higher number of cardiovascular events as well as other conditions, such as cognitive impairment, as the cohort ages from the mid-50s to the mid-60s. Consequently, over the following 10 years, the CARDIA study will offer a distinctive resource for understanding how the women's reproductive life course epidemiology informs cardiovascular risk as well as reproductive and chronological aging.

COMMENT

"The impact of womens' reproductive milestones on cardiovascular disease risk: Crystal ball gazing into the CARDIA study!!!"

The physiological effects of the female reproductive system on the cardiovascular system have been a topic generating great discussion amongst the cardiologists and physicians alike for the last four decades. These benefits of the female reproductive health as well as the perils due to her ill health have been studied extensively in the past.[38] However, there are very few studies that have studied these changes prospectively over decades. The major difficulty in prospective studies is the significant amount of attrition in the follow-up of study subjects. However, the data generated from these studies is pristine and plays a vital component in understanding the disease as well as developing management strategies. The historical Framingham Heart Study is the shining example of such a study.

However, when it comes to studying a woman's reproductive milestones in a similar fashion, the Coronary Artery Risk Development in Young Adults (CARDIA) study is beyond any comparison. The CARDIA study was carried out as a multicenter prospective study over four sites in the United States of America in 1985–1986.[39] It enrolled about 2,788 lady participants of Black as well as White race aged 18–30 years and were followed up for more than three decades. Most participants were assessed longitudinally with medical and reproductive history records, nutritional information, body composition, ectopic fat imaging, medication, imaging, and cardiovascular disease (CVD) event recording. It was one of the first studies to show a significant difference between the incidence of cardiovascular disorders between the races and age of presentation. The findings of the study led to nearly 77 publications assessing the impact of various reproductive parameters on a woman's cardiovascular health.

The authors of this review have very elegantly discussed the various key points of the CARDIA study as well as the group of studies which came out of it. They have extensively reviewed the literature and have tried to ascertain the basic pathophysiological mechanism responsible for the deterioration of cardiovascular health among women with reproductive disorders. Each attribute has been discussed in detail by the authors with the available data being discussed at the start and the authors' own opinion being conveyed at the last of each attribute. This provides a holistic approach to the entire review and imparts knowledge in an easily palatable form to the readers.

The attributes that were discussed were menarche, contraception, polycystic ovarian disease, lactation, and reproductive aging with menopause. Several important key points were brought out by the authors in the discussion. The fact that early menarche was associated with poorer cardiovascular risk profiles has been a common observation with a very elusive pathophysiology.[40] The authors have discussed two possible hypotheses for this phenomenon, namely the Barker Thrifty Phenotype and the Pederson Hypothesis, which discuss the effect of fetal and late childhood nutrition impact on menarche and future cardiovascular disease. The authors also concluded that the initial observation of oral contraception having a higher incidence of cardiovascular events was possibly due to higher dosage of estrogens and an earlier generation of progestins.[41] The current dose of oral contraceptives has not been associated with a higher CVD risk. The beneficial effects of lactation on cardiovascular health have been highlighted in this article and are a very important take-home message for the physicians and patients alike.[42] The practice of lactation has to be reinforced in the present times.

To conclude, this review article is a comprehensive review of all the available literature on the CARDIA study, which has been prospectively studying women from menarche to menopause and has been effective in filling the knowledge gaps and lacunae in the assessment of cardiovascular disease risk in women in the reproductive age group.

REFERENCES

1. Eaker ED, Chesebro JH, Sacks FM, Wenger NK, Whisnant JP, Winston M. Cardiovascular disease in women. Circulation. 1993;88(4 Pt 1):1999-2009.
2. Canoy D, Beral V, Balkwill A, Lucy Wright F, Kroll ME, Reeves GK, et al. Age at menarche and risks of coronary heart and other vascular diseases in a large UK cohort. Circulation. 2015;131(3):237-44.
3. Grandi SM, Smith GN, Platt RW. The relative contribution of pregnancy complications to cardiovascular risk prediction: are we getting it wrong? Circulation. 2019;140(24):1965-7.
4. Arnott C, Patel S, Hyett J, Jennings G, Woodward M, Celermajer DS. Women and cardiovascular disease: pregnancy, the forgotten risk factor. Heart Lung Circ. 2020;29(5):662-7.
5. O'Leary DH, Bots ML. Imaging of atherosclerosis: carotid intima–media thickness. Eur Heart J. 2010;31(14):1682-9.
6. Gill D, Georgakis MK, Zuber V, Karhunen V, Burgess S, Malik R, et al. Genetically predicted midlife blood pressure and coronary artery disease risk: Mendelian randomization analysis. J Am Heart Assoc. 2020;9(14):e016773.
7. Xu L, Borges MC, Hemani G, Lawlor DA. The role of glycaemic and lipid risk factors in mediating the effect of BMI on coronary heart disease: a two-step, two-sample Mendelian randomisation study. Diabetologia. 2017;60(11):2210-20.
8. Gartlehner G, Patel SV, Viswanathan M, Feltner C, Weber RP, Lee R, et al. Hormone therapy for the primary prevention of chronic conditions in postmenopausal women: an evidence review for the U.S. Preventive Services Task Force. Rockville: Agency for Healthcare Research and Quality (US); 2017.
9. Gasevic D, Ross ES, Lear SA. Ethnic differences in cardiovascular disease risk factors: a systematic review of North American Evidence. Can J Cardiol. 2015;31(9):1169-79.
10. Magnus MC, Iliodromiti S, Lawlor DA, Catov JM, Nelson SM, Fraser A. Number of offspring and cardiovascular disease risk in men and women: the role of shared lifestyle characteristics. Epidemiology. 2017;28(6):880-8.
11. Chung MK, Eckhardt LL, Chen LY, Ahmed HM, Gopinathannair R, Joglar JA, et al. Lifestyle and risk factor modification for reduction of atrial fibrillation: a scientific statement from the American Heart Association. Circulation. 2020;141(16):e750-72.
12. Expert Panel on Detection, Evaluation, and Treatment of High Blood Cholesterol in Adults. Executive Summary of The Third Report of The National Cholesterol Education Program (NCEP) Expert Panel on Detection, Evaluation, And Treatment of High Blood Cholesterol In Adults (Adult Treatment Panel III). JAMA. 2001;285(19):2486-97.
13. O'Neill S, O'Driscoll L. Metabolic syndrome: a closer look at the growing epidemic and its associated pathologies. Obes Rev. 2015;16(1):1-12.
14. Mottillo S, Filion KB, Genest J, Joseph L, Pilote L, Poirier P, et al. The metabolic syndrome and cardiovascular risk a systematic review and meta-analysis. J Am Coll Cardiol. 2010;56(14):1113-2.
15. Festa A, D'Agostino Jr R, Howard G, Mykkanen L, Tracy RP, Haffner SM. Chronic subclinical inflammation as part of the insulin resistance syndrome: the Insulin Resistance Atherosclerosis Study (IRAS). Circulation. 2000;102(1):42-7.
16. Yudkin JS, Stehouwer CD, Emeis JJ, Coppack SW. C-reactive protein in healthy subjects: associations with obesity, insulin resistance, and endothelial dysfunction: a potential role for cytokines originating from adipose tissue? Arterioscler Thromb Vasc Biol 1999;19(4):972-8.
17. Miranda PJ, DeFronzo RA, Califf RM, Guyton JR. Metabolic syndrome: Definition, pathophysiology, and mechanisms. Am Heart J. 2005;149:33-45.
18. Levy D, Larson MG, Vasan RS, Kannel WB, Ho KK. The progression from hypertension to congestive heart failure. JAMA. 1996;275:1557-62.
19. Vounzoulaki E, Khunti K, Abner SC, Tan BK, Davies MJ, Gillies CL. Progression to type 2 diabetes in women with a known history of gestational diabetes: Systematic review and meta-analysis. BMJ. 2020;369:m1361.
20. Lauenborg J, Mathiesen E, Hansen T, Glumer C, Jorgensen T, Borch-Johnsen K, et al. The prevalence of the metabolic syndrome in a Danish population of women with previous gestational diabetes mellitus is three-fold higher than in the general population. J Clin Endocrinol Metab. 2005;90:4004-10.
21. Wekker V, van Dammen L, Koning A, Heida KY, Painter RC, Limpens J, et al. Long-term cardio-metabolic disease risk in women with PCOS: asystematic review and meta-analysis. Hum Reprod Update. 2020;26(6):942-60.

22. Mu F, Rich-Edwards J, Rimm EB, Spiegelman D, Missmer SA. Endometriosis and risk of coronary heart disease. Circ Cardiovasc Qual Outcomes. 2016;9(3):257-64.
23. Shufelt CL, Torbati T, Dutra E. Hypothalamic amenorrhea and the long-term health consequences. Semin Reprod Med. 2017;35(3):256-62.
24. Pinola P, Lashen H, Bloigu A, Puukka K, Ulmanen M, Ruokonen A, et al. Menstrual disorders in adolescence: a marker for hyperandrogenaemia and increased metabolic risks in later life? Finnish general population-based birth cohort study. Hum Reprod. 2012;27(11):3279-86.
25. Regitz-Zagrosek V, Lehmkuhl E, Weickert MO. Gender differences in the metabolic syndrome and their role for cardiovascular disease. Clin Res Cardiol. 2006;95:136-47.
26. Avis NE, McKinlay SM. A longitudinal analysis of women's attitudes toward the menopause: Results from the Massachusetts Women's Health Study. Maturitas. 1991;13:65-79.
27. Rodriguez-Cano A, Mier-Cabrera J, Balas-Nakash M, Muñoz-Manrique C, Legorreta-Legorreta J, Perichart-Perera O. Dietary changes associated with improvement of metabolic syndrome components in postmenopausal women receiving two different nutrition interventions. Menopause. 2015;22:758-64.
28. Abuful A, Gidron Y, Henkin Y. Physicians' attitudes toward preventive therapy for coronary artery disease: is there a gender bias? Clin Cardiol. 2005;28:389-93.
29. Mosca L, Linfante AH, Benjamin EJ, Berra K, Hayes SN, Walsh BW, et al. National study of physician awareness and adherence to cardiovascular disease prevention guidelines. Circulation. 2005;111:499-510.
30. Han E, Lee Y, Kim Y, Kim B, Park J, Kim D, et al. Nonalcoholic fatty liver disease and sarcopenia are independently associated with cardiovascular risk. Am J Gastroenterol. 2020;115(4):584-95.
31. Aminde LN, Dzudie A, Mapoure YN, Tantchou JC, Veerman JL. Estimation and determinants of direct medical costs of ischaemic heart disease, stroke and hypertensive heart disease: evidence from two major hospitals in Cameroon. BMC Health Serv Res. 2021; 21(1):1-3.
32. Hayes L, White M, Unwin N, Bhopal R, Fischbacher C, Harland J, et al. Patterns of physical activity and relationship with risk markers for cardiovascular disease and diabetes in Indian, Pakistani, Bangladeshi and European adults in a UK population. J Public Health. 2002;24(3):170-8.
33. Irfan M, Jabbar M, Hameed S. Dietary habits and prevalence of underweight/obesity in students of university of Gujrat, Pakistan. J Liaquat Uni Med Health Sci. 2019;18(02):175-80.
34. Hu LT, Bentler PM, Kano Y. Can test statistics in covariance structure analysis be trusted? Psychol Bull. 1992;112(2):351-62.
35. Mulaik SA. Linear Causal Modeling with Structural Equations. Boca Ratom FL: CRC Press; 2009.
36. Hu LT, Bentler PM. Cutoff criteria for fit indexes in covariance structure analysis: conventional criteria versus new alternatives. Struct Equ Modeling: A Multidisciplinary J. 1999;6(1):1-55.
37. Hosmer Jr DW, Lemeshow S, Sturdivant RX. Applied Logistic Regression. New York: Wiley; 2013.
38. Wuest J Jr, Dry T, Edwards J. The degree of coronary atherosclerosis in bilaterally oophorectomized women. Circulation. 1953;7:801-9.
39. Friedman G, Cutter G, Donahue R, Hughes G, Hulley S, Jacobs D Jr, et al. CARDIA: study design, recruitment, and some characteristics of the examined subjects. J Clin Epidemiol. 1988;41:1105-16.
40. Lakshman R, Forouhi N, Sharp S, Luben R, Bingham S, Khaw K, et al. Early age at menarche associated with cardiovascular disease and mortality. J Clin Endocrinol Metab. 2009;94:4953-60.
41. Brabaharan S, Veettil S, Kaiser J, Rao V, Wattanayingcharoenchai R, Maharajan M, et al. Association of hormonal contraceptive use with adverse health outcomes: an umbrella review of meta-analyses of randomized clinical trials and cohort studies. JAMA Netw Open. 2022;5:e2143730.
42. Stuebe A, Rich-Edwards J, Willett W, Manson J, Michels K. Duration of lactation and incidence of type 2 diabetes. JAMA. 2005;294:2601-10.

SECTION 6

CVD in Women: Acute Coronary Syndrome

Section Editor: **Sarita Rao**

Associate Editors: Roshan Rao, Roopali Khanna, Hema S, Pankaj Manoria, Prerna Goyal, Priya Palimkar, Amjad Ali, Abha Pandit, Mahpaekar Mashhadi, Harsh A Chaudhary, Achukatla Kumar

ARTICLE 1

Gender Disparities in Prevalence by Diagnostic Criteria, Treatment and Mortality of Newly Diagnosed Acute Myocardial Infarction in Korean Adults

Kim SR, Bae S, Lee JY, Kim MS, Kim MN, Chung WJ, et al. Gender disparities in prevalence by diagnostic criteria, treatment and mortality of newly diagnosed acute myocardial infarction in Korean adults. *Sci Rep.* 2023;13(1):4120.

Abstract

Objective: Acute myocardial infarction (AMI) is the leading cause of morbidity and mortality. AMI in women is under-recognized and undermanaged. This study was aimed to evaluate long-term data with respect to prevalence, management, and mortality in AMI by gender.

Material and methods: The study included 633,097 patients hospitalized for AMI [Code "121" of International Classification of Diseases, 10th revision (ICD-10)] according to Korean National Health Insurance Service (KNHIS) Claims Database from 2002 to 2018, out of which 40% were women. The KNHIS database includes almost all medical procedures done in Korea since 2002. Those who received only outpatient treatment were excluded. Also, patients who did not underwent cardiac enzymes testing were excluded. Those requiring readmission due to relapse or complications were not included subsequently, if their initial episode of first hospitalization was included.

Demographic data and performance rates of coronary angiography (CAG) and percutaneous transluminal coronary angioplasty (PTCA) were assessed. Medications prescribed during discharge were also assessed. In-hospital 3-day, 7-day, 30-day, and 1-year mortality rates were assessed.

Results: The occurrence rates of AMI have risen between 2011 and 2018, with an increase from 71 cases per 100,000 individuals to 110 cases per 100,000 individuals. Nonetheless, women exhibited lower hospitalization rates for AMI compared to men (53 vs. 88 per 100,000 individuals in 2011 and 82 vs. 139 per 100,000 individuals in 2018) ($p \leq 0.0001$). There was a consistent increase in the rates of CAG in male patients (44.6% in 2003, 68.4% in 2010, 73.6% in 2018), but the same was not seen in women (30.7% in 2003, 46.0% in 2010, 45.7% in 2018). More than 85% of patients who were advised to undergo CAG opted for percutaneous coronary intervention (PCI). However, women exhibited a lower propensity for undergoing PCI compared to men. Since 2011, there has been a lower rate of PCI in women compared to men (81.1% vs. 88.3% in 2011 and 77.5% vs. 85.8% in 2018, $p < 0.0001$). Additionally, there has been an increase in-hospital mortality from 2.2 to 5.3% since 2003 along with increased 30-day mortality (6.9% in 2018). Age-adjusted short-term mortality (at 3 and 7 days) was higher in women, but there was no significant difference in 30-day mortality. Further, age-adjusted 1-year mortality was lower in women than men.

Conclusion: This long-term study from the KNHIS database shows that for years, women have been under-recognized, underdiagnosed, and undertreated, be it revascularization or medical therapy, and necessary action needs to be taken to close the gender gap.

COMMENT

What was Known Prior to this Study?

Coronary artery disease (CAD) is regarded as a disease mainly affecting male population. Woman are underdiagnosed and undertreated.[1] Underdiagnosis can be due to relatively less prevalence of obstructive CAD[2] (because of probable hormonal protection) or due to atypical presentation. Undertreatment can be due to social/financial reasons or due to under-recognition of a nonobstructive cause of ischemic heart disease (IHD) in women.

What this study adds? The present study included 633,097 patients hospitalized for acute myocardial infarction (AMI) according to Korean National Health Insurance Service (KNHIS) database from 2002 to 2018. The aim of the study was to investigate the long-term trends of prevalence, treatment methodologies, and mortality of AMI by gender. Out of those hospitalized, 40% were women. Although the incidence of hospitalized patients has been increasing since 2011, women are less likely to be hospitalized than men. Women with AMI had increased short-term as well as long-term mortality than men. Age-adjusted mortality was higher in women for 3- and 7-day mortalities. There was no significant difference in 30-day mortality. However, 1-year mortality was lower in women compared to men. The prescription rate of blockers and statins was also lower in women similar to previous studies.[3]

Knowledge gaps identified: Long-term data should also include other components of major adverse cardiac and cerebrovascular events (MACCE) such as target vessel revascularization (TVR), nonfatal myocardial infarction (MI), and nonfatal stroke. Similar studies must be done in other developing countries.

ARTICLE 2

Sex-specific and Hormone-related Differences in Vascular Remodeling in Atherosclerosis

Yerly A, van der Vorst EPC, Baumgartner I, Bernhard SM, Schindewolf M, Döring Y. Sex-specific and hormone-related differences in vascular remodelling in atherosclerosis.
Eur J Clin Invest. 2023;53(1):e13885.

Abstract

Cardiovascular diseases (CVDs) attributing to global mortality and morbidity have shown a complexity of pathophysiological mechanisms, affecting the final pathway to atherosclerosis and its complications. Sexual dimorphisms in CVD presentation and outcomes have unfolded some of the interesting sex-related differences in vascular remodeling in atherosclerosis. A greater number of men have been reported to have cardiovascular (CV) risk factors compared to women, which explains the greater prevalence and early onset of CVDs in men whereas women present with CVDs more commonly post menopause and they are more adversely affected by various risk factors. These biological sex-related disparities in CVDs could be partly explained by understanding the effects of sex hormones on immune expression, endothelial dysfunction, vascular smooth muscle cell proliferation, and plaque formation. Plaque morphological characteristics such as size, number, inflammation, composition, and stability have been shown to be modulated under the influence of sex hormones. Estrogens in women protect against atherosclerosis, thus decreasing the risk of CVDs whereas androgens in men act like a double-edged sword. Decreasing levels of estrogens with aging have been found to be associated with an increased risk of atherosclerotic CVDs; at the same time, they have also been implicated in promoting inflammatory cells recruitment at the site of endothelial injury. Though we have come a way long in delineating the mechanistic pathways involved in atherosclerosis, still a lot more needs to be explored to completely understand the sex as a biological variable of atherosclerosis. This review article is an attempt to highlight the role of sex hormones in the process of atherosclerotic vascular remodeling which can be harnessed for future therapeutics in CVDs.

COMMENT

Atherosclerotic cardiovascular disease (CVD), being the leading cause of death in both men and women at a global level, has always been an area of research since decades. Recently, there has been a tremendous enhancement in our knowledge about gender disparities in different cardiovascular (CV) risk factors, clinical presentation, immune expression, and hormonal impact on vascular remodeling in atherogenesis. This article provides a blanket review on sex as a biological determinant of atherosclerosis, which can affect its development and progression in various ways.[4-7]

ARTICLE 3

Incidence and Outcomes of Cardiogenic Shock Among Women with Spontaneous Coronary Artery Dissection

Osman M, Syed M, Simpson TF, Bhardwaj B, Kheiri B, Divanji P, et al. Incidence and outcomes of cardiogenic shock among women with spontaneous coronary artery dissection.
Catheter Cardiovasc Interv. 2022;100(4):530-4.

Abstract

Background: Spontaneous coronary artery dissection (SCAD) is not an uncommon cause of acute myocardial infarction (AMI) in female patients. Although most SCAD can be treated conservatively, few patients can develop cardiogenic shock (CS) and may require mechanical circulatory support. But the incidence of cardiogenic shock and outcome in SCAD patients is not much studied.

Method: Data pertaining to women admitted with AMI with and without SCAD from October 1, 2015, to December 31, 2018, in the United States National Readmission Database was analyzed. After adjusting the baseline characteristics, the incidence of CS among women with AMI with and without SCAD and odds for developing CS were calculated. In addition to this, the research also calculated the utilization of percutaneous coronary intervention, need for mechanical circulatory support, severe disability surrogates, and 30-day readmission rates.

Results: In this study 664,292 patients admitted with AMI were analyzed, out of which 6,643 patients had SCAD. SCAD patients were younger {57 years [interquartile range (IQR) 48–68] vs. 71 years (IQR 60–81), $p < 0.01$}. Patients with SCAD had fewer comorbidities but had a higher incidence of CS compared to patients without SCAD (9% vs. 5%, $p < 0.01$) and remained at an increased risk after adjusting for baseline comorbidities {adjusted odds ratio 1.5 [95% confidence interval (CI) 1.2–1.7]}. Among the cardiogenic shock group, patients with SCAD had better survival (rate) compared to non-SCAD patients (39% vs. 31%, $p < 0.01$) and were more likely to receive mechanical circulatory support.

Conclusion: The study shows that women with AMI due to SCAD had a higher risk of developing CS and needed more frequent use of mechanical circulatory support. Interestingly, the SCAD group has better survival rate at discharge compared to non-SCAD women patients.

COMMENT

The incidence of spontaneous coronary artery dissection (SCAD) is higher in young and middle-aged women acute myocardial infarction (AMI) patients, especially in the peripartum period. Mostly, SCAD publications in the past include case reports and small case series. In the general population, the incidence of SCAD is between 0.28% and 1.1%,[8] but there is a paucity of data regarding SCAD in women. The incidence of SCAD has increased significantly in the recent years, due to the increased use of coronary angiography in patients presented with AMI, as well as the use of high-resolution intracoronary imaging like intravascular ultrasound (IVUS) and especially optical coherence tomography

(OCT) that enhances the diagnosis of SCAD more precisely than coronary angiogram.[9,10]

The sample statistics of the study was good enough to yield reliable results. It shows the real-world data regarding the incidence and prevalence of SCAD in women AMI patients. The present study corroborates the findings of previous such studies which support that there is a higher incidence of SCAD in young and middle-aged women AMI patients and establishes that the same trend continues to exists.

The incidence of cardiogenic shock (CS) varies from 1 to 16% in SCAD patients and even higher in peripartum cases (20–24%).[11] In accordance with previous such studies, this study also illustrates that the CS incidence in the SCAD group is 9% as compared to 5% in the non-SCAD group.

As per the previous recommendation, SCAD patients with CS require early hemodynamic support with inotropes and vasopressors, intra-aortic balloon pump (IABP), extracorporeal membrane oxygenation (ECMO), left ventricular (LV) assist device, and Impella. This study also puts forth the trend of more frequent use of mechanical circulatory support in SCAD CS patients compared to SCAD with no CS. Despite more frequent use of mechanical circulatory support, the SCAD group has a better survival rate upon discharge compared to non-SCAD women patients. It is mostly because of the less comorbidities and younger age of the presentation in SCAD women. Therefore, this study demonstrates that although CS incidence is high in SCAD women, these patients have better survival if treated judiciously with revascularization and mechanical circulatory support. Mechanical circulatory support provides sufficient time for healing of intramural hematoma and makes weaning easy in the SCAD group.

ARTICLE 4

Sex-related Differences in Thrombus Burden in STEMI Patients Undergoing Primary Percutaneous Coronary Intervention

Manzi MV, Buccheri S, Jolly SS, Zijlstra F, Frøbert O, Lagerqvist B, et al. Sex-related differences in thrombus burden in STEMI Patients undergoing primary percutaneous coronary intervention.
JACC Cardiovasc Interv. 2022;15(20):2066-76.

Abstract

Background: Women after ST-segment elevation myocardial infarction (STEMI) have a poorer prognosis in comparison to men. After STEMI, the predictive role of thrombus burden (TB) in influencing sex-related differences in clinical outcomes has not been understood well.

Objectives: The present study was designed to evaluate the sex-related differences in TB and its clinical implications in STEMI patients.

Methods: From the three major randomized clinical trials of manual thrombus aspiration, individual patient data were collected and analyzed, including overall 19,047 STEMI patients; out of them 13,885 (76.1%) were men and 4,371 (23.9%) were women. The primary endpoints of the study consisted of 1-year cardiovascular (CV) death outcomes. The secondary endpoints consisted of parameters including recurrent myocardial infarction, heart failure, all-cause mortality, stroke, stent thrombosis (ST), and target vessel revascularization at 1-year outcomes.

Results: Worse 1-year outcomes were noted in patients with high TB (HTB) when compared with patients who were presented with low TB [adjusted hazard ratio (HR) for CV death: 1.52; 95% confidence interval (CI) 1.10–2.12; $p = 0.01$]. Female sex was found to be associated with an increased risk for 1-year CV death irrespective of TB, in unadjusted analyses. But in women with HTB, the risk for 1-year CV death was noted to be higher (HR 1.23; 95% CI 1.18–1.28; $p < 0.001$); they also showed an increased risk for all-cause death and ST than men, after adjustment analysis.

Conclusion: Angiographic evidence suggestive of HTB negatively affects prognosis in patients with STEMI. Here, women had shown an increased risk for ST, CV, and all-cause mortality when compared to men, among patients presented with HTB. For a better understanding of the pathophysiological mechanisms leading to excess mortality in women with STEMI and HTB in the future, more research is required.

COMMENT

STEMI with high thrombus burden and women: A double whammy: ST-elevation myocardial infarction (STEMI) in women is associated with poorer short- and long-term outcomes compared to men.[12] Various factors such as old age, delayed presentation, undertreatment, smaller vessel diameter, and more comorbidities have been contributed to poorer outcomes in women. High thrombus burden (TB) in STEMI leads to distal embolization and increased slow-flow or no-reflow leading to increased cardiac events. STEMI in women has already been associated with high mortality, but whether it is primarily due to high TB or due to some other factor is not clear.

In this study, authors have analyzed data from three major trials: (i) TAPAS (Thrombus Aspiration during Percutaneous coronary intervention in Acute myocardial infarction Study), (ii) TASTE (Thrombus Aspiration in ST-Elevation myocardial infarction in Scandinavia), and (iii) TOTAL (Thrombectomy with PCI vs. PCI Alone in Patients with STEMI) trials, focusing on the outcome depending upon sex and TB. A total of 18,256 patients were included in the study, women comprising 4,371 (23.9%). When compared to men, women were more elderly and hypertensive and had a longer median ischemic time. High TB was defined as Thrombolysis in Myocardial Infarction (TIMI) thrombus grade ≥3 and low TB as TMI thrombus grade <3. High TB was seen less frequently in women (71.4%) when compared to men (75.5%). There was no significant difference in treatment given among women and men.[13] The use of newer P2Y12 inhibitors was <40% in both groups. The incidence of cardiovascular death in patients categorized by sex and TB showed the highest mortality in females with high TB followed by females with low TB, followed by men with high TB, and the lowest seen in men with low TB. After adjusting the confounding factors, the difference between mortality among women and men was found not significant in the low TB group but higher in women in the high TB group. Women with high TB had significantly higher rates of cardiovascular death, all-cause death, stent thrombosis, and heart failure, with the highest frequency during the first 30 days. Though overall women had a low incidence of high TB compared to men, in women the prognosis was poorer in the presence of high TB. The reason for the low thrombus burden in women compared to men can be postulated due to the protective effect of estrogens which decreases the risk of thrombus formation.

The challenge is how to address this high TB. The trials have shown that routine thrombus aspiration has no benefit in terms of cardiovascular mortality and event rate but increases the risk of stroke. The antithrombotic agent and timely intervention have been shown to decrease the event rate, but various trials have shown that they are underprescribed in women in view of the high bleeding risk. Guideline-directed medical therapy (GDMT) should be strictly followed in women, especially with high TB. Further studies are warranted to address this issue of high thrombus burden and its treatment in women.

Key messages

- Women with STEMI are older, have more comorbidities, are late presenters, are undertreated, and have a lower incidence of high TB compared to men.
- In STEMI with high TB, women have worse outcomes in terms of cardiovascular mortality, all-cause mortality, and stent thrombosis compared to men.
- Antithrombotic treatment should be prescribed more aggressively in women to decrease this gap of event rates compared to men.

ARTICLE 5

Ischemia with No Obstructive Coronary Arteries (INOCA): A Review of the Prevalence, Diagnosis and Management

Hansen B, Holtzman JN, Juszczynski C, Khan N, Kaur G, Varma B, et al. Ischemia with No Obstructive Arteries (INOCA): A review of the prevalence, diagnosis and management.
Curr Probl Cardiol. 2023;48(1):101420.

Abstract

Ischemia with No Obstructive Coronary Artery Disease (INOCA) refers to patients who exhibit ischemia during coronary angiography but do not have any evidence of obstructive coronary artery disease (CAD). INOCA is estimated to be prevalent in approximately 3–4 million individuals, with a higher occurrence among females. It comprises various endotypes, which include microvascular dysfunction, vasospasm, and a combination of both conditions. The diagnosis of INOCA necessitates the use of noninvasive or invasive techniques to evaluate coronary flow reserve (CFR), the Index of Microcirculatory Resistance (IMR), and the presence of spasm induced by acetylcholine injection. Despite the fact that INOCA is linked to a higher risk of major adverse cardiovascular event (MACE) and a decline in quality of life, it is concerning that less than half of the patients receive appropriate treatment. The treatment of INOCA remains challenging, as current therapeutics are customized to target specific endotypes. Ongoing clinical trials are being conducted to evaluate the effectiveness of traditional medications used for CAD.

COMMENT

Ischemia with No Obstructive Coronary Artery Disease (INOCA) is an important entity which was previously denied its due place in the myriad array of cardiovascular diseases.[14] Women are more at risk and have been undertreated and misdiagnosed to a great degree. Awareness and proper testing can promote better identification and treatment of INOCA. This is imperative to reduce the morbidity and mortality of this disease. The present article comprehensively guides the approach to and management of INOCA.[15] With the existing treatments and drugs available, symptom control and disease modification should be attempted. Cardiac rehabilitation is an effective nonpharmacological therapy which should be widely used for all patients with INOCA.

A recent study has classified four different endotypes of INOCA:[16]
1. Coronary microvascular disease
2. Epicardial vasospastic angina
3. Microvascular vasospastic angina
4. Masked diffuse disease

Identification of the endotypes by invasive and noninvasive tests is a requirement to a methodical approach to managing INOCA.

European Society of Cardiology chronic coronary syndromes (ESC CCS) 2019 guidelines indicate noninvasive methods as first-line testing for anginal patients. It is imperative to stress the utility of echocardiograms due to the wider availability and lesser costs. Transthoracic Doppler–coronary flow reserve (TTD-CFR) is known to reflect the presence of macrovascular as well as microvascular disease in the coronary circulation.[17] Most frequently, the technique is used with an adenosine/dipyridamole protocol in conjunction with a stress echocardiography examination. Mid and distal left anterior descending (LAD) and right coronary artery posterior/descending artery (RCA/PDA) vessels are imaged and assessed.[18]

The results of ongoing trials such as the INOCA IT, WARRIOR, EXAMINE-CAD, iCorMicA, and DISCOVER INOCA are awaited for more understanding and effective strategies to deal with patients living with INOCA.

ARTICLE 6

Less Revascularization in Young Women but Impaired Long-term Outcomes in Young Men after Myocardial Infarction

Kerola AM, Palomäki A, Rautava P, Kyto V. Less revascularization in young women but impaired long-term outcomes in young men after myocardial infarction.
Eur J Prevent Cardiol. 2022;29:1437-45.

Abstract

Aim: Female gender has been linked to worse poor outcomes following a myocardial infarction (MI); however, there is limited evidence available for young patients. Our research aimed to investigate disparities in cardiovascular outcomes between sexes after MI in the young patient population.

Methods and results: We conducted a study on consecutive young patients aged 18–54 years who experienced out-of-hospital myocardial infarction (MI). These patients were admitted to 20 hospitals in Finland, totaling 8,934 cases, of which 17.3% were women. The data were collected from national registries from 2004 to 2014. The median duration of follow-up for the participants was 9.1 years, with a maximum period of 14.8 years. Young women who experienced MI had a higher number of comorbidities at baseline. Additionally, they underwent revascularization procedures less frequently compared to young men with MI. Moreover, after the MI event, young women received fewer evidence-based secondary prevention medications, including P2Y12 inhibitors, renin–angiotensin signaling pathway inhibitors, and statins. There were no significant differences observed between the sexes regarding long-term mortality or the occurrence of major adverse cardiovascular events (MACE, recurrent MI, stroke, or cardiovascular-related death) in the unadjusted analysis,

However, men had poorer outcomes after MI after baseline feature and treatment-difference adjustment. Adjusted long-term mortality was 21.3% in men versus 17.2% in women [hazard ratio (HR) 1.29; 95% confidence interval (CI) 1.10–1.53; $p = 0.002$]. The cumulative MACE rate was 33.9% in men versus 27.9% in women during follow-up (HR 1.23; 95% CI 1.09–1.39; $p = 0.001$) Among the participants, the frequency of recurrent MI and cardiovascular-related deaths was higher in men compared to women. However, there were no significant differences in the occurrence of stroke between the two genders.

Conclusion: In our study, we observed that young women received less active treatment after experiencing MI compared to young men. We found that male sex was associated with worse long-term cardiovascular outcomes in young patients who had suffered an MI after adjusting for baseline features.

COMMENT

The incidence of myocardial infarction (MI) has decreased in older populations; however, it remains a significant cause of morbidity and mortality among young individuals.[19] The risk-factor profile differs significantly from that of older adults compared to younger patients with MI. Some traditional cardiovascular risk factors, such as smoking and having a family history of premature coronary artery disease (CAD), are more prevalent in this younger population. Additionally, women in this group are more likely to be premenopausal. On the other hand, many comorbidities and frailties, which are more commonly seen in older adults, are less frequent among younger MI patients. These variations in risk factors and health characteristics underscore the need for tailored approaches in managing and preventing MI in the younger population.[20,21]

Based on previous studies, the prevailing perception has been that women tend to experience worse outcomes after suffering a MI compared to men.[22] Indeed, it is crucial to highlight that the majority of studies indicating worse MI prognoses in women has primarily focused on short-term outcomes following the MI event. The available evidence regarding sex differences in long-term outcomes after MI among young is limited and contradictory. More extensive and focused studies are needed to gain comprehensive insights into the impact of MI in young patients.

This nationwide study that involved linking various registers investigated the potential sex differences in early mortality and long-term outcomes among Finnish patients who experienced a MI and were under the age of 55 years. The study followed these patients for a maximum period of 14.8 years.

To account for a wide array of potential confounding factors, such as various comorbidities and the type and treatment of MI, the authors employed two effective methods: (i) Propensity scoring and (ii) inverse probability weighting (IPW). These methods are valuable tools in observational studies as they help control for confounding variables and enhance the validity of the study's findings.[23] After accounting for various confounding factors, it became evident that young men had poorer long-term outcomes following MI compared to young women. Surprisingly, there were no significant sex differences in short-term survival rates. Despite these findings, it was observed that young women with MI were less likely to receive guideline-recommended pharmacological therapies and were less frequently subjected to revascularization procedures. These results suggest that although young women may have received less aggressive treatment, they still exhibited better long-term outcomes compared to young men after an MI event.

The study has certain limitations, including the absence of data on laboratory results, angiographical data, and more detailed clinical information (e.g., Killip class, heart rate, blood pressure). Additionally, the study lacks data on socioeconomic status, delays in care, and sex-specific risk factors such as early menarche or menopause, adverse pregnancy outcomes, or lifestyle-related factors. These missing data points may lead to residual confounding, meaning that some unmeasured or unaccounted factors could still influence the observed outcomes, potentially affecting the study's conclusions.

Indeed, based on the results of this study, it is imperative to give equal attention to coronary procedures for both men and women. The findings highlight the significance of providing timely and appropriate coronary interventions to young patients of all genders who experience an MI.

ARTICLE 7

Updates on MINOCA and INOCA through the 2022 Publications in the International Journal of Cardiology

Pelliccia F, Camici PG. Updates on MINOCA and INOCA through the 2022 publications in the International Journal of Cardiology.
Int J Cardiol. 2023;374:8-11.

Abstract

In recent times, there has been growing interest in the syndromes of Myocardial Infarction or Ischemia with No Obstructive Coronary Artery Disease (referred to as MINOCA and INOCA). Several diagnostic uncertainties related to these conditions have been addressed and better understood. Contrary to initial beliefs, there is now evidence indicating that patients with MINOCA and INOCA experience major adverse cardiovascular events (MACE) that are not less serious than those seen in patients with obstructive coronary artery disease (CAD). Several articles published in the International Journal of Cardiology in 2022 have contributed significant and valuable insights into the intricate puzzle of MINOCA and INOCA.

COMMENT

Graziani and colleagues conducted a study involving almost 3,000 patients with hypertrophic cardiomyopathy (HCM) and Fabry's disease. Their research revealed that electrocardiographic left ventricular hypertrophy (LVH) and echocardiographic left ventricular (LV) wall thickness were independently linked to Myocardial Infarction with No Obstructive Coronary Artery Disease MINOCA.[24] In an Italian study conducted by Magnani et al. focusing on early myocardial infarction (MI), it was found that the mortality rate was lower in the MINOCA group. However, the incidences of nonfatal reinfarction, ischemic stroke, and all-cause mortality were found to be similar.[25]

Recent research focusing on MINOCA has examined the prognosis of affected patients, revealing a 12-month all-cause mortality rate of 4.7% (with a 95% confidence interval ranging from 2.6 to 6.9%). Comparative studies consistently indicate that individuals experiencing MINOCA tend to have a more favorable prognosis compared to those who suffer from acute myocardial infarction (AMI) associated with obstructive coronary artery disease.[26]

In the study conducted by Williams et al., the impact of sex on MINOCA was studied, and it was found that men were more susceptible to MINOCA caused by myocarditis and Takotsubo syndrome, while women were more prone to stroke. Additionally, the study identified age and left ventricular ejection fraction (LVEF) as independent predictors of mortality.[27]

As of now, there have been no randomized controlled trials conducted specifically on secondary treatment preventions for MINOCA. Indeed, the SWEDEHEART registry, which included data from over 9,000 patients, demonstrated a decrease in major adverse cardiovascular event (MACE) in patients who received treatment with statins or angiotensin-converting enzyme inhibitors (ACEIs). Treatment with beta-blockers demonstrated a positive trend in improving outcomes for MINOCA patients. On the other hand, the use of dual antiplatelet therapy 1 year after diagnosis did not show a significant impact on patient outcomes. However, it is crucial to note that this study was retrospective and observational in nature, which means that there is a risk of residual confounding.

In the context of Ischemia with No Obstructive Coronary Artery Disease (INOCA), Mehta et al. conducted an insightful review.[28] Their analysis revealing a substantial number of patients with suspected CAD exhibiting INOCA and highlights the prevalence of INOCA. Importantly, INOCA is linked to recurrent hospital admissions due to episodes of severe chest pain, reduced functional capacity, diminished health-related quality of life, and substantial healthcare costs.

ARTICLE 8

Updates on Pharmacologic Management of Microvascular Angina

Soleymani M, Masoudkabir F, Shabani M, Vasheghani-Farahani A, Behnoush AH, Khalaji A. Updates on pharmacologic management of microvascular angina.
Cardiovasc Ther. 2022:6080258.

Abstract

Anginal chest pain in absence of significant coronary obstruction is gaining recognition with microvascular angina (MVA) being a key contributor. Previously thought to be a benign entity, MVA is now known to be associated with higher incidences of major adverse cardiac events. Due to lack of evidence-based guidelines for management, the therapy is mainly empirical. In this review article, authors have discussed about various suspected mechanisms behind the development of MVA and targeted therapies.

COMMENT

Microvascular angina (MVA) refers to symptomatic myocardial ischemia without evidence of coronary obstruction or impedance to coronary circulation. The incidence has increased over the past decades probably due to better understanding of the pathophysiology and diagnostic testing available. Previously thought to be benign, this is associated with a three to six-fold higher incidence of major adverse cardiac events over 5 years[15] and is far more common in women.[29]

Pathophysiology: Mechanisms contributing to MVA are thought to be multifactorial. There is impaired vasodilatation of coronary arteries consequent to endothelial dysfunction[30] and proinflammatory and coagulative factors.[31] A high incidence in menopausal women suggests a role of estrogen deficiency causing endothelial dysfunction.[29] As intravascular ultrasound studies have shown coronary atherosclerosis in majority of MVA cases,[32] aggressive check on atherosclerotic risk factors and treatment of related morbidities is therefore crucial.

Diagnosis: As per the Coronary Vasomotion Disorders International Study Group, a definitive diagnosis of MVA can be made if the following criteria are met:
- Presence of anginal symptoms or angina equivalents Absence of obstructive/flow limiting coronary stenosis
- Objective evidence of myocardial ischemia on noninvasive testing
- Evidence of coronary microvascular dysfunction (CMD) on coronary function testing (CFT)

Management: There is a lack of evidence-based guidelines for the management of MVA, but various approaches have been proposed on the basis of the pathophysiological mechanisms involved.
- *Pharmacotherapy*: It aims at control of symptoms and improvement of quality of life. Due to involvement of many factors in the pathogenesis of MVA, any simple regimen therapy may not always yield success.
- *Statins, angiotensin-converting enzyme inhibitors, and aspirin (anti-atherosclerotic therapy)*: Because of the anti-atherosclerotic and anti-thrombotic effects, the potential to counteract oxidative stress on a cellular level, and anti-inflammatory effects, these drugs can improve both endothelial and microvascular function.[33,34]
- *Beta-blockers, calcium channel blockers, and nitrates (anti-anginal therapy)*: These agents work by improving coronary flow rate, improve the vasodilatory response, and help in ameliorating the anginal pain, thereby improving symptoms and exercise tolerance.[35]
- *Other strategies*: Various new pharmacotherapeutic strategies are being tried for symptom control and modulation of the factors responsible:
    ○ Ranolazine (improves ventricular relaxation and oxygen consumption)[36]
    ○ Ivabradine (decreases heart rate through blocking the If channels)[37]
    ○ Low-dose tricyclic antidepressants (modulate cardiac pain perception)[38]
    ○ Aminophylline (blocks mediation of nociception as well as has an effect of attenuating the excess dilation of the microcirculation in relatively well-perfused areas, thereby shunting blood to poorly perfused areas)
    ○ Phosphodiesterase inhibitors, e.g., cilostazol and sildenafil (improve coronary flow rate)[39,40]
    ○ Rho-kinase inhibitors, i.e., fasudil (prevents acetylcholine-induced coronary spasm)[41,42]
    ○ Antihyperglycemic agents, sodium–glucose cotransporter 2 inhibitors (SGLT-2Is), and metformin (improve the endothelial dysfunction)
    ○ 17-beta estradiol (in postmenopausal women)
    ○ Vitamin D supplements (if deficient)
    ○ Omega-3 fatty acids

- Proton-pump inhibitors [in patients with gastroesophageal reflux disease (GERD)]
- N-acetyl-l-cysteine (NAC)

These agents, though promising, have lower levels of evidence as of now and need to be studied further.

To sum up, though MVA is gaining recognition, the pathophysiological mechanisms may differ case to case. There is a need for large randomized clinical trials to form evidence-based guidelines for the management.

ARTICLE 9

Association between Hormone Therapy and Short-term Cardiovascular Events in Women with Spontaneous Coronary Artery Dissection

Mori R, Macaya F, Giacobbe F, Moreno V, Quadri G, Chipayo D, et al. Association between hormone therapy and short-term cardiovascular events in women with spontaneous coronary artery dissection.
Rev Esp Cardiol (Engl Ed). 2023;76(3):165–72.

Abstract

Background: Spontaneous coronary artery dissection (SCAD) is a cause of acute coronary syndrome that has a clear female preponderance (81–92%). Changes in sex hormone levels are a known triggering factor for SCAD in women. Hypotheses regarding the potential role of sex hormones in SCAD are supported by the clear female preponderance of the disease and its relationship with pregnancy. However, clinical data on how hormonal therapy (HT) impacts the outcome in women diagnosed with SCAD are lacking. This study aimed at finding the association between HT and clinical outcome in women presenting with SCAD.

Method: The study enrolled consecutive patients presenting with SCAD from the DISCO-IT/SPA (dissezioni spontanee coronariche Italian-Spanish) registry. DISCO-IT/SPA is an observational, international, multicenter, retrospective registry that enrolled SCAD patients from 26 centers. Patients were enrolled in the registry from January 1, 2009, to December 31, 2019. All enrolled patients suffice angiographic criteria for SCAD. Patients with >50% atherosclerotic disease in the culprit or the other vessels were excluded. Treatment with HT was assessed via direct patient interview and/or by checking the electronic prescription system but not necessarily both. HT could include estrogens, progestogens, or gonadotropins and the patient had to have been on it at the time of the SCAD event, with an undefined onset time.

The primary composite outcome was nonfatal myocardial infarction (MI) (fourth universal definition of MI) and/or unplanned percutaneous coronary intervention (PCI) at any point after the index catheterization and until 28 days of follow-up (4 weeks). Given that HT was discontinued in most patients on this therapy, we decided to analyze the primary outcome at 28 days to examine a more direct relationship with the exposure. The 12-month outcomes are also reported.

Results: 224 women with complete data and follow-up at a minimum of 28 days were included in this study. Overall, the mean age was 52.0 ± 10.0 (range 29–84) years. A total of 39 patients (17.4%) were receiving HT for a median time of 3 years, which in most cases was oral contraception (51.3%). Only three patients had an intrauterine device. Baseline characteristics of patients with and without HT at the time of the event were similar, except for a higher prevalence of migraines and a lower prevalence of dyslipidemia in the HT group. In terms of clinical presentation, 47.8% presented with ST-elevation MI (STEMI) and 47.3% with non–ST-elevation MI (NSTEMI). The main angiographic features of both groups, including SCAD angiotype, did not differ significantly. Most patients ($n = 142$; 63.4%) were managed conservatively as the initial strategy, without significant differences among groups. The primary composite outcome following the index catheterization and during the first 28 days of follow-up occurred in a higher proportion in the HT group: 7 (17.9%) versus 14 (7.6%) patients, $p = 0.0386$. More patients on HT required unplanned PCI: 7 (17.9%) versus 10 (5.4%), $p = 0.007$, and the most common indication was chest pain with evidence of ischemia on electrocardiogram (87.5%).

Looking at 12-month outcomes, although the absolute difference in the composite outcome remained large between patients with and without HT, it was no longer statistically significant (20.5% vs. 10.8%, $p = 0.095$). The incidence of nonfatal MI was also not statistically different (15.4% vs. 8.1%, $p = 0.156$). In contrast, the difference in unplanned PCI remained significant (20.5% vs. 7.0%, $p = 0.008$). No deaths were recorded during the first year of follow-up in the study population.

Conclusion: The study shows that women diagnosed with SCAD and being treated with hormonal therapy have a statistically significant higher incidence of nonfatal MI and/or unplanned PCI at any point after the index catheterization and until 28 days of follow-up. At 12 months of follow-up, an insignificant difference was found in the incidence of non-fatal MI but a statistically significant number of patients required revascularization in the HT group.

COMMENT

The effects of estrogen on arteries vary with the stage of reproductive life, being protective against the development of atherosclerosis in premenopausal women.[43] On the other hand, we know that patients on hormonal therapy (HT) (estrogen and progesterone) may experience subtle alterations of the arterial wall caused by fragmentation of the reticulin fibers, degeneration of collagen, loss of normal corrugation of elastic fibers, hypertrophy of the smooth muscle cells, and changes in the mucopolysaccharide content and protein composition of the media.[44,45] This study shows that the exogenous hormones cause alterations in the arterial wall and impact negatively on women with spontaneous coronary artery dissection (SCAD).

Still, a larger number of patients on hormonal therapy (HT) need to be studied for proper establishment of the relationship. This study does not check the institution of optimum medical therapy for the patients as it can alter the outcome for either group. There were very few patients of SCAD treated with Gp IIb/IIIa inhibitors, so their role in the treatment and impact on outcome needs to be studied further. How helpful are the newer drugs [angiotensin receptor-neprilysin inhibitor (ARNI) and sodium-glucose cotransporter-2 inhibitor (SGLT-2I)] for patients with SCAD is yet to be evaluated.

ARTICLE 10

Sex Differences in 10-year Outcomes Following STEMI: A Subanalysis from the EXAMINATION-EXTEND Trial

Gabani R, Spione F, Arevalos V, Grima Sopesens N, Ortega-Paz L, Gomez-Lara J, et al. Sex differences in 10-year outcomes following STEMI: A subanalysis from the EXAMINATION-EXTEND trial.
JACC Cardiovasc Interv. 2022;15(19):1965–73.

Abstract

Background: Women experience poorer short-term results after ST-segment elevation myocardial infarction (STEMI) compared to men, displaying a higher mortality rate. The influence of gender on extremely long-term outcomes remains uncertain.

Objective: The objective of this study was to evaluate if gender has an impact on extremely prolonged outcomes subsequent to STEMI treatment.

Methods: EXAMINATION-EXTEND, a study that followed up for 10 years on the EXAMINATION trial, which originally investigated the use of everolimus-eluting coronary stents for treating patients with STEMI, assigned 1,498 participants in a 1:1 ratio to receive either everolimus-eluting stents or bare-metal stents. This recent investigation specifically focused on the role of gender and was a subset analysis. The primary endpoint was to evaluate the composite patient-oriented outcome (including all-cause mortality, any occurrence of myocardial infarction, or any instance of revascularization) at the 10-year mark. Secondary endpoint included examining the separate components of the primary endpoint. Adjustments for age were made for all measured outcomes.

Result: Out of the total 1,498 STEMI patients, 254 (17%) were women. When considering the entire group, women were comparatively older and had a higher prevalence of arterial hypertension but a lower history of smoking compared to men. Over the 10-year period, there was no significant contrast between women and men concerning the patient-oriented combined outcome (40.6% for women vs. 34.2% for men; adjusted hazard ratio 1.14; 95% confidence interval 0.91–1.42; *p*-value = 0.259). However, there was a tendency toward a slightly elevated all-cause mortality rate in women in comparison to men (27.6% for women vs. 19.4% for men; adjusted hazard ratio 1.30; 95% confidence interval 0.99–1.71; *p*-value = 0.063), while no distinctions were observed in cardiac death or other endpoints.

Conclusion: During an extensive follow-up period, there were no notable distinctions in the comprehensive patient-centered outcome between women and men. Nevertheless, there was a tendency toward increased all-cause mortality in women, a phenomenon unrelated to cardiac death. These current results emphasize the necessity for tailored personalized medical approaches for women following percutaneous revascularization. These strategies should encompass cardiovascular and sex-specific risk factor management as well as precise targeted treatments.

COMMENT

Coronary artery disease (CAD) stands as the leading cause of mortality for both males and females. Yet, there exist divergent consequences for men and women dealing with symptomatic CAD. On average, CAD tends to manifest in women roughly a decade later than in men. Some indications also point toward women experiencing higher mortality rates compared to men.[46,47] More precisely, within a population experiencing ST-segment elevation myocardial infarction (STEMI), it is established that women exhibit higher mortality rates than men, both while being hospitalized and in the period following discharge, extending up to 1 year.[48-50]

This study's findings reveal that women experiencing STEMI did not exhibit worse very long-term outcomes in terms of the patient-oriented composite endpoint (POCE) when compared to men. However, women did show a slightly higher incidence of all-cause mortality, with this increase not being driven by deaths related to cardiac causes. Notably, women demonstrated a lower risk of target vessel revascularization (TVR) in the initial 5 years following STEMI in comparison to men, although this difference diminished beyond that period. Additionally, age emerged as an independent predictor of the POCE for both men and women.

In the 10-year assessment of patients who underwent primary percutaneous coronary intervention (PCI) for STEMI, gender did not emerge as a significant factor affecting POCE events. Despite this, there existed a nonsignificant tendency toward elevated all-cause mortality among women compared to men, and this contrast was not attributed to cardiac-related deaths. Furthermore, it is noteworthy that men exhibited a higher rate of repeat revascularizations within the initial 5 years of follow-up, although this gap leveled out by the 10-year mark, resulting in no discernible difference at that point.

The study comes with certain limitations. We were unable to incorporate certain potential variables into our analysis, including factors related to outcomes and patient care, like the long-term adherence of patients to drug treatments. It is important to note that our subanalysis encompassed a smaller portion of women with STEMI in comparison to men. Consequently, our ability to effectively examine variations in outcomes was restricted, and thus, our results should be viewed as generating hypotheses rather than definitive conclusions.

REFERENCES

1. Gholizadeh L, Davidson P. More similarities than differences: An international comparison of CVD mortality and risk factors in women. Health Care Women Int. 2008;29:3-22.
2. Park SM, Merz CN. Women and ischemic heart disease: Recognition, diagnosis and Management. Korean Circ J. 2016;46:433-42.
3. Blomkalns AL, Chen AY, Hochman JS, Peterson ED, Trynosky K, Diercks DB, et al. Gender disparities in the diagnosis and treatment of non-ST-segment elevation acute coronary syndromes: large-scale observations from the CRUSADE (Can Rapid Risk Stratification of Unstable Angina Patients Suppress Adverse Outcomes With Early Implementation of the American College of Cardiology/American Heart Association Guidelines) National Quality Improvement Initiative. J Am Coll Cardiol. 2005;45:832-7.

4. Aggarwal NR, Patel HN, Mehta LS, Sanghani RM, Lundberg GP, Lewis SJ, et al. Sex differences in ischemic heart disease: Advances, obstacles, and next steps. Circ Cardiovasc Qual Outcomes. 2018;11(2):e004437.
5. Libby P, Buring JE, Badimon L, Hansson GK, Deanfield J, Bittencourt MS, et al. Atherosclerosis. Nat Rev Dis Primers. 2019;5(1):56.
6. Jang IK, Bouma BE, Kang DH, Park SJ, Park SW, Seung KB, et al. Visualization of coronary atherosclerotic plaques in patients using optical coherence tomography: comparison with intravascular ultrasound. J Am Coll Cardiol. 2002;39(4):604-9.
7. Folsom AR, Aleksic N, Sanhueza A, Boerwinkle E. Risk factor correlates platelet and leukocyte markers assessed by flow cytometry in a population-based sample. Atherosclerosis. 2009;205(1):272-8.
8. Jacqueline S, Mancini GBJ, Humphries KH. Contemporary review on spontaneous coronary artery dissection. J Am Coll Cardiol. 2016;68(3)297-312.
9. Poon K, Bell B, Raffel OC, Walters DL, Jang IK, et al. Spontaneous coronary artery dissection: utility of intravascular ultrasound and optical coherence tomography during percutaneous coronary intervention. Circ Cardiovasc Interv. 2011;4:e5-e7.
10. Saw J. Spontaneous coronary artery dissection. Can J Cardiol. 2013;29:1027-33.
11. Hayes SN, Kim ESH, Saw J, Adlam D, Arslanian-Engoren C, Economy KE, et al. Spontaneous coronary artery dissection: current state of the science: a scientific statement from the American Heart Association. Circulation 2018;137:e523-57.
12. Shah T, Haimi I, Yang Y, Gaston S, Taoutel R, Mehta S, et al. Meta-analysis of gender disparities in in-hospital care and outcomes in patients with ST-segment elevation myocardial infarction. Am J Cardiol. 2021;147:23-32.
13. Fadini GP, de Kreutzenberg S, Albiero M, Coracina A, Pagnin E, Baesso I, et al. Gender differences in endothelial progenitor cells and cardiovascular risk profile: the role of female estrogens. Arterioscler Thromb Vasc Biol. 2008;28:997-1004.
14. Pacheco Claudio C, Quesada O, Pepine CJ, Merz CNB. Why names matter for women: MINOCA/INOCA (myocardial infarction/ischemia and no obstructive coronary artery disease). Clin Cardiol. 2018;41(2):185-93.
15. Gulati M, Cooper-DeHoff RM, McClure C, Johnson BD, Shaw LJ, Handberg EM, et al. Adverse cardiovascular outcomes in women with non obstructive coronary artery disease: a report from the Women's Ischemia Syndrome Evaluation Study and the St James Women Take Heart Project. Arch Intern Med 2009;169(9):843-50.
16. Hwang D, Park SH, Koo BK. Ischemia with non obstructive coronary artery disease, concept, assessment, and management. JACC Asia. 2023;3(2):169-84.
17. Aggarwal NR, Wood MJ. Sex differences in the pathophysiology, presentation, diagnosis and management of cardiac disease, 1st edition. Waltham: Elsevier; 2021.
18. Sicari R, Nihoyannopoulos P, Evangelista A, Kasprzak J, Lancellotti P, Poldermans D, et al. Stress echocardiography expert consensus statement: European Association of Echocardiography (EAE) (a registered branch of the ESC). Eur J Echocardiogr. 2008;9:415-37.
19. Gupta A, Wang Y, Spertus JA, Geda M, Lorenze N, Nkonde-Price C, D'Onofrio G, et al. Trends in acute myocardial infarction in young patients and differences by sex and race, 2001 to 2010. J Am Coll Cardiol. 2014;64:337-45.
20. Gulati R, Behfar A, Narula J, Kanwar A, Lerman A, Cooper L, et al. Acute myocardial infarction in young individuals. Mayo Clin Proc. 2020;95:136-56.
21. Shah N, Kelly AM, Cox N, Wong C, Soon K. Myocardial infarction in the "young": risk factors, presentation, management and prognosis. Heart Lung Circ. 2016;25:955-60.
22. Bugiardini R, Manfrini O, Cenko E. Female sex as a biological variable: a review on younger patients with acute coronary syndrome. Trends Cardiovasc Med 2019;29:50-5.
23. Deb S, Austin PC, Tu JV, Ko DT, Mazer CD, Kiss A, et al. A review of propensity-score methods and their use in cardiovascular research. Can J Cardiol. 2016;32:259-65.
24. Graziani F, Lillo L, Biagini E, Limongelli G, Autore C, Pieroni M, et al. Myocardial infarction with non-obstructive coronary arteries in hypertrophic cardiomyopathy vs Fabry disease. Int J Cardiol. 2022;369:29-32.
25. Magnani G, Bricoli S, Ardissino M, Maglietta G, Nelson A, Tagliazucchi GM, et al. Long-term outcomes of early-onset myocardial infarction with non-obstructive coronary artery disease (MINOCA). Int J Cardiol. 2022;354:7-13.
26. Pasupathy S, Air T, Dreyer RP, Tavella R, Beltrame JF. Systematic review of patients presenting with suspected myocardial infarction and nonobstructive coronary arteries. Circulation. 2015;131:861-70.
27. Williams MGL, Dastidar A, Liang K, Johnson TW, Baritussio A, et al. Sex differences in patients with acute coronary syndromes and non-obstructive coronary arteries: presentation and outcome, Int J Cardiol. 2022;372:15-22.

28. Mehta PK, Quesada O, Al-Badri A, Fleg JL, Volgman AS, Pepine CJ, et al. Ischemia and no obstructive coronary arteries in patients with stable ischemic heart disease. Int J Cardiol. 2022;348:1-8.
29. Kaski JC. Overview of gender aspects of cardiac syndrome X. Cardiovasc Res. 2002;53(3):620-6.
30. Bottcher M, Botker HE, Sonne H, Nielsen TT, Czernin J. Endothelium-dependent and -independent perfusion reserve and the effect of L-arginine on myocardial perfusion in patients with syndrome X. Circulation. 1995;91(9):2345-52.
31. Schroder J, Zethner-Moller R, Bove KB, Mygind ND, Hasbak P, Michelsen MM. Protein biomarkers and coronary microvascular dilatation assessed by rubidium-82 PET in women with angina pectoris and no obstructive coronary artery disease. Atherosclerosis. 2018;275:319-27.
32. Khuddus MA, Pepine CJ, Handberg EM, Noel Bairey Merz C, Sopko G, Bavry AA, et al. An intravascular ultrasound analysis in women experiencing chest pain in the absence of obstructive coronary artery disease: a substudy from the National Heart, Lung and Blood Institute-Sponsored Women's Ischemia Syndrome Evaluation (WISE). J Interv Cardiol. 2010;23(6):511-9.
33. Kayikcioglu M, Payzin S, Yavuzgil O, Kultursay H, Can LH, Soydan I. "Benefits of statin treatment in cardiac syndrome-X1. Eur Heart J. 2003;24:1999-2005.
34. Pizzi C, Manfrini O, Fontana F, Bugiardini R. Angiotensin-converting enzyme inhibitors and 3-hydroxy-3-methylglutaryl coenzyme A reductase in cardiac syndrome X: role of superoxide dismutase activity. Circulation. 2004;109:53-8.
35. Togni M, Vigorito F, Windecker S, Abrecht L, Wenaweser P, Cook S, et al. Does the beta-blocker nebivolol increase coronary flow reserve? Cardiovascular Drugs Ther. 2007;21:99-108.
36. Hasenfuss G, Maier LS. Mechanism of action of the new anti-ischemia drug ranolazine. Clin Res Cardiol. 2008;97:222-6.
37. Villano A, Di Franco A, Nerla R, Sestito A, Tarzia P, Lamendola P, et al. Effects of ivabradine and ranolazine in patients with microvascular angina pectoris. Am J Cardiol. 2013;112:8-13.
38. Phan A, Shufelt C, Merz CN. Persistent chest pain and no obstructive coronary artery disease. JAMA. 2009;301:1468-274.
39. Yoo SY, Song SG, Lee JH, Shin ES, Kim JS, Park YH, et al. Efficacy of cilostazol on uncontrolled coronary vasospastic angina: a pilot study. Cardiovascular Ther. 2013;31;179-85.
40. Denardo SJ, Wen X, Handberg EM, Noel Bairey Merz C, Sopko GS, Cooper-DeHoff RM, et al. Effect of phosphodiesterase type 5 inhibition on microvascular coronary dysfunction in women: a Women's Ischemia Syndrome Evaluation (WISE) ancillary study. Clin Cardiol. 2011;34:483-7.
41. Masumoto A, Mohri M, Shimokawa H, Urakami L, Usui M, Takeshita A. Suppression of coronary artery spasm by the Rho-kinase inhibition fasudil in patients with vasospastic angina. Circulation. 2002;105:1545-7.
42. Mohri M, Shimokawa H, Hirakawa Y, Masumoto A, Takeshita A. Rho-kinase inhibition with intracoronary fasudil prevents myocardial ischemia in patients with coronary microvascular spasm. J Am Coll Cardiol. 2003;41:15-9.
43. Clarkson TB. Estrogen effects on arteries vary with stage of reproductive life and extent of subclinical atherosclerosis progression. Menopause. 2018;25:1262-74.
44. Tweet MS, Miller VM, Hayes SN. The evidence on estrogen, progesterone, and spontaneous coronary artery dissection. JAMA Cardiol. 2019;4:403-4.
45. Macaya F, Garcia-Arribas D, Escaned J. Reply. Ann Thorac Surg. 2020;109:1308.
46. Anand SS, Islam S, Rosengren A, Franzosi MG, Steyn K, Yusufali AH, et al. Risk factors for myocardial infarction in women and men: Insights from the INTERHEART study. Eur Heart J. 2008;29:932-40.
47. Yusuf S, Hawken S, Ôunpuu S, Dans T, Avezum A, Lanas F, et al. Effect of potentially modifiable risk factors associated with myocardial infarction in 52 countries (the INTERHEART study): case-control study. Lancet. 2004;354:937-52.
48. Fang J, Alderman MH, Keenan NL, Ayala C. Acute myocardial infarction hospitalization in the United States, 1979 to 2005. Am J Med. 2010;123:259-66.
49. Norris CM, Ghali WA, Galbraith PD, Graham MM, Jensen LA, Knudtson ML. Women with coronary artery disease report worse health-related quality of life outcomes compared to men. Health Qual Life Outcomes. 2004;1:21.
50. de Boer SP, Roos-Hesselink JW, van Leeuwen MA, Lenzen MJ, van Geuns RJ, Regar E, et al. Excess mortality in women compared to men after PCI in STEMI: an analysis of 11,931 patients during 2000-2009. Int J Cardiol. 2014;176:456-63.

SECTION 7

Coronary Artery Disease and CVD in Women

Section Editor: Bhupinder Singh

Associate Editors: Suraj Kumar, Surender Deora

ARTICLE 1

Sex Differences in the Clinical Presentation of Acute Coronary Syndromes

de Abreu M, Zylberman M, Vensentini N, Villarreal R, Zaidel E, Antonietti L, et al. Sex differences in the clinical presentation of acute coronary syndromes.
Curr Probl Cardiol. 2022;47(10):101300.

Abstract

Background: There exists a gender difference in the type of clinical presentation of the acute coronary syndrome (ACS) either as ST-segment elevation ACS (STEACS) or non-ST segment elevation ACS (NSTEACS). This study aimed to find out the variation in the clinical presentation of ACS between both genders.

Methods: From the Epi-Cardio Registry, the data of 10,019 patients were analyzed.

Result: Compared to men (46.7%), women (60.3%) had a higher proportion of ACS patients presenting as NSTEACS with a statistically significant p-value of <0.001. This gender difference in the clinical presentation was dominantly attributed to the higher prevalence of non-obstructive coronary artery disease (CAD) among ACS patients (20.9% vs. 6.6%) and the majority of the patients without significant CAD had NSTEACS at presentation (77.7% vs. 22.3%). Among the patients with significant CAD, there was no gender difference in the type of presentation of ACS.

Conclusion: In patients with ACS, compared to men women at younger ages had a higher likelihood to have nonobstructive CAD. On the contrary, this gender difference in the presentation of ACS was not found in patients with obstructive CAD.

COMMENT

As noted in the above study that there is a gender difference in the type of clinical presentation in patients with acute coronary syndrome (ACS) having nonobstructive coronary artery disease (CAD) on coronary angiogram. This difference is more so in young females. A study by Berger et al. had shown that men have a higher proportion of STEACS than women.[1] There was found to be an interaction between age and gender for the presentation of ACS. In men, the non-ST segment elevation ACS (NSTEACS) was more likely a presentation compared to women as age increases. On the contrary, this association was not observed in women. Studies have documented the gender differences in the risk factors of CAD. Hypertension, chronic stable angina, and dyslipidemia were more frequent in women and all these factors are more associated with the clinical presentation of NSTEACS. Smoking, on the other hand, was found to be the major risk factor in men. Smoking is strongly linked with ST-segment elevation ACS (STEACS) as a clinical presentation. These gender differences in risk factors were more divergent at younger ages and continued to converge as the age of presentation increased.

This study appropriately highlighted the gender disparity in the clinical presentation of ACS in relation to the age, presence or absence of obstructive CAD on angiogram, and the extent of CAD.

ARTICLE 2

Sex-related Differences in Plaque Characteristics and Endothelial Shear Stress-related Plaque-progression in Human Coronary Arteries

Wentzel JJ, Papafaklis MI, Antoniadis AP, Takahashi S, Cefalo NV, Cormier M, et al. Sex-related differences in plaque characteristics and endothelial shear stress related plaque-progression in human coronary arteries. *Atherosclerosis. 2022;342:9-18.*

Abstract

Background and aims: Clinical manifestation of atherosclerosis is variable in women compared to men. Endothelial shear stress (ESS) plays a pivotal role in the initiation, progression, and related complications of atherosclerosis. To understand the altered expression of atherosclerosis in women, this study did a comparison of the anatomical variables and ESS-related plaque growth in human coronary arteries between both genders.

Methods: From the PREDICTION study, data of 1,183 coronary arteries were studied in terms of the difference in coronary artery plaque, EES characteristics, and progression of plaque among men and women. The study group was male-dominated (male/female: 944/239). The study group was stratified by age also. The coronary artery plaque-related characteristics were obtained using the intravascular ultrasound (IVUS)-based vascular profiling and data were reported per 3 mm coronary artery segment [13,030 3-mm segments (male/female: 10,465/2,565)]. A follow-up at 6–10 months was done to look for the plaque progression.

Result: It was found that the coronary artery and atherosclerotic plaque size were significantly smaller in females compared to men. The other parameters such as plaque burden, ESS, and progression rate of plaque were similar in both genders. The increase in plaque burden was associated with less ESS (inversely related) with *p*-value of <0.001. This inverse relation was the same in both genders (β: −0.62 ± 0.13 vs. −0.68 ± 0.05, *p* = 0.62). However, in the age group <55 years, the ESS-related plaque growth was significantly more in women compared to men (<55 years, β: −2.02 ± 0.61 vs. −0.33 ± 0.10, *p* = 0.007). The gender difference in plaque growth reduced in magnitude in the other age categories till age 75 years.

Conclusion: Women have smaller size of coronary arteries and plaque compared to men. However, the ESS and ESS-related progression of coronary plaque were similar. The gender difference in the ESS-related plaque progression was noted when age stratification was done.

COMMENT

Coronary artery disease (CAD) presentation is variable between men and women. This is dominantly attributed to the gender-mediated difference in the pathophysiology of atherosclerosis. Previous studies have shown that generally, the plaque size is smaller in women.[2] Endothelial shear stress (ESS) is considered to be a major determinant of endothelial cell injury and the formation of plaque and its future progression.[3]

The above study demonstrated the intravascular ultrasound (IVUS)-based characterization of the coronary artery plaque and confirmed that the coronary plaques are of smaller size in females and more importantly the inverse relation of ESS-related plaque progression was more evident in females compared to men at age <55 years in the earlier studies on the sex-related difference in cardiovascular diseases. Although estrogen hormone in premenopausal women is expected to improve endothelial function, there was ESS-related plaque progression was noted at age < 55 years in females. These gender-related differences at the younger age could be attributed to the altered lifestyle, other confounding risk factors, and early catch-up phenomenon[4] after menopause.

ARTICLE 3

Sex-specific Associations of Myocardial Perfusion Imaging with Outcomes in Patients with Suspected Chronic Coronary Syndrome

Georgiopoulos G, Mavraganis G, Aimo A, Giorgetti A, Cavaleri S, Fabiani I, et al. Sex-specific associations of myocardial perfusion imaging with outcomes in patients with suspected chronic coronary syndrome.
Hellenic J Cardiol. 2023;71:8-15.

Abstract

Background: Myocardial perfusion scintigraphy (MPS) is a well-established noninvasive technique for ischemia assessment and prognosticating patients with suspected chronic coronary syndrome (CCS). Identifying the ischemic extent of >10% on MPS is one of the important findings to optimize the anti-ischemic treatment and opt for revascularization strategies.

Methods: This is a prospectively done study. A total of 1229 consecutive patients without known coronary artery disease (CAD) were taken and underwent stress-rest MPS. All patients were followed up for a mean duration of 4.6 years.

Result: The mean age of the study group was 70 ± 9.5 years and had male dominance (73.5% males). The clinical profile of males and females was comparable. The incidence rate of cardiovascular (CV) events was similar in both genders (6.6% vs. 4.6% respectively, $p = 0.186$). In men, the primary endpoints such as CV death and/or nonfatal myocardial infarction (MI) [adjusted hazard ratio (HR) 3.13; 95% confidence interval (CI) 1.79–5.46; $p = 0.001$], all-cause mortality (HR 3.01; 95% CI 1.31–6.93; $p = 0.01$), and incidence of late revascularization (HR 1.84; 95% CI 1.22–2.78; $p = 0.004$) were significantly higher among patients with a summed stress score (SSS) > 7 on MPS. This finding was not observed in women. Similarly, a summed difference score (SDS) > 6 was significantly associated with higher primary endpoints in the male gender only.

Conclusion: Among patients who are being evaluated for suspected CCS, an abnormal stress test on MPS independently predicts poor outcome in the male gender. However, the results were not predictive for female gender. This calls for the development of gender-specific cut-offs to provide appropriate care to women as well.

COMMENT

The risk stratification of a patient with chronic coronary syndrome (CCS) can be done by various noninvasive modalities, out of which myocardial perfusion scintigraphy (MPS) is one of the modalities. A threshold of SSS > 12 on stress MPS is considered to be a major prognostic marker among patients with CCS.[5] The above study identified that a moderate amount of inducible ischemia such as SSS > 7 and SDS > 6 was associated with increased cardiovascular (CV) events and/or non-fatal myocardial infarction in men not in women. In large studies studying the role of revascularization strategies in CCS patients, females are underrepresented.

These gender differences in the MPS predictability are partially explained by the relatively lower prevalence of significant coronary artery disease (CAD) among females, technical limitations in females such as breast tissue-related attenuation, smaller left ventricular dimensions, regional obesity, and body habitus. This study highlights the importance of having a sex-specific cut-off for the MPS which should be validated in multiple cohorts for wider acceptability.

ARTICLE 4

The Prevalence of Risk Factors and Pattern of Obstructive Coronary Artery Disease in Young Indians (<45 Years) Undergoing Percutaneous Coronary Intervention: A Gender-based Multicenter Study

Jariwala P, Padmavathi A, Patil R, Chawla K, Jadhav K. The prevalence of risk factors and pattern of obstructive coronary artery disease in young Indians (<45 years) undergoing percutaneous coronary intervention: A gender-based multicenter study.
Indian Heart J. 2022;74(4):282-8.

Abstract

Objective: A significant proportion of patients are presenting at a very early age which is probably attributable to the changing lifestyle. This study aimed to assess the prevalence of risk factors and clinical outcomes of obstructive coronary artery disease among young (<45 years) females undergoing percutaneous coronary intervention (PCI) compared to males of the same age group.

Material and methods: The study was multicentric, retrospective, and observational in design. The data of all patients at age <45 years undergoing PCI was taken and stratified according to gender. As per the guidelines, three high-volume centers were included in the study.

Result: Out of a total of 3,656 patients undergoing PCI, 3.1% ($n = 113$) and 6.9% ($n = 254$) were young (<45 years age) females and males, respectively. Traditional risk factors such as smoking ($p = 0.004$), dyslipidemia ($p < 0.001$), alcoholism ($p < 0.001$), and overweight ($p < 0.001$) were significantly higher in young males compared to females. The other risk factors such as diabetes mellitus, high blood pressure, and family history of premature CAD were similar between males and females. The most common clinical manifestation for the genders was acute coronary syndrome (95.6% in young females vs. 95% in young males). The pattern of obstructive CAD was similar in both genders with single-vessel disease as the most common type. The occurrence of cardiogenic shock was 4.4% and in-hospital mortality was 1.7% for young females. This was similar to young males.

Conclusion: Among all patients undergoing PCI, young patients (both males and females) contributed to 10% of the cases with obstructive CAD. Though the males contributed more proportion of cases, the obstructive CAD is not uncommon in young females.

COMMENT

The incidence of young coronary artery disease (CAD), usually defined as CAD occurring at age <45 years, is rising due to the higher incidence of traditional risk factors such as diabetes, hypertension, obesity, and sedentary lifestyle. Indian data for young CAD is less. Published literature has shown that the average age of presentation of young CAD is 36.11 years,[6] and young CAD has got a male preponderance and a better clinical outcome compared to the elderly subgroups.[7]

The present study also showed male dominance in young patients with obstructive CAD. Even though the hormonal interplay should be providing the protective benefit for young females for the development of obstructive CAD but the increasing prevalence of traditional risk factors such as diabetes and hypertension is nullifying the protective effect. As shown in the present study and also well evident from previous studies as well that the younger patients are found to have less complex coronary anatomy like the majority have single-vessel disease. The complexity of coronary anatomy is the same for both genders.

Therefore, the need of the hour is to give utmost attention to the screening protocols and counseling for young patients so that the modifiable risk factor can be regulated in order to reduce the occurrence of CAD in young and the mortality associated with it.

ARTICLE 5

Sex Difference in the Association of the Triglyceride Glucose Index with Obstructive Coronary Artery Disease

Lu YW, Tsai CT, Chou RH, Tsai YL, Kuo CS, Huang PH, et al. Sex difference in the association of the triglyceride glucose index with obstructive coronary artery disease.
Sci Rep. 2023;13(1):9652.

Abstract

Aims and objectives: Metabolic syndrome is linked with the development of coronary artery disease (CAD). Insulin resistance is an important link between these. In this study, we studied the association triglyceride-glucose (TyG) index, a surrogate marker of insulin resistant, with the obstructive CAD and sex difference for the same.

Material and methods: Between January, 2010 and December, 2018, all patients requiring invasive coronary angiography for the evaluation of stable angina pectoris formed the study population. The study group was stratified according to TyG index. The angiographic review of obstructive CAD was done by two interventional cardiologists independently. Demographic profiles of the two groups were compared in term of characteristics and clinical outcomes.

Result: The patients with higher TyG (≥ 8.60) had a higher body mass index (BMI) (26.84 ± 4.14 vs. 24.91 ± 3.97; $p < 0.001$) and higher prevalence of diabetes mellitus (42.8% vs. 18.6%; $p < 0.001$), hypertension (70% vs. 61.9%; $p = 0.028$), and elevated lipid profile compared to lower TyG. On multivariate logistic regression analysis, the higher TyG value was found to be the independent predictor of the obstructive CAD risk for nondiabetic women [adjusted odds ratio (aOR) 2.15, 95% confidence interval (95% CI) 1.08–4.26, $p = 0.02$] compared to men. Coronary anatomy was more complex in patients with higher TyG.

Conclusion: Though the sex difference was not observed for diabetic patients, a higher TyG predicted the risk of obstructive CAD for nondiabetic and overall females.

COMMENT

Insulin resistance (IR) is associated with increased cardiovascular disease risk among patients without diabetes mellitus due to direct consequences of increased glucose concentration, procoagulant properties, and oxidative stress.[8-10] A higher triglyceride-glucose (TyG) index is considered as a surrogate marker of IR. Several studies have demonstrated the predictive role of TyG in acute coronary syndrome (ACS), or nonalcoholic fatty liver disease subjects, major adverse cardiac event (MACE) in ACS patients, arterial stiffness, etc. This study further strengthens the data for TyG association with obstructive coronary artery disease (CAD). It adds to the literature for its predictive role among nondiabetic females for CAD.

Apart from the traditional risk factors such as hypertension, diabetes, obesity, and lifestyle, the TyG could add to the risk stratification of the patients, especially female gender.

ARTICLE 6

Relationship between Breast Arterial Calcification and Coronary Artery Disease by Invasive Coronary Angiography in Postmenopausal Women

Gardinalli-Filho G, Dantas JV, Nahas GP, Brito Buttros DA, Carvalho FC, Carvalho-Pessoa E, De Luca Vespoli H, Petri Nahas EA. Relationship between breast arterial calcification and coronary artery disease by invasive coronary angiography in postmenopausal women.
Eur J Radiol. 2022;157:110606.

Abstract

Purpose: Coronary artery calcification in a well-known risk factor of coronary artery disease (CAD). This study aimed to find the association of breast arterial calcification (BAC) and coronary angiography-proven CAD among postmenopausal females.

Methods: This was a cross-sectional study. In this study, postmenopausal females (age ≥45 years) who underwent invasive coronary angiogram (ICA) for evaluation of CAD and digitalized mammography, within 6 months of each other, formed the study group. Females who either had evidence of breast cancer/exhibited grade-D breast density (BI-RADS®) upon mammography or had undergone prior percutaneous coronary intervention were excluded. An electronic medical record system was used to obtain digital mammograms and interpretations for the BAC were done by two independent and experienced physicians without knowledge of the ICA results. Similarly, coronary angiograms were reviewed independently and categorized into single-vessel disease, two-vessel disease, and multivessel disease (≥3 vessels).

Result: Total 183 postmenopausal females were evaluated, 39 (21.3%) had BAC. Females with BAC were older and had a longer time gap after menopause compared to females without BAC (68.2 ± 9.6 vs. 59.6 ± 10.0 years of age and 19 ± 10.1 vs. 13.5 ± 8.2 years, respectively) with a significant p-value of <0.0001). Clinical risk factor-wise, only smoking was found to be significantly higher in women without BAC ($p = 0.007$). In terms of the complexity of coronary anatomy, no significant difference was observed in both groups ($p = 0.683$). On multivariate logistic regression analysis, after adjustment for age, time since menopause, and smoking, the presence of BAC was not associated with a significant risk of observing a greater number of affected vessels upon ICA (OR 1.07; 95% CI 0.41–2.76; $p = 0.609$).

Conclusion: Among postmenopausal females, the presence of BAC was not associated with the severity and extent of CAD.

COMMENT

Coronary artery calcification is a well-established marker of coronary artery disease (CAD).[11] Similarly, other vessel calcification has been studied as a marker of CAD and breast arterial calcification (BAC) has recently emerged as a potential marker for cardiovascular disease in postmenopausal females. In the published literature, it was observed that the incidence of BAC was about 10% in 40-year aged females and increased to about 50% in 80-year aged females.[12] The present study results were consistent with the already published literature. The inverse relation between smoking (a known risk factor for CAD) and BAC seems paradoxical but is partially explained on the basis of the type of peripheral calcification which involves the middle layer of the arteries (compared to intimal calcification in atherosclerosis) and has an inverse relation with smoking.[13]

The results of various studies, which have studied the association of BAC with CAD, are heterogeneous. The present study did not find any significant association of BAC with the extent and severity of CAD in invasive coronary angiogram (ICA). As discussed previously, the pathophysiology of the type and site of calcification of the arterial wall is different in coronary calcification (intimal calcification) and other vessel calcification wherein deeper layers of the arterial wall are involved. Thus, two findings of BAC and CAD probably reflect two different processes, which could explain our results.

Due to the huge heterogeneity of the results, a large population-based prospective trial is needed to further study this association.

ARTICLE 7

Early Coronary Atherosclerosis in Women with Previous Preeclampsia

Hauge MG, Damm P, Kofoed KF, Ersbøll AS, Johansen M, et al. Early coronary atherosclerosis in women with previous preeclampsia.
J Am Coll Cardiol. 2022;79(23):2310-21.

Abstract

Background: In women, a history of preeclampsia is considered one of the risk factors for coronary artery disease (CAD) later in life.

Objective: To compare the prevalence of CAD in young females with previous preeclampsia and women from the general population.

Methods: Women between the age of 40 and 55 years with previous preeclampsia were compared with women from the general population of matched age and parity. The study population was evaluated by an extensive clinical questionnaire, a clinical examination, and a coronary computed tomography angiography (CTA). The main study outcome assessed was the prevalence of any coronary atherosclerosis on coronary CTA or a calcium score > 0 in case of a nondiagnostic coronary CTA.

Result: Total 1,417 women were studied. The mean age was 47 years. 708 women had previous preeclampsia and 709 subjects from the general population formed the control group. Compared to the control group, women with previous preeclampsia have higher chances of dyslipidemia [338 (47.7%) vs. 296 (41.7%); $p = 0.023$], diabetes mellitus [24 (3.4%) vs. 8 (1.1%); $p = 0.004$], hypertension [284 (40.1%) vs. 162 (22.8%); $p = 0.001$], and high body mass index (27.3 ± 5.7 kg/m^2 vs. 25.0 ± 4.2 kg/m^2; $p = 0.001$). On multivariate logistic regression analysis after adjustment for age, diabetes mellitus, smoking, dyslipidemia, menopause, body mass index, and parity, the prevalence of any coronary atherosclerosis was higher in the preeclampsia group [193 (27.4%) vs. 141 (20.0%); $p = 0.001$] with an OR 1.41 [95% CI 1.08–1.85; $p = 0.012$].

Conclusion: Women aged 40–55 years of age, with previous preeclampsia, had a slightly higher prevalence of coronary atherosclerosis compared with age- and parity-matched women from the general population. Preeclampsia was found to be the independent cardiovascular risk factor after adjustment for traditional risk factors.

COMMENT

There is an increased prevalence of cardiovascular diseases in young. Early-onset development of coronary artery disease (CAD) is seen in the female gender as well.[14,15] This early onset of CAD in the Indian subcontinent is probably attributed to the increased prevalence of traditional risk factors and lifestyle changes. There have been few studies identifying preeclampsia as one of the cardiovascular risk factors in young females. The present study has clearly demonstrated that young women with previous preeclampsia have a higher prevalence of coronary atherosclerosis compared with age- and parity-matched women from the general population. The coronary computed tomography angiography (CTA) may be appropriate in risk stratification in young females especially so with a previous history of preeclampsia for identification of early-onset atherosclerosis and timely initiation of risk-modifying therapy.

ARTICLE 8

Comparative Effectiveness of Initial Computed Tomography and Invasive Coronary Angiography in Women and Men with Stable Chest Pain and Suspected Coronary Artery Disease: Multicenter Randomized Trial

DISCHARGE Trial Group. Comparative effectiveness of initial computed tomography and invasive coronary angiography in women and men with stable chest pain and suspected coronary artery disease: Multicentre randomised trial. *BMJ. 2022;379:e071133.*

Abstract

Objective: To determine the gender-based comparative effectiveness of coronary computed tomography angiography (CCTA) and invasive coronary angiography (ICA) in patients with suspected stable coronary artery disease (CAD).

Design: This trial had a prospective design. It was multicenter, randomized pragmatic trial.

Setting: This study was conducted at 26 hospitals across 16 European countries.

Participants: A total of 3,561 patients of suspected CAD with pretest probability of 10–60% were referred for ICA. 2,002 (56.2%) were women and 1,559 (43.8%) were men.

Intervention: Both the genders were randomized 1:1 to receive a strategy of either CCTA (1,019 and 983 women) or ICA (789 and 770 men) as the initial diagnostic modality and intention-to-treat analysis was performed. The blinded randomized allocation could not be performed while investigators assessing the outcomes were blinded to the randomization group. Both groups were stratified based on gender and center.

Main outcome measures: The primary endpoint was major adverse cardiovascular events (MACE) which included cardiovascular death, nonfatal myocardial infarction, or nonfatal stroke. Secondary endpoints included an expanded MACE composite (cardiovascular death, nonfatal myocardial infarction, nonfatal stroke, transient ischemic attack, or major procedure-related complications).

Results: A median follow-up of the study population was of 3.5 years. A complete follow-up was obtained for 98.9% (1,979/2,002) of women and 99.0% (1,544/1,559) of men. The gender interaction between CCTA and ICA group was not found to be statistically significant for MACE ($p = 0.29$), the expanded MACE composite ($p = 0.45$), or major procedure-related complications ($p = 0.11$). For women and men, the rate of MACE did not differ between the CCTA and ICA groups. Compared to women, men had a significantly less occurrence of the expanded MACE composite endpoint in the CCTA group than in the ICA group (2.8% vs. 5.3%; hazard ratio 0.52; 95% confidence interval, 0.31–0.87). Compared to men, women had a lower risk of having a major procedure-related complication in the CCTA group than in the ICA group (0.3% vs. 2.1%; hazard ratio 0.14; 95% confidence interval 0.04–0.46).

Conclusion: In this study, no gender difference was evident in terms of the benefit of using CCTA over ICA as the initial diagnostic modality for the evaluation of suspected stable CAD patients with an intermediate pretest probability of CAD. An initial CCTA scan was associated with fewer major procedure-related complications in women and a lower frequency of the expanded MACE composite in men.

COMMENT

This was a well-conducted prospective, multicentric, randomized trial. It concluded that there was no gender difference in terms of the advantage of one over the other diagnostic modality for the initial evaluation of an intermediate pretest probability patient for suspected coronary artery disease (CAD). The results of this study are in accordance with the results of the gender-based posthoc analysis of previously conducted studies such as PROMISE, ISCHEMIA, and SCOT-HEART trials.[16-18] The frequency of nondiagnostic CCTA was the same for both genders (ranging from 5 to 6%) when done with 64 or higher-slice CT. It was as low as 3.7% if 320 slice CT was used for the test. In this study, women who received coronary computed tomography angiography (CCTA) as an initial diagnostic strategy had a significantly lower risk of a major procedure-related complication than women who received invasive coronary angiography (ICA). This observation is probably attributed to the lower prevalence of CAD requiring invasive investigation and coronary revascularization, especially in women. Therefore, it highlights the important contribution of CCTA as a gatekeeper for invasive investigation and treatment in women.

ARTICLE 9

Sex Difference in Coronary Artery Spasm Tested by Intracoronary Acetylcholine Provocation Test in Patients with Nonobstructive Coronary Artery Disease

Park JY, Choi SY, Rha SW, Choi BG, Noh YK, Kim YH. Sex difference in coronary artery spasm tested by intracoronary acetylcholine provocation test in patients with nonobstructive coronary artery disease.
J Interv Cardiol. 2022;2022:5289776.

Abstract

Introduction: The presentation and outcome of cardiovascular diseases are variable in men and women. This study aimed to compare the gender difference in the features of coronary artery spasm (CAS) in patients with nonobstructive coronary disease (NOCD) and their clinical outcomes.

Methods: Between November, 2004 and May, 2014, a total of 5,491 patients with NOCD were enrolled in the study. All of these patients underwent an acetylcholine provocation test for the evaluation of chest pain. CAS was defined if >70% of the luminal narrowing of the artery was observed on coronary angiogram during the acetylcholine provocation test.

Result: In the study population 2,506 were men and 2,985 were women. Patients were followed up for a mean duration of $1,218 \pm 577$ days. A propensity score matching (PSM) analysis was performed to adjust for confounding factors in all patients. After propensity matching, 1,201 pairs in all patients and 713 pairs in patients with CAS were generated. In all patients, compared with men, women had significantly less incidence of CAS (62.3% vs. 50.9%; $p < 0.01$). Compared to men, the incidence of myocardial bridge (MB) and moderate stenosis was less in women, while the incidence of ischemic chest pain and transient ST-segment elevation was more in women. Among the patients with CAS, the incidence of multivessel spasm was higher in men than women (35.7% vs. 29.7%, $p < 0.01$). On multivariate logistic regression analysis, dyslipidemia, elderly age subset, and MB were found to be the independent risk factors of CAS in both genders. In CAS patients, various individual and composite major outcomes for up to 5 years were not statistically different in both genders. In men with CAS, major adverse cardiac events (MACE) at 5 years were significantly higher in the elderly subgroup, and both MACE and recurrent angina at 5 years were significantly higher in patients with moderate stenosis. In women with CAS, mild stenosis was a risk factor of 5-year MACE, while myocardial bridge was a risk factor of 5-year recurrent angina.

Conclusion: In this study, the angiographic and clinical parameters such as incidence of coronary spasm, risk factors, 5-year MACE, and recurrent angina during the acetylcholine provocation test were different in both genders. In both genders, the elderly age group, dyslipidemia, and MB were the independent risk factors of CAS. However, major clinical outcomes up to 5 years in CAS patients were not different according to sex.

COMMENT

Coronary artery spasm is a pathophysiological condition, usually associated with nonobstructive coronary artery disease that is linked with various clinical syndromes including arrhythmia, angina, acute coronary syndrome, and sudden cardiac death.[19] Females undergoing coronary angiogram for the evaluation of chest pain are more likely to have normal coronaries or nonobstructive coronary artery disease (CAD) compared to males. A study had shown about 40% incidence of coronary artery spasm (CAS) on acetylcholine provocation testing among symptomatic females with nonobstructive CAD on coronary angiography.[20] The present study showed a significantly higher incidence of CAS in males (63%) compared to females (51%). A disproportionately high incidence of CAS in male has been attributed to the presence of myocardial bridge (MB) which was found more frequently in males. MB is considered an important risk factor for CAS.[21] It is observed in the literature that around 25–35% of the patients with CAS have associated microvascular dysfunction rather than epicardial coronary spasm. In the present study, even though the incidence of CAS was low in females, the incidence of transient ST-T changes and angina was high. This is likely to be linked with the microvascular dysfunction especially so in females. Another phenomenon peculiar to females is the estrogen protection against endothelial dysfunction; therefore, the incidence of CAS is low in the present study. However, this association of hormonal effect with CAS needs further studies.

ARTICLE 10

Psychosocial Well-being and Progression of Coronary Artery Calcification in Midlife Women

Janssen I, Powell LH, Everson-Rose SA, Hollenberg SM, El Khoudary SR, Matthews KA. Psychosocial well-being and progression of coronary artery calcification in midlife women.
J Am Heart Assoc. 2022;11(5):e023937.

Abstract

Background: Prevention of cardiovascular disease (CVD) plays an important role in reducing the burden of noncommunicable diseases. CVD is a major public health concern. The well-known risk factors including physical activity, a healthy diet, and tobacco cessation undoubtedly have a major role in CVD prevention while psychosocial well-being as a risk factor is less well studied. This study aimed to find association of the combination of psychosocial well-being indices and the progression of coronary artery calcium (CAC).

Methods and results: The study participants were taken from the SWAN (Study of Women's Health Across the Nation) ancillary Heart Study. A total of 312 women (mean age 50.8 years) with no clinical CVD at baseline were taken for the study. Six validated psychosocial questionnaires for the assessment of life engagement, optimism, life satisfaction, vitality, positive affect, and rewarding multiple roles were used to create a composite psychosocial well-being score. Electron beam tomography (EBT) was used to calculate the CAC. Subclinical CAC progression was defined if Agatston units increased by ≥10 over 2.3. Relative risk (RR) regression models examined the effect of psychosocial well-being on CAC progression, progressively adjusting for healthy lifestyle behaviors, sociodemographic factors, depression, and standard CVD risk factors. At baseline, CAC score > 0 was found in 42.9% of the study participants. The CAC progression was noted in 17.6% of the cases. Psychosocial well-being was associated with less progression (RR 0.909; 95% CI 0.843–0.979; $p = 0.012$), and it was significant even after adjustment for the potential confounders, health behaviors, and depression. For the overall study population, this association was weakened (RR 0.943; 95% CI 0.871–1.020; $p = 0.142$) after adjustment for standard CVD risk factors but it remained significant for the subgroup of women ($n = 134$) with baseline CAC > 0 (RR 0.921; 95% CI 0.852–0.995; $p = 0.037$).

Conclusion: Psychosocial well-being and mind side of the mind-heart-body continuum play an additional role in optimum early prevention of CVD.

COMMENT

Coronary artery calcium (CAC) score is one of the quantitative, subclinical markers of atherosclerotic coronary artery disease and its complications. Very little is known about the effect of psychosocial well-being or behavior of middle-aged women on atherosclerotic disease progression. Psychosocial well-being is not just the absence of mental disorders such as depression, and anxiety, but it has an independent impact on cardiovascular outcomes.[22] Even after adjustment of the traditional cardiovascular disease (CVD) risk factors, the present study found a strong association between psychosocial well-being and CAC progression in a subgroup of women with prevalent CAC at the baseline.

These results highlight that not only health behaviors but also general well-being should be considered in the early preventive measures in middle-aged women for the progression of atherosclerotic coronary artery disease (CAD).

REFERENCES

1. Berger J, Elliott L, Gallup D, Roe M, Granger CB, Armstrong PW, et al. Sex differences in mortality following acute coronary syndromes. JAMA. 2009;302:874-82.
2. Ten Haaf ME, Rijndertse M, Cheng JM, de Boer SP, Garcia-Garcia HM, van Geuns RJM, et al. Sex differences in plaque characteristics by intravascular imaging in patients with coronary artery disease. EuroIntervention. 2017;13(3):320-8.
3. Wentzel JJ, Chatzizisis YS, Gijsen FJH, Giannoglou GD, Feldman CL, Stone PH Endothelial shear stress in the evolution of coronary atherosclerotic plaque and vascular remodelling: current understanding and remaining questions, Cardiovasc Res. 2012;96: 234-43.
4. Mosca L, Barrett-Connor E, Wenger NK Sex/gender differences in cardiovascular disease prevention: what a difference a decade makes, Circulation. 2011;124:2145-54.
5. Uebleis C, Becker A, Griesshammer I, Cumming P, Becker C, Schmidt M, et al. Stable coronary artery disease: prognostic value of myocardial perfusion SPECT in relation to coronary calcium scoring–long-term follow-up. Radiology. 2009;252(3):682e690.
6. Tammiraju I, Radhakrishna T, Jagadish BK, Sanghamitra R. Acute coronary syndrome in young - A tertiary care centre experience with reference to coronary angiogram. Journal of practices of cardiovascular sciences. 2019;5(1):18-25.
7. Singh B, Singh A, Goyal A, Chhabra S, Tandon R, Aslam N, et al. The Prevalence, Clinical Spectrum and the Long Term Outcome of ST-segment Elevation Myocardial Infarction in Young - A Prospective Observational Study. Cardiovasc Revasc Med. 2019;20(5):387-91.
8. Adeva-Andany MM, Martínez-Rodríguez J, González-Lucán M, Fernández-Fernández C, Castro-Quintela E. Insulin resistance is a cardiovascular risk factor in humans. Diabetes Metab Syndr. 2019;13(2):1449-55.
9. Won K-B, Park G-M, Lee S-E, Cho I-J, Kim HC, Lee BK et al. Relationship of insulin resistance estimated by triglyceride glucose index to arterial stiffness. Lipids Health Dis. 2018;17(1):268.
10. Wang L, Cong H-L, Zhang J-X, Hu Y-C, Wei A, Zhang Y-Y, et al. Triglyceride-glucose index predicts adverse cardiovascular events in patients with diabetes and acute coronary syndrome. Cardiovasc Diabetol. 2020;19(1):80.
11. Jin H-Y, Weir-McCall JR, Leipsic JA, Son J-W, Sellers SL, Shao M, et al. The relationship between coronary calcification and the natural history of coronary artery disease. JACC Cardiovasc Imaging. 2021;14(1):233-42.
12. Kamel SI, Redfield RL, Rajaram B, Anderson KM, Lev Y. Potential clinical impact of reporting breast arterial calcifications on screening mammograms in women without known coronary artery disease. Breast J. 2021;27(9):706-14.
13. Zuin M, Rigatelli G, Scaranello F, Ribecco SG, Picariello C, Zuliani G, et al. Breast arterial calcifications on mammography and coronary artery disease: A new screening tool for cardiovascular disease? Inter J Cardiol. 2016;220:310-1.
14. Arora S, Stouffer GA, Kucharska-Newton AM, Qamar A, Vaduganathan M, Pandey A, et al. Twenty year trends and sex differences in young adults hospitalized with acute myocardial infarction. Circulation. 2019;139(8):1047-56.
15. Gabet A, Danchin N, Juillière Y, Olié V. Acute coronary syndrome in women: rising hospitalizations in middle-aged French women, 2004-14. Eur Heart J. 2017;38(14):1060-5.
16. Pagidipati NJ, Hemal K, Coles A, Mark DB, Dolor RJ, Pellikka PA, et al. Sex differences in functional and CT angiography testing in patients with suspected coronary artery disease. J Am Coll Cardiol. 2016;67:2607-16.
17. Reynolds HR, Shaw LJ, Min JK, Spertus JA, Chaitman BR, Berman DS, et al.; ISCHEMIA Research Group. Association of sex with severity of coronary artery disease, ischemia, and symptom burden in patients with moderate or severe ischemia: Secondary analysis of the ISCHEMIA randomized clinical trial. JAMA Cardiol. 2020;5:773-86.
18. Mangion K, Adamson PD, Williams MC, Hunter A, Pawade T, Shah ASV, et al. Sex associations and computed tomography coronary angiography-guided management in patients with stable chest pain. Eur Heart J. 2020;41:1337-45.
19. Ong P, Athanasiadis A, Hill S, Vogelsberg H, Voehringer M, Sechtem U. Coronary artery spasm as a frequent cause of acute coronary syndrome: The CASPAR (Coronary Artery Spasm in Patients With Acute Coronary Syndrome) study. J Am Coll Cardiol. 2008;52(7):523-7.
20. Ong P, Athanasiadis A, Borgulya G, Vokshi I, Bastiaenen R, Kubik S, et al. Clinical usefulness,

angiographic characteristics, and safety evaluation of intracoronary acetylcholine provocation testing among 921 consecutive white patients with unobstructed coronary arteries. Circulation. 2014; 129(17):1723-30.
21. Teragawa H, Fukuda Y, Matsuda K, Hirao H, Higashi Y, Yamagata T, et al. Myocardial bridging increases the risk of coronary spasm. Clin Cardiol. 2003;26(8):377-83.
22. Levine GN, Cohen BE, Commodore-Mensah Y, Fleury J, Huffman JC, Khalid U, et al. Psychological health, well-being, and the mind-heart- Body connection: a scientific statement from the American Heart Association. Circulation. 2021;143:e763-83.

SECTION 8

Miscellaneous

Section Editors: Kunal Mahajan, J Cecily Mary Majella, Ankur Goyal

Associate Editors: Jai Bharat Sharma, Rahul Yadav, Surender Kumar, Suresh Kumar P, Raghothaman Sethumadhavan, Raagini Gupta, Nikita Sharma, Zoofi Shan, Muzammil Farooqi, Rabia Aggarwal, Khushi Goyal, Anshdeep Saluja, Harsh Kishore, Samman Verma, Akash Batta

ARTICLE 1

Gender Differences in Benefits of Empagliflozin in Patients with HFpEF

Butler J, Filippatos G, Siddiqi TJ, Ferreira JP, Brueckmann M, Bocchi E, et al. Effects of empagliflozin in women and men with heart failure and preserved ejection fraction.
Circulation. 2022;146(14):1046-55.

Abstract

Background: The study aimed to assess how gender impacts the response to empagliflozin treatment in patients with heart failure and preserved ejection fraction (HFpEF) enrolled in the EMPEROR-Preserved trial (Empagliflozin Outcome Trial in Patients With Chronic Heart Failure With Preserved Ejection Fraction). It aimed to explore potential differences in clinical characteristics between women and men and their respective therapeutic outcomes.

Methods: The primary outcome of this study was a combined endpoint of cardiovascular death or hospitalization for heart failure. Secondary outcomes included total heart failure hospitalization, cardiovascular and all-cause mortality, and scores from the Kansas City Cardiomyopathy Questionnaire. The comparison was conducted in the entire study population with subgroup analysis based on left ventricular ejection fraction. Additionally, the study examined the effects of empagliflozin on various physiological variables, such as changes in systolic blood pressure, uric acid, hemoglobin, body weight, and natriuretic peptide levels.

Results: Out of the total 5,988 patients, 2,676 (44.7%) were women. In the placebo group, women showed a tendency toward a lower risk of adverse outcomes, including a decreased risk of all-cause mortality [hazard ratio 0.69 (95% CI 0.56, 0.84)].

Empagliflozin, when compared to placebo, exhibited a similar reduction in the risk of cardiovascular death or hospitalization for heart failure in both men [hazard ratio 0.81 (95% CI 0.69, 0.96)] and women [hazard ratio 0.75 (95% CI 0.61, 0.92)], with no statistically significant interaction based on sex. Moreover, the relationship between empagliflozin and outcomes across different ejection fraction groups was not influenced by gender.

The study also found similar results for secondary outcomes and physiological measures. In both men and women, empagliflozin improved the Kansas City Cardiomyopathy Questionnaire

Clinical Summary Score to a comparable extent (1.38 for men vs. 1.63 for women at 52 weeks), with similar findings for the Kansas City Cardiomyopathy Questionnaire scores.

Conclusion: Empagliflozin yielded comparable advantages in terms of outcomes and health status for patients of both sexes diagnosed with HFpEF.

COMMENT

Women are more likely than men to be affected by heart failure and preserved ejection fraction (HFpEF). Despite having multiple comorbidities and symptoms, and having worse health-related quality of life as opposed to men, women with HFpEF have lower rates of heart failure hospitalizations and mortality.[1] This could be attributed to differences between men and women in the way their left ventricles remodel in response to end-diastolic stretch and age, resulting in smaller left ventricular volumes and higher left ventricular ejection fractions (LVEFs) in women. Women also demonstrate greater increases in left ventricular filling pressures to increased venous return and exhibit higher arterial stiffness. Additionally, women are more prone to epicardial and intramyocardial fat deposition, thus leading to increased adipocyte-associated inflammation.[2,3] These disparities suggest that the response to treatments for HFpEF may differ between the two sexes.

In the landmark trial demonstrating the benefit of sacubitril/valsartan in HFpEF, the PARAGON-HF trial (Efficacy and Safety of LCZ696 Compared to Valsartan, on Morbidity and Mortality in Heart Failure Patients With Preserved Ejection Fraction), it was seen that women receiving treatment with sacubitril/valsartan had significantly reduced risk of HF hospitalization but the improvement in health status was smaller.[4]

The EMPEROR-Preserved (Empagliflozin Outcome Trial in Patients With Chronic Heart Failure With Preserved Ejection Fraction) trial investigated the effects of the sodium-glucose cotransporter-2 inhibitor empagliflozin in patients diagnosed with HFpEF and a LVEF > 40%. The trial demonstrated a notable decrease in the risk of cardiovascular death or hospitalization due to heart failure in the empagliflozin-cohort. However, the sex differences of these outcomes were not reported. This study concluded that the benefits of empagliflozin were across the spectrum of patients with HFpEF, irrespective of sex and baseline LVEF (41–49%, 50–59%, and ≥60%). It showed that empagliflozin reduced the risk of the primary outcome of cardiovascular death or hospitalization for HF to a similar degree in both women and men. This benefit was also demonstrated on secondary outcomes (total HF hospitalizations, cardiovascular death, and all-cause mortality), physiological measures, and health status.

Clinical implications: It worthwhile to note that the benefit of empagliflozin is in contrast to sacubitril/valsartan, which seems to have a sex difference in its effect on patients with HFpEF. The clinical benefits of empagliflozin are consistent in both sexes, hence patients with HFpEF may be prescribed empagliflozin, irrespective of their sex.

ARTICLE 2

Sex Differences in Bleeding Events in Patients Receiving Aspirin and P2Y12 Inhibitor after Percutaneous Coronary Intervention for Acute Coronary Syndrome

Ten Haaf ME, van Geuns RJ, van der Linden MMJM, Smits PC, de Vries AG, Doevendans PA, et al. Sex-related bleeding risk in acute coronary syndrome patients receiving dual antiplatelet therapy with aspirin and a P2Y12 inhibitor. *Med Princ Pract. 2023;32(3):200-8.*

Abstract

Objective: This study aimed to evaluate the sex differences in bleeding events in patients receiving aspirin and a P2Y12 inhibitor after percutaneous coronary intervention (PCI) done for acute coronary syndrome (ACS).

Methods: This trial enrolled 1,172 women (median age 67.5 years) and 3,087 men (median age 62.2 years) with ACS/PCI receiving either prasugrel or clopidogrel between August, 2011 and June, 2013.

Results: In this trial, 52.6% of women and 66.9% of men received prasugrel as their primary P2Y12 inhibitor, along with aspirin. Women had more frequency of contraindications for prasugrel use than men (47.9% vs. 26.9%, $p < 0.001$) hence received clopidogrel. Femoral access was preferred for PCI in women compared to men (47.6% vs. 38.1%, $p < 0.001$). At the 1-year mark, women had a higher incidence of major bleeding than men (2.6% vs. 1.6%, $p = 0.018$). Female had a more than double risk of thrombolysis in myocardial infarction (TIMI) major bleeding (adjusted hazard ratio 2.33; 95% CI 1.26–4.32). These observations were derived after adjusting for established bleeding risk factors. This two-fold risk was also evident at discharge and was related to access-site bleedings (0.9% vs. 0.1%, $p < 0.001$). No significant sex differences were observed in major bleeding after 1-year follow-up.

Conclusion: Women with ACS undergoing PCI and on dual antiplatelet therapy (DAPT) are at an increased risk of bleeding as compared to men. This excess risk was attributable to access-site bleeding, especially with the femoral approach.

COMMENT

The use of both aspirin and a P2Y12 receptor antagonist is a fundamental approach in the contemporary management of acute coronary syndrome (ACS). The dual antiplatelet therapy (DAPT) with above two drugs effectively reduces the incidence of stent thrombosis; however, it increases the bleeding risk. Moreover, women who present with ACS are generally older and have a more unfavorable cardiovascular risk profile compared to men, thus, making them more susceptible to both thrombotic and bleeding events following PCI.[5,6]

Existing guidelines, primarily derived from randomized controlled trials (RCTs), do not offer gender-specific recommendations regarding the choice, dosage, and durations of antithrombotic regimens.[7] The RCTs forming the basis of these guidelines may not represent the real-world population as they have highly selected participants with a lower cardiac risk profile. Hence, this registry study including patients of daily life was planned to establish convincing evidence of sex-related differences.

What Does this Study Add?

This study added to the gender-specific evidence for the use of DAPT in patients with ACS/PCI. It showed that women had a higher occurrence of access-site TIMI major bleedings compared to men; however, no significant sex differences in bleedings were observed from the time of the procedure until the 1-year follow-up after adjusting for other bleeding risk factors. Additionally, there were no discernible disparities in ischemia-related outcomes between women and men, and overall event rates remained low.

The excess bleeding events in women may be due to their higher age and prevalence of other risk factors for bleeding. However, even after adjusting for these factors, the excess risk remained high among women. In this context, it is worth mentioning that the higher occurrence of bleeding complications in women was primarily due to femoral access-site bleeds. This is in line with existing evidence which shows higher numbers of access-site bleedings in women than in men.[8] This can be overcome by opting radial approach. It can be challenging in females due to small caliber of radial artery and increased vulnerability to spasm, thus limiting the efficacy of transradial PCI.[9] The results of this study indicate that radial access should be prioritized as the primary choice, even in women, whenever it is technically feasible. This is also in consensus with recent guidelines which advocate for radial access instead of femoral access in coronary angiography and PCI, particularly when performed by experienced operators.[5,6]

Inappropriate dosing of antithrombotic drugs, especially in women with lower body volume, is a risk factor for bleeding. It is imperative to give optimal dose of DAPT without reducing the anti-ischemic effect and lowering the bleeding risk.[10] This study revealed no association between body weight and bleeding risk in both men and women. Hence, it seems that the weight criterion is suitable and requires no adjustment.

Limitations: This registry study had a few limitations. There were limited number of bleeding events noted in this study hence it lacks sufficient statistical power to adequately establish relationship between gender and bleeding tendency. Secondly, the TIMI definition relies on the cause and timing of bleeding, but in practical terms, these aspects can be rather ambiguous. Thirdly, due to a limited sample, the effect of inappropriate dosing on bleeding cannot be thoroughly determined. Lastly, this registry reports data from a single country between 2011 and 2013, and the pharmacological options for ACS/PCI patients have evolved in the last decade, including use of newer P2Y12 inhibitors such as ticagrelor and direct-acting oral anticoagulants; thus, these observations may not accurately reflect current day practice in many countries.

ARTICLE 3

Gender Differences in Mortality Rate after Surgical Aortic Valve Replacement

Kang HU, Nam JS, Kim D, Kim K, Chin JH, Choi IC. Impact of Sex on Mortality in Patients Undergoing Surgical Aortic Valve Replacement.
J Pers Med. 2022;12(8):1203.

Abstract

Background: Aortic stenosis (AS) ranks as the second most prevalent valvular heart disease in the United States. While the occurrence of AS does not show significant variation between genders, there is debate surrounding whether sex differences influence the long-term mortality of patients with severe AS who undergo surgical aortic valve replacement (SAVR).

Methods: This study retrospectively analyzed the electronic medical record data of 917 patients [female, $n = 424$ (46.2%)] with severe AS who underwent isolated SAVR at a tertiary center in Korea between January 2005 and December 2018.

Results: Over a median follow-up period of 5.2 years, 74 male patients (15.0%) and 41 female patients (9.7%) passed away. The 10-year mortality rate was significantly higher in male patients compared to female patients (24.7% vs. 17.9%, $p = 0.005$). On evaluating the probability of long-term mortality 10 years after surgery, it was found that the adjusted hazard ratio for mortality in males was 1.93 (95% CI 1.28–2.91; $p = 0.002$). Subgroup analyses indicated that the association between male sex and long-term mortality after surgery remained significant, unaffected by any demographic or clinical factors.

Conclusion: Female patients with severe AS undergoing SAVR showed an improved long-term survival as opposed to male patients.

COMMENT

At present, aortic stenosis (AS) ranks as the second most prevalent valvular heart disease in the United States. It impacts approximately 12.4% of individuals aged over 75 years and its incidence tends to rise with increasing age.[11] While the occurrence of AS does not show sex-specific significant variation, there are differences between the sexes in terms of valvular anatomy and physiological response to ventricular pressure overload. Male hearts as opposed to female hearts typically exhibit increased fibrosis of the myocardium secondary to collagen deposition thereby leading to increased left ventricular volume, mass and mass/volume index. Female hearts on the other hand respond to pressure overload with concentric left ventricular hypertrophy, and less chamber dilation than male hearts, thus leading to delayed onset of AS symptoms.[12]

In contrast to the results of this trial females with severe AS have been considered to have a higher risk of mortality after SAVR than males because of older age, additional comorbidities, and higher frailty at diagnosis.[13] Even though the female patients in this study were also characterized by advanced age, elevated EuroSCORE II scores, lower preoperative hematocrit levels, and higher prevalence of concurrent conditions, including hypertension, heart failure, and cerebrovascular disorders, they still showed an improved long-term survival as opposed to male patients.

The impact of sex differences on the long-term mortality rate in severe AS patients undergoing SAVR continues to be uncertain and subject to controversy. Several studies have suggested that sex may not significantly affect the mortality of severe AS treated with SAVR.[13] In contrast, certain studies have found an association between female sex and a lower survival rate following SAVR and some also suggest that females have better outcomes after SAVR due to predisposition and hormonal factors.[14,15]

Limitations: This was a single-center retrospective study, hence has the risk of potential selection bias. The results of this study are limited to Korean population and could be a reflection of differences in the natural human lifespan between the sexes, with more life expectancy in females.

ARTICLE 4

Sex Differences in Outcomes after Single Antiplatelet Maintenance Therapy after Percutaneous Coronary Intervention

Shin ES, Jun EJ, Kim B, Won KB, Koo BK, Kang J, et al; HOST-EXAM Investigators. Association of clinical outcomes with sex in patients receiving chronic maintenance antiplatelet monotherapy after percutaneous coronary intervention: A post hoc gender analysis of the HOST-EXAM study.
J Am Heart Assoc. 2023;12(8):e026770.

Abstract

Background: The HOST-EXAM (Harmonizing Optimal Strategy for Treatment of Coronary Artery Stenosis–Extended Antiplatelet Monotherapy) trial concluded that single antiplatelet therapy (SAPT) with clopidogrel effectively reduces risk of adverse clinical events as opposed to SAPT with aspirin in patients undergoing percutaneous coronary intervention (PCI) with drug eluting stent (DES). The difference of gender on this result remains elusive.

Methods: This was a post hoc analysis of the HOST-EXAM trial. Patient who well tolerated dual antiplatelet therapy (DAPT) for 6–18 months post PCI without any significant adverse event were included. The primary endpoint of analysis was composite of all-cause mortality, nonfatal myocardial infarction, stroke, acute coronary syndrome, or Bleeding Academic Research Consortium (BARC) bleeding type ≥3 at 24 months post randomization. The bleeding endpoint was a BARC bleeding type 2 to 5.

Results: The primary endpoint was similar between males and females [adjusted hazard ratio (HR) 0.79 (95% CI 0.62–1.02); $p = 0.067$], and the bleeding end point [adjusted HR 0.79 (95% CI 0.54–1.17); $p = 0.240$] was also comparable. Male patients receiving SAPT with clopidogrel had lower risk of primary composite end point [adjusted HR 0.70 (95% CI 0.55–0.89); $p = 0.004$] and bleeding endpoint [adjusted HR 0.65 (95% CI 0.44–0.96); $p = 0.031$] as opposed to SAPT with aspirin. This difference was not there in female patients.

Conclusion: In men, clopidogrel monotherapy was superior to aspirin and there was significant reduction in the risk of the primary composite endpoint and bleeding events. However, in women, the favorable effect of clopidogrel over aspirin was diminished due to the higher all-cause mortality in clopidogrel monotherapy group.

COMMENT

Despite the availability of modern treatment options, aspirin continues to be the mainstay of choice for single antiplatelet therapy (SAPT) after percutaneous coronary intervention (PCI) with a drug eluting stent (DES) and clopidogrel has been considered as a second choice for patients who are unable to tolerate aspirin. HOST-EXAM (Harmonizing Optimal Strategy for Treatment of Coronary Artery Stenosis-Extended Antiplatelet Monotherapy) trial showed that SAPT with clopidogrel after dual antiplatelet therapy (DAPT) is associated with less mortality, nonfatal myocardial infarction (MI), stroke, readmission due to acute coronary syndrome (ACS), and Bleeding Academic Research Consortium (BARC) bleeding type ≥3 as compared to SAPT with aspirin.[16] Additionally, it is known that women are predisposed to ischemic and bleeding events after the early period of PCI as opposed to men.[17] However, the importance risk during the chronic maintenance period with SAPT remains unclear.

What Does this Study Add?

In this post hoc subgroup analysis, significant variations in baseline characteristics were noted between males and females. Women exhibited substantially older age and a higher prevalence of cardiovascular risk factors compared to men. Throughout the period of chronic maintenance SAPT after PCI with DES, there were no significant differences in the incidences of the primary composite endpoint and bleeding events between males and females. Even after accounting for baseline and procedural characteristics, the results remained consistent. It was concluded that in men, clopidogrel monotherapy was superior to aspirin and there was significant reduction in the risk of the primary composite endpoint and bleeding events. This benefit was not observed in female patients possibly due to low enrollment of women (25% of women in this trial). Instead, SAPT with clopidogrel was associated with significantly higher total mortality in women, and not in men. This may be due to their older age at baseline and increased prevalence of cardiovascular risk factors.

Further studies are warranted to investigate these findings and to formulate sex-specific recommendations for the choice of antiplatelet therapy in chronic maintenance period after PCI with a DES.

Limitations: This was a subgroup analysis, hence was predisposed to a few limitations. The randomization was not stratified according to the gender, and may have caused multiplicity and statistical error. The number of female participants in the trial was modestly low. There were substantial differences in age, presence of cardiovascular risk factors (diabetes, hypertension, or chronic kidney disease) at baseline in two groups. Hence, the subgroups were not individually powered to draw definitive conclusions. The results of this substudy are limited to the South Korean population included in the HOST-EXAM trial; thus, it may be difficult extrapolate these results to a broader population. Additionally, this study included patients who well tolerated DAPT for 6–18 months before the SAPT switchover; however, in real-world patients DAPT may be prescribed for a duration shorter than 6 months or may be associated with an adverse event within 6 months. The validity of these results in this subset of patients remains less clear.

ARTICLE 5

Sex Differences in Quality of Life of Heart Failure Patients

Tapia J, Basalo M, Enjuanes C, Calero E, José N, Ruíz M, et al. Psychosocial factors partially explain gender differences in health-related quality of life in heart failure patients.
ESC Heart Fail. 2023;10(2):1090-102.

Abstract

Background: The effect of gender on quality of life (QoL) in heart failure (HF) remains less researched. This study aimed to evaluate gender-specific differences in health-related QoL among real-world chronic HF patients and their psychosocial and clinical determinants.

Methods: This study was a single-center, observational, prospective cohort study that included 1,236 consecutive patients diagnosed with chronic HF. Demographic data and baseline characteristics were noted using a semi-structured questionnaire and Minnesota Living with Heart Failure Questionnaire (MLHFQ) was used to assess health-related QoL.

Results: Female patients with HF exhibited lower scores in global QoL compared to males. (MLHFQ overall summary score: 49 ± 23 vs. 43 ± 24; p value < 0.001, respectively). Additionally, females also had poorer scores in both physical and emotional dimensions. However, they scored better on the social dimension compared to males. On performing univariate analysis and multivariate analysis after adjusting for clinical determinants, females had worse global, physical and emotional QoL, and better social QoL compared with men. However, these differences were mitigated in multivariate analysis with adjustment for psychosocial determinants alone, or both psychosocial and clinical determinants.

Conclusion: This demonstrates that there is disparity in health-related QoL between men and women with chronic HF with women having worse QoL. It can be attributed to the interaction between both biological and psychosocial factors. Although, biological factors are important and evident, psychosocial factors also remain vital and need to be addressed.

COMMENT

Heart failure is a multifaceted clinical syndrome, and its burgeoning prevalence, mortality rates, and consumption of healthcare resources make it a significant concern for community health. The prevalence of heart failure (HF) in the general adult population is estimated to be around 1-2%, but this figure is likely underestimated and, is on the rise due to the aging population.[18] The 5-year survival rates have shown improvement, reaching 60%, although it remains notably higher compared to other chronic illnesses.[19] HF-related hospitalizations account for approximately 1-2% of all hospital admissions, and HF stands as the most frequent diagnosis in hospitalized patients over the age of 65 years.[20]

The primary objectives of chronic HF care revolve around improving the hard endpoints of mortality and hospitalization rates. However, soft targets which include patient reported outcomes play a vital role in the health-related quality of life (QoL) of a chronic HF patient. This health-related QoL is useful in assessment of patient perspective and is a predictor of both mortality and hospitalization. There have been disease-specific instruments designed to capture health-related QoL in different aspects including physical, emotional, social and global domains. They have been well recognized and are endorsed for use in routine practice by international institutions.[21]

The literature about gender-specific differences in QoL of patient with chronic HF is divided. While several studies have indicated women to have a poorer QoL compared to men, even after accounting for biological factors such as age, ejection fraction; and the New York Heart Association (NYHA) classification and others reported no major gender-based difference.[22] Psychosocial variations between males and females with chronic HF have also been documented. Most of these disparities tend to lead to unfavorable outcomes in women compared to men.[23]

In this study of chronic HF patients, conducted at a single center through observational and prospective analysis, it was shown that the disparity in health-related QoL between men and women might be partially attributed to the interaction of biological and psychosocial factors. While clinical factors predominantly influence QoL in HF patients, the contribution of psychosocial factors is crucial to comprehensively comprehend the role of gender.

Limitations: This study had intrinsic limitations of a single center cross sectional study design. Hence, it does not establish a causal relationship or a temporal association between changing determinants and health related QoL. The population studied included patients in a hospital setting and it may not be appropriate to generalize these findings to real-world HF patients. The participants included in this study were recruited between 2004 and 2014, almost a decade back. Numerous newer therapies for chronic HF have emerged since then, hence it is not prudent to generalize this data to current chronic HF patients.

ARTICLE 6

Gender Differences in Heart Failure Trends in China from 1990 to 2019

Peng X, Wang J, Li J, Li Y, Wang X, Liu X, et al. Gender-specific prevalence and trend of heart failure in China from 1990 to 2019.
ESC Heart Fail. 2023;10(3):1883-95.

Abstract

Background: Heart failure (HF) stands as a major contributor to the worldwide burden of morbidity and mortality. Nevertheless, the complete extent of the HF epidemic in China remains less understood. There is a lack of gender-specific registry data regarding the prevalence of HF. The current study's objective was to analyze the sex-specific prevalence and temporal trends of HF in China and evaluate the respective causes and risk factors.

Methods: Data from the Global Burden of Diseases, Injuries, and Risk Factors Study 2019, segmented by gender was used to assess the age-standardized prevalence and years lived with disability of HF. Joinpoint research models were used to derive temporal trend of HF and attributable risk factors from 1990 to 2019.

Results: There was a steady decline in the age-standardized prevalence rate of HF from 1,079.4 in 1990 to 1,032.8 per 100,000 individuals in 2019. The prevalence of HF had a steep rise since 2017, which more pronounced in females [annual percentage change (APC) of 2.72 for females and 0.61 for males, $p < 0.05$] and by 2019, there were more females with HF than males. The predominant cause of HF was hypertensive heart disease (42.65% of cases in females, 41.19% of cases in males).

Conclusion: Heart failure has shown a consistent decline over the past two decades, a noteworthy increase has been observed since 2017, particularly among females. Hypertensive heart disease has emerged as the primary cause of HF. Metabolic risk factors, especially elevated systolic pressure triggers the cascade of events that lead to HF; hence it is crucial to prioritize HF screening and implement measures to control these metabolic risk factors. Additionally, gender differences in HF prevalence should be taken into account when addressing these issues.

COMMENT

Heart failure (HF) is a highly prevalent condition with significant mortality and disability rates in both men and women. Studies have reported a gender disparity in the prevalence of HF, with males being at a higher risk.[24,25] Despite the decreasing HF incidence, this gender gap has steadily increased over recent years.[26]

This study showed that an increasing trend of HF prevalence, particularly in females [annual percent change (APC) of 2.72] and to a lesser extent in males (APC of 0.61) since 2017. By 2019, the age-standardized rate of HF prevalence in females exceeded that of males. Hypertensive heart disease (HHD) was predominant etiology of HF in both females

(42.65% of cases) and males (41.19% of cases). Uncontrolled high systolic blood pressure was shown to be major cause of HF-related HHD from 2017 to 2019, with an APC of 2.68 for females and 0.48 for males ($p < 0.05$).

The increasing prevalence of HF as demonstrated by this study coincides with the global trend. The prevalence HF in United States is expected to increase by 46% from 2012 to 2030, with increase in total HF patients to 3.0% from 2.4% of total population.[27] The etiology of HF has also dramatically changed in the last few decades. Rheumatic heart disease (RHD) was the leading cause of HF in the last century; however, now the prevalence has decreased from 34.4% in 1980 to 18.6% in 2000.[28] Currently, after ischemic heart disease (IHD), hypertension is the most common cardiovascular risk factor with high morbidity, low awareness, and control rate. Data from this study demonstrated that the most common cardiac-specific causes of HF were HHD (42.7% for females and 41.2% for males), followed by IHD, and RHD. This order was similar to previously published results; however, data from China indicates that IHD is the leading contributor to HF.[29]

Over the years, the cardiovascular risk factor profile has undergone rapid changes. Favorable improvements in the natural environment, lifestyles, and economy have significantly reduced China's HF burden associated with malnutrition and inadequate healthcare. However, with the aging population growing and unhealthy lifestyles prevailing, metabolic syndrome, including hypertension, high blood glucose, dyslipidemia, and high body mass index (BMI) have emerged as the major risk factors for HF.[30] Gender disparities in prevalence of these risk factors remains less addressed; however, due to their strong association with IHD, HHD, and eventually HF, it becomes crucial to investigate this gap.

Limitations: Due to the fact that the data used in the Global Burden of Disease Study 2019 (GBD 2019 study) were estimated from both published and unpublished sources, the prevalence of HF was indirectly measured, potentially leading to confounding in the data. A comprehensive analysis of phenotypes of HF was not done which would have beneficial for both clinicians and researchers. The annual percentage change model might be susceptible to ecological fallacies as the data were aggregated at the population level. Hence, to validate our findings, and further establish causal relationships and temporal trends, additional research is warranted.

ARTICLE 7

Gender Disparities after Transcatheter Aortic Valve Replacement with Newer-generation Transcatheter Heart Valves: A Systematic Review and Meta-analysis

Trongtorsak A, Thangjui S, Adhikari P, Shrestha B, Kewcharoen J, Navaravong L, et al. Gender disparities after transcatheter aortic valve replacement with newer generation transcatheter heart valves: A systematic review and meta-analysis.
Med Sci. 2023;11:33.

Abstract

Background: Transcatheter aortic valve replacement (TAVR) with early-generation transcatheter heart valves (THVs) in previous studies delineated gender disparity in mortality and vascular complications. This study was contemplated to determine if gender-related differences persisted with THVs of newer generation.

Aims and objective: The aim of this study was to assess gender differences after TAVR with newer-generation THVs.

Methods: The researchers thoroughly searched MEDLINE and Embase databases since beginning to April 2023 for identifying studies reporting gender-specific outcomes with newer-generation THVs (Sapien 3, Corevalve Evolut R, and Evolut Pro) implantation in TAVR. The major outcomes studied were 30-day mortality, 1-year mortality, and vascular complications.

Results: Five studies (four databases) were included which comprised of 47,933 patients (21,073 females and 26,860 males). Transfemoral approach for TAVR was used in 96% of patients. Higher 30-day mortality [odds ratio (OR) 1.53; 95% confidence interval (CI) 1.31–1.79; p-value < 0.001) and vascular complications (OR 1.43; 95% CI 1.23–1.65; $p < 0.001$) was observed in female patients. Nonetheless, both gender had similar 1-year mortality (OR 0.78; 95% CI 0.61–1.00; $p = 0.28$).

Conclusion: Although 1-year mortality was similar between the genders, 30-day mortality rates and vascular complications are still higher even with newer-generation THVs for TAVR. More research and innovations are warranted to improve outcomes of TAVR in females.

COMMENT

This first of its kind systematic review and meta-analysis for assessing gender disparity with newer generation of transcatheter heart valves (THVs) for transcatheter aortic valve replacement (TAVR) revealed higher risk of 30-day mortality and vascular complications. Despite higher rate adverse early outcomes, 1-year mortality showed no difference between genders. Several factors in development of newer-generation THVs have brought down complication rates such as sheath size decreasing vascular complications, outer skirt decreasing paravalvular leaks, higher implantation decreasing high-grade atrioventricular (AV) block, and concomitant cerebral protection for stroke reduction.[31-33] Nevertheless, gender disparity persists because of higher vascular complication ascribed to higher sheath-to-femoral artery ratio, greater technique difficulty due to anatomy, and root size. Higher 30-day mortality is possibly due to higher periprocedural bleed, vascular complications, pulmonary hypertension, greater wall thickness and smaller left ventricular (LV) cavity.[34] However, longer follow-up studies have shown better survival in females and are encouraging.

Impact of findings: Periprocedural complications reduction can have instrumental role in narrowing the gender-specific disparity in TAVR outcomes. Other than sheath size, better pre-procedural access-site planning, alternate site selection where appropriate and good closure may help. Peripheral artery disease and chronic kidney disease (CKD) are significant major factor predicting adverse outcome of TAVR in females.[35] Continuous innovations in THVs, technique and more research in understanding gender-specific challenges are required to narrow the gender difference in early outcomes after TAVR.

ARTICLE 8

Gender Differences in Atrial Fibrillation: From the Thromboembolic Risk to the Anticoagulant Treatment Response

Rago A, Pirozzi C, D'Andrea A, Di Micco P, Papa AA, D'Onofrio A, et al. Gender differences in atrial fibrillation: From the thromboembolic risk to the anticoagulant treatment response.
Medicina (Kaunas). 2023;59(2):254.

Abstract

Background: Atrial fibrillation (AF) is the most common sustained arrhythmia and has risk of thromboembolism. The female gender is an independent risk factor for thromboembolic events in atrial fibrillation. This review intends to learn gender disparities in cardioembolic risk and response to anticoagulation amidst AF patients.

Objective: The author aims to evaluate the gender-disparity in cardioembolic risk and anticoagulant response in patients with AF.

Materials and methods: The researcher reviewed the reports about gender difference and thromboembolic risk in AF in PubMed database.

Results: The gold standard treatment for thromboembolic risk prevention in nonvalvular AF patients is nonvitamin K oral anticoagulants (NOACs). There is similar rate of stroke and systemic embolism (SE) amidst men and women on NOACs and vitamin K antagonists (VKAs); however, there was lower risk of intracranial bleeding, major bleeding, and all-cause mortality in women compared to men.

Conclusion: The thromboembolic risk increases in female patients mainly in the presence of other factors and hence is an important risk modifier than a risk factor. There is need for appropriate and tailored anticoagulant therapy in AF patients; however, gender-specific efficacy and safety profile of NOACs and VKAs need further research.

COMMENT

Gender differences in atrial fibrillation (AF) epidemiology, pathophysiology, clinical presentation, outcomes, and therapeutic response have been well described in various studies. Women has higher risk of stroke than in men with multiple mechanisms like hormonal, electrical and structural characteristics explained in literature.[36] The gender-specific risk of stroke in females vary across age groups and hence CHA_2DS_2-VASc score came in practice for better prediction of stroke events. Nevertheless in women aged <65 years, evidence for gender-specific risk is unclear and hence the concept of risk modifier arose.[37] Females with AF have higher risk of heart failure, stroke, and mortality than male counterparts due to advanced age and presence of more comorbidities such as hypertension, diabetes, renal dysfunction, and prior stroke.[38] It is very intriguing to note that some authors have found that non vitamin K oral anticoagulants (NOACs) have similar overall efficacy, lesser risk of intracranial hemorrhage, or major bleeding and may balance the gender disparity in outcome.[39]

Impact of review: The researchers have put in great effort to highlight gender difference through the spectrum of AF in women. Nonetheless, the gaps in understanding the underlying mechanisms persist and further longitudinal studies evaluating prothrombotic state, genetic predisposition, sociocultural causes, gender differences in pharmacokinetics and pharmacodynamics of NOACs may add to our comprehension. A gender-sensitive tailored approach may be helpful in optimizing anticoagulant therapy in AF.

ARTICLE 9

Sex Differences in Characteristics, Outcomes, and Treatment Response with Dapagliflozin Across the Range of Ejection Fraction in Patients with Heart Failure: Insights from DAPA-HF and DELIVER

Wang X, Vaduganathan M, Claggett BL, Hegde SM, Pabon M, Kulac IJ, et al. Sex differences in characteristics, outcomes, and treatment response with dapagliflozin across the range of ejection fraction in patients with heart failure: Insights from DAPA-HF and DELIVER.
Circulation. 2023;147(8):624-34.

Abstract

Background: Gender is an effect modifier for heart failure (HF) therapies. Sodium-glucose cotransporter-2 inhibitors (SGLT-2Is) have proved to be essential pharmacotherapeutic agent across the spectrum of HF. However the gender disparity in treatment effect and safety profile of SGLT-2Is is still vague. The researchers aim to assess the effect of gender on safety and efficacy of dapagliflozin.

Methods: The researchers performed patient-level pool analysis of DAPA-HF (Dapagliflozin and Prevention of Adverse Outcomes in Heart Failure) and DELIVER (Dapagliflozin Evaluation to Improve the Lives of Patients With Preserved Ejection Fraction Heart Failure) trials. Gender differences in clinical outcomes were assessed. The primary outcome was a composite of worsening HF or cardiovascular death and secondary outcomes included cardiovascular death, all-cause death, HF hospitalization, urgent HF visits total events (first and recurrent HF hospitalization and cardiovascular death), and Kansas City Cardiomyopathy Questionnaire (KCCQ) scores across the range of left ventricular ejection fraction.

Results: In this analysis, there were 11,007 patient comprising 1,356 (35%) women. The female patients were older, with higher body mass index, higher prevalence of hypertension, and atrial fibrillation. Nonetheless, women had lower prevalence of diabetes and stroke or myocardial infarction. The baseline ejection fraction was higher in women and KCCQ score was worse. Women had lesser cardiovascular death [adjusted hazard ratio 0.69 (95% CI 0.60–0.79)], all-cause death [adjusted hazard ratio 0.69 (95% CI 0.62–0.78)], HF hospitalizations [adjusted hazard ratio 0.82 (95% CI 0.72–0.94)], and total events [adjusted rate ratio 0.77 (95% CI 0.71–0.84)] than men after adjusting for baseline differences. Primary endpoints were reduced by dapagliflozin similarly in both men and women (p interaction = 0.77). There were no gender differences in secondary outcome (all p interaction > 0.35) as well as safety events. The patients in the entire spectrum of ejection fraction were benefitted with dapagliflozin with no gender-related effect modification (p interaction > 0.40). Neither there were gender-related differences in serious adverse events and adverse events nor adverse reactions leading to drug discontinuation.

Conclusion: Gender did not modify the effect of dapagliflozin across the spectrum of ejection fraction. There was similar benefit of dapagliflozin in DAPA HF and DELIVER trial, irrespective of gender.

COMMENT

Female gender as effect modifier in response to heart failure (HF) pharmacotherapies has recently been reported wherein women appear to derive more benefit from neurohormonal modulators (namely angiotensin receptor blockers, mineralocorticoid receptor antagonists, and angiotensin receptor-neprilysin inhibitors) across a wider HF ejection fraction (EF) range compared with men.[40] This patient-level pooled meta-analysis of DAPA-HF (Dapagliflozin and Prevention of Adverse Outcomes in Heart Failure) and DELIVER (Dapagliflozin Evaluation to Improve the Lives of Patients With Preserved Ejection Fraction Heart Failure) trials delineates that both genders across the range of EF-derived homogenous benefits from dapagliflozin in HF. Dapagliflozin not only reduced the primary composite outcome of cardiovascular (CV) death or a worsening HF event, but also reduced all-cause death, total events and improved KCCQ (Kansas City Cardiomyopathy Questionnaire) scores, irrespective of gender. Furthermore, dapagliflozin had similar safety profile compared with placebo in both genders in these two trials. These findings are also consistent with other sodium-glucose cotransporter-2 inhibitors (SGLT-2Is), suggesting that it is a class effect for these drugs.

Impact of findings: Definitely, the results of this analysis are comforting and reassuring to female patients and physicians alike that benefits of dapagliflozin have been explored in women and men and gender did not modify the effect of dapagliflozin or empagliflozin on outcomes.[41] This consistency will not only enhance our data but also further reinforce support to the American Heart Association (AHA)/American College of Cardiology (ACC)/ Heart Failure Society of America (HFSA) guidelines, indicating a class effect of SGLT-2 inhibitors across the spectrum of EF in HF.

ARTICLE 10

Gender Differences in Acute Aortic Dissection

Bossone E, Carbone A, Eagle KA. Gender differences in acute aortic dissection.
J Pers Med. 2022;12(7):1148.

Abstract

Objective: The main aim of this study is to evaluate the gender difference in acute aortic dissection. Gender differences in both type A and type B acute aortic dissection were analyzed.

Methods: Statistics from various studies and Registries were analyzed for gender differences in etiology, risk factors, clinical presentation, diagnosis and management of acute aortic dissection.

Results: The incidence of acute aortic dissection in population-based studies is 2.6–3.5 cases per 100,000 person-years (67% type A; 33% type B). Women were affected less frequently than men in most of the studies and Registries (31–48% vs. 52–69%). In terms of numbers, men are involved more than women (9.1 vs. 5.4 per 100,000 men and women, respectively; $p < 0.001$). Women were older by about 6–7 years than men at the time of diagnosis. However, Chinese study does not show gender difference in age at presentation. In German Registry for Acute Aortic Dissection Type A (GERAADA), women were older than men (65.5 ± 12.7 vs. 59.2 ± 13.3 years; $p < 0.001$) but the incidence is lesser than men. The involvement of abdomen aorta in acute aortic dissection was more in men than in women (43% vs. 39%; $p = 0.01$). Renal and visceral malperfusion were higher in men than women (38.5% vs. 32.8% $p = 0.001$). Aortic root replacement was less frequent in women (21.6% vs. 17.7%; $p < 0.001$). Aortic arch repairs were equal in both sexes. The incidence of neurological events such as hemiparesis and hemiplegia after surgery were equal among men and women (women 11.5% vs. men 10.1%; $p = 0.240$). In Nordic Consortium for Acute Type A Aortic Dissection (NORCAAD), women contributed 32% of acute aortic dissection and were older by 5 years. Women were more hypertensive than men (58% vs. 48%; $p = 0.001$) and had chronic obstructive pulmonary disease (COPD) and less body mass index (26 ± 5 vs. 27 ± 4 kg/m^2; $p < 0.001$). Intraoperative mortality and 30-day death were equal among both the gender (women 9.1% vs. men 6.7%; $p = 0.17$). In the meta-analysis of about nine studies, the in-hospital and 30-day mortality was similar between women and men ($p = 0.67$). The incidence of dialysis and postsurgical stoke were equal in both gender. Women had lower risk of reintervention for bleeding (RR 0.84; 95% CI 0.75–0.94; $p < 0.01$).

Only few studies had compared the gender difference in type B acute aortic dissection. Women contributed about 43.6% in women in study by Liang et al. Women presented at later age and were managed medically than men (87.4% vs. 81.8%; $p < 0.001$). In-hospital mortality [OR 0.91; 95% confidence interval (CI) 0.79–1.00; $p = 0\,0.2$] and stroke (OR 0.91; 95% CI 0.51–1.57; $p = 0.7$) did not differ significantly between men and women. Women are less prone to acute kidney injury (OR 0.68; 95% CI 0.60–0.70; $p < 0.001$) but more prone for cardiac events during procedure (OR 1.45; 95% CI 1.01–2.11; $p = 0.04$). Takahashi et al. analyzed patients with type B acute aortic dissection. In this study, women represented 29.3%, were older, and presented later in life. Intramural hematomas were more common in women (63.7% vs. 53.7%, $p < 0.001$).

Conclusion: A comprehensive understanding of gender differences in AAD is lacking. For both type A and B AAD, women, at the time of diagnosis, are older than men and complain less frequently about abrupt onset of pain, with delayed presentation to the emergency department. In type A AAD, women less frequent surgical treatment. In type B AAD, no significant differences are registered for in-hospital mortality between the two genders.

COMMENT

Acute aortic dissection is dangerous disease with high mortality. The mortality is reduced when compared to olden days. The gender difference in acute aortic dissection is less discussed in major guidelines and studies. Overall, the incidence of acute aortic dissection is low among the women compared to men.[42,43] The age at which the women presents are older than men by about 6–7 years.[44] However, Chinese study does not shows gender difference in age at presentation.[45] This shows demographic difference in the presentation of acute aortic dissection. Indian studies are needed to establish the gender difference in acute aortic dissection. Women had chronic obstructive pulmonary disease (COPD), hypertension than men.[46] Men were obese than women. Intraoperative mortality and 30-day mortality are equal between both genders in spite of older presentation of women. However, when only type A aortic dissection is considered women had higher mortality than men. This increase in mortality may be due to older presentation of women. Postoperative complications such as stroke, need for dialysis was equal among the genders.

Since the symptoms are nonspecific, usually diagnosis of acute aortic dissection is delayed and sometimes missed which is more common in women. Imaging modalities, particularly computer tomography, are used in the diagnosis of acute aortic dissection. In India, access to computer tomography is limited which once again leads to missing the diagnosis of acute aortic dissection. High index of suspicion is needed to diagnose acute aortic dissection in women. Once diagnosis is made, immediate treatment saves the life. In Type A acute aortic dissection, an emergency surgery is indicated whereas medical management is of choice in type B acute aortic dissection, which are not complicated. In complicated type B dissection, the management is thoracic endovascular repair (TAVER). Blood pressure control of below 120/80 mm Hg and heart rate below 60 bpm are the crux of medical management for both genders.

More studies are needed to increase our knowledge about the gender difference in clinical presentation, diagnosis, and management of acute aortic dissection. This may lead to increase in diagnostic accuracy and reduction in morbidity and mortality due acute aortic dissection.

ARTICLE 11

Sex and Gender Differences in the use of Oral Anticoagulants for Non-valvular Atrial Fibrillation: A Population-based Cohort Study in Primary Health Care in Catalonia

Giner-Soriano M, Prat-Vallverdú O, Ouchi D, Vilaplana-Carnerero C, Rosa M. Sex and gender differences in the use of oral anticoagulants for non-valvular atrial fibrillation: A population-based cohort study in primary health care in Catalonia.
Front Pharmacol. 2023;14:1110036.

Abstract

Objectives: This study aimed to describe the sex and gender differences in the treatment initiation and in the sociodemographic and clinical characteristics of all patients initiated on an oral anticoagulant (OAC), and the sex and gender differences in prescribed doses and adherence and persistence to the treatment of those receiving direct oral anticoagulants (DOAC).

Material and methods

Study design: This study was a population-based cohort study including adults with nonvalvular atrial fibrillation (NVAF) who initiated OAC treatment.

Inclusion criteria: They included all individuals who were ≥18 years-old with an active diagnosis of NVAF registered in electronic records who initiated treatment with OAC from January 2011 to December 2020. Patients were followed-up from the day one up to death, disenrollment from the database, end of treatment or end of study period.

Exclusion criteria: In this study, they excluded people with valvular AF and people using DOAC for indications other than NVAF: Those diagnosed with pulmonary embolism or deep vein thrombosis (DVT) during the previous 12 months to the OAC initiation, and those receiving OAC for surgical prophylaxis of hip or knee replacement during the last 6 months.

Data source: The data source is the Information System for Research in Primary Care (SIDIAP).[47]

Variables: The variables assessed at baseline were—socioeconomic characteristics, bad habits, comorbidities, body mass index (BMI), CHA_2DS_2-VASc (score C; congestive heart failure, H; hypertension, A2; age ≥75 years, D; diabetes, S2; prior stroke, V; vascular disease, A; age 65–75 years, Sc: sex category),[48] HAS-BLED (Hypertension, Abnormal renal/liver function, Stroke, Bleeding history, Labile INR, Elderly, Drugs/alcohol).

Drug exposure: Patients with NVAF were considered as new user or naïve patient if they started a new OAC prescription during the study period (2011–2020). If they had received any other OAC in the prior 12 months, different to the prescription given now, they were defined as prevalent users or non-naïve patients.

Those people receiving the full dose were defined as "overdosed", and those receiving the reduced dose were defined as "underdosed."

Discontinuation was defined as no dispensing of OAC during >2 months after having initiated treatment.

Adherence was measured by Medication Possession Ratio (MPR), which is the quotient between the drug amount dispensed and the drug amount prescribed. A patient was considered adherent to the treatment when medication possession ratio (MPR) ≥ 80%.

Statistical analysis: The baseline characteristics of the cohort in the study were described as relative and absolute frequencies for categorical variables and with mean and standard deviation (SD) or median and interquartile range (IQR) for quantitative variables. They performed a bivariate analysis across genders using the Chi-square test for categorical data and the Kaplan–Meier curves to estimate the mean survival time for time to event variables.

The smooth algorithm was used to model the drug exposure. All statistical analyses were conducted with R software.

Results: During the study period, 123,250 people with NVAF were initiated on OAC treatment; 57,832 (46.9%) of them were women and 65,418 (53.1%) were men **(Flowchart 1)**. Most patients (94.3% women and 94.5% men) were new users, and the OAC prescribed was Vitamin K antagonist (VKA) in 62.4% of patients. Patients were followed-up during a mean of 45.6 months (SD 31.5); 45.7 months for women and 45.4 for men ($p = 0.143$).

Women in the study were older than men, had higher BMI, and worse kidney function, whereas men were more frequently smokers and drinkers. HAS-BLED score—there were more men than women with scores 0–1 and more women than men with scores ≥2. Cancer, diabetes, ischemic heart disease/previous stroke were more frequent in men, while dyslipidemia and hypertension were more frequent in women.

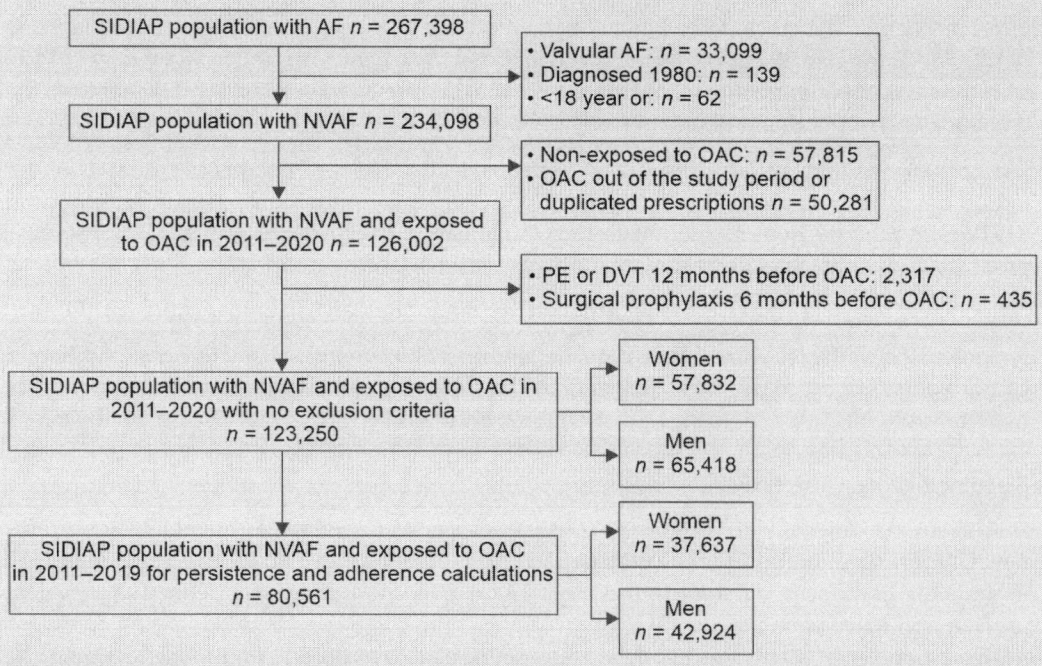

FLOWCHART 1: Flowdiagram of population included.
(AF: atrial fibrillation; DVT: deep venous thrombosis; NVAF: nonvalvular AF; OAC: oral anticoagulant; PE: pulmonary embolism; SIDIAP: Information System for Research in Primary Care)

Women who were initiated on DOAC had a mean CHA_2DS_2-VASc score of 3.9 (SD 1.4) and men 2.6 (1.6), whereas it was 3.9 (1.2) in women and 2.7 (1.4) in men initiating VKA. In **Figure 1**, we see that 87.6% of women had a CHA_2DS_2-VASc score ≥ 3, and there were 12.4% of women with a score ≤2 receiving OAC treatment. Apixaban showed the highest frequency of women with score ≥3 (90.3%) and dabigatran, the lowest (82%). CHA_2DS_2-VASc score was lower in men; 79.4% of men had CHA_2DS_2-VASc ≥ 2 and 20.6%, <2. Also, apixaban had the highest percentage of men with high stroke risk (82.5%) and dabigatran the lowest (69.5%).

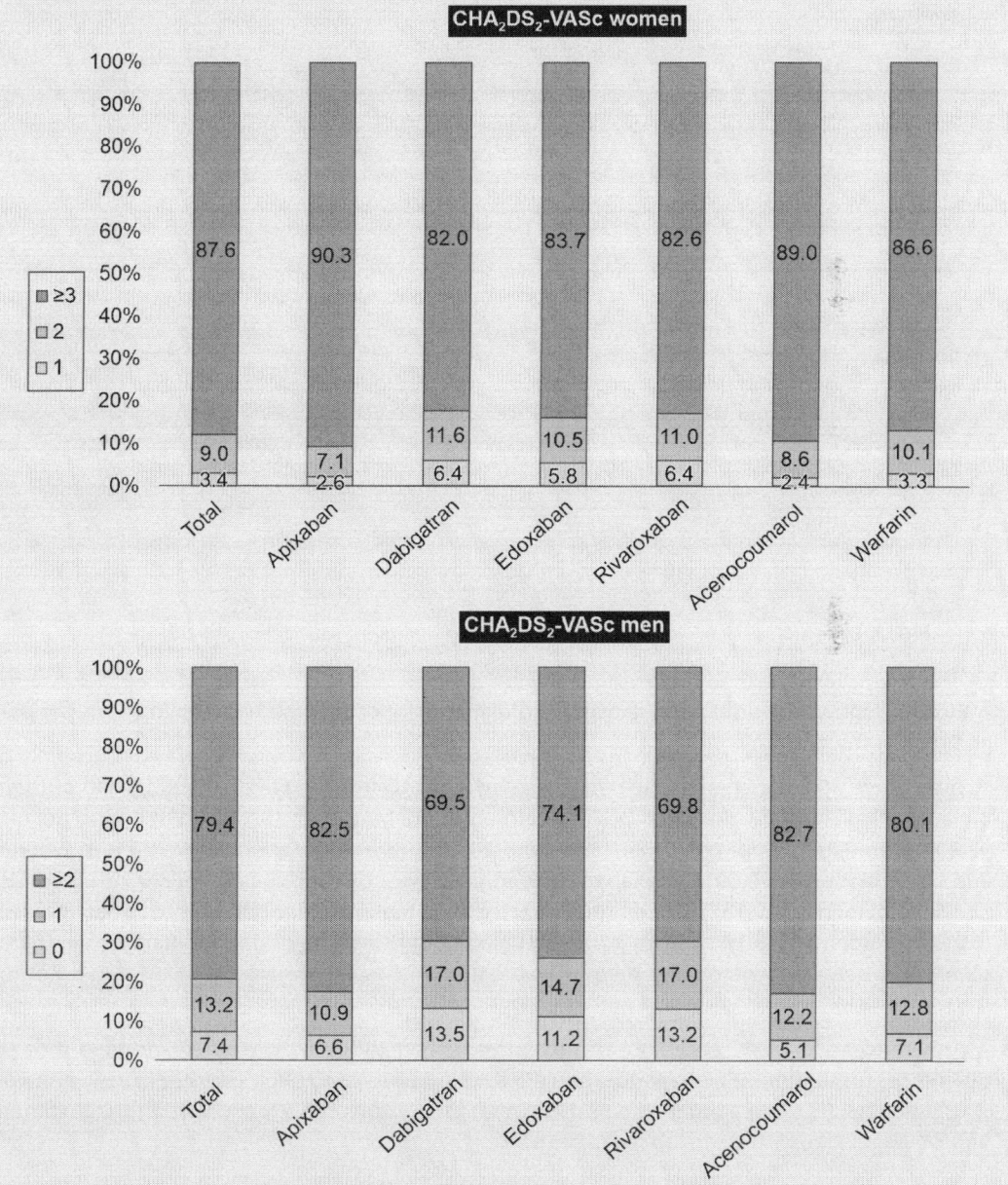

FIG. 1: Baseline CHA_2DS_2-VASc in women and men treated with oral anticoagulants.

The **Figure 1** shows the CHA_2DS_2-VASc scores in all women receiving anticoagulants and by substance: 1, 2, and ≥3.

Regarding the dose adequacy, women were more frequently underdosed than men for all DOAC, except for edoxaban ($p = 0.355$), apixaban being the DOAC with the highest frequency of underdosing; 39% of women and 27.4% of men ($p < 0.001$) were receiving a reduced dose. Men were more frequently overdosed than women, **(Fig. 2)**.

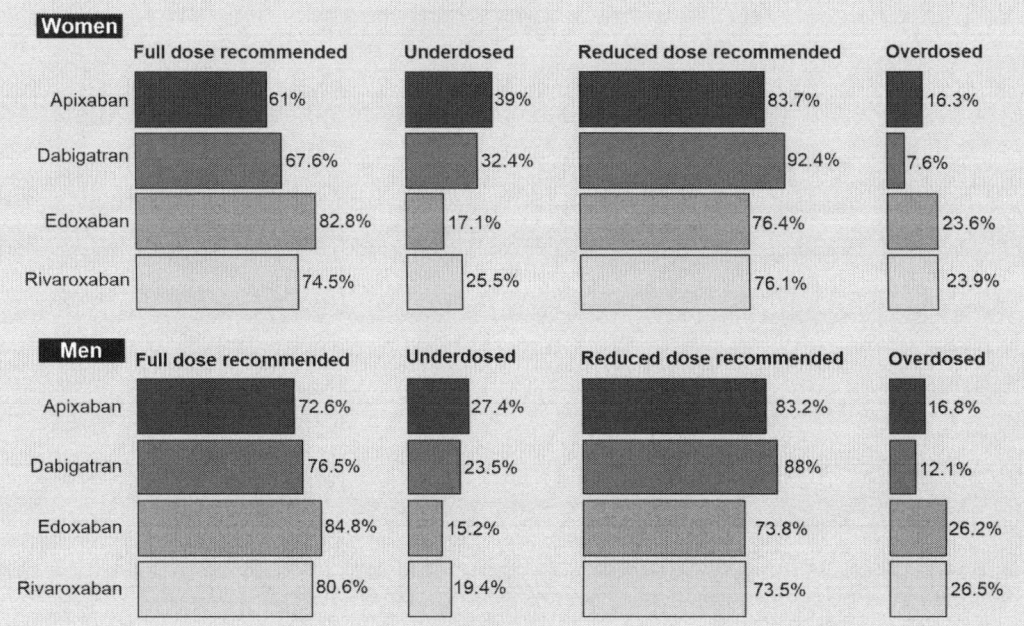

FIG. 2: Dose adequacy in women and men initiating treatment with direct oral anticoagulants.

Figure 2 shows the dose adequacy for all direct oral anticoagulants, women at the upper part and men at the bottom.

There were 80,561 patients who were initiated on OAC from 2011–2019 and 28,840 of them initiated DOAC. Men discontinued DOAC treatment more frequently than women during the first year after initiation. Dabigatran had the highest frequency of discontinuation (8.7% in women and 11.4% in men, $p < 0.001$). Edoxaban showed the lowest discontinuation rate (5.2% in women and 6.9% in men, $p = 0.106$). Discontinuations for apixaban were not different between genders (6.2% in women and 6.3% in men, $p = 0.901$). Regarding the time of discontinuation, we found differences between women and men for dabigatran (4.4 vs. 4.7 months, $p = 0.014$), but not for the rest of DOAC.

Adherence to all DOAC was high, as most patients had MPR ≥ 80%. Women and men showed differences for treatment with rivaroxaban (85.8% vs. 83.8%; $p = 0.006$). The other DOAC showed no differences; 83.6% in women and 82.4% in men for apixaban, 85.9% and 86.7% for dabigatran, and 84.9% and 85.3% for edoxaban **(Table 1)**.

TABLE 1: Discontinuation and adherence to direct oral anticoagulants.

n (%)	Apixaban				Dabigatran				Edoxaban				Rivaroxaban			
	Overall	Women	Men	p-value	Overall	Women	Men	p-value	Overall	Women	Men	p-value	Overall	Women	Men	p-value
All DOAC n = 28,840	n = 10,184	n = 4,931 (48.4)	n = 5,253 (51.6)		n = 6,123	n = 2,539 (41.5)	n = 3,584 (58.5)		n = 3,233	n = 1,535 (47.5)	n = 1,698 (52.5)		n = 9,300	n = 4,117 (44.3)	n = 5,183 (55.7)	
1st year discontinuation	635 (6.2)	305 (6.2)	330 (6.3)	0.901	629 (10.3)	221 (8.7)	408 (11.4)	0.001	197 (6.1)	80 (5.2)	117 (6.9)	0.106	803 (8.6)	328 (8.0)	475 (9.2)	0.038
Months to discontinuation	—	—	—	0.695	—	—	—	0.014	—	—	—	0.324	—	—	—	0.155
Mean (SD)	5.0 (3.1)	5.0 (3.1)	5.0 (3.1)		4.6 (2.8)	4.4 (2.8)	4.7 (2.8)		5.0 (2.9)	4.5 (2.7)	5.4 (3.1)		4.6 (2.9)	4.5 (2.9)	4.7 (2.8)	
Median (IQR)	4.1 (2.3–7.2)	4.0 (2.3–7.0)	4.2 (2.3–7.4)		3.9 (2.2–6.5)	3.5 (1.9–6.4)	4.2 (2.4–6.5)		4.2 (2.7–6.9)	3.7 (2.6–6.1)	4.7 (3.1–7.6)		3.8 (2.2–6.3)	3.6 (2.0–5.9)	4.0 (2.3–6.5)	
MPR	—	—	—	0.142	—	—	—	0.104	—	—	—	0.708	—	—	—	0.006
≥80% (adherent)	8,451 (83.0)	4,124 (83.6)	4,327 (82.4)		5,257 (85.9)	2202 (86.7)	3,055 (85.2)		2,745 (84.9)	1309 (85.3)	1,436 (84.6)		7375 (84.7)	3,532 (85.8)	4,343 (83.8)	
<80% (nonadherent)	1,733 (17.0)	807 (16.4)	926 (17.6)		866 (14.1)	337 (13.3)	529 (14.8)		488 (15.1)	585 (14.2)	262 (15.4)		1,425 (15.3)	585 (14.2)	8–10 (162)	

Note: p-values for the comparison between genders. Chi-square test for categorical variables, and Kaplan–Meier curves to compare the restricted mean survival time to discontinuation (in months).
(IQR: interquartile range; MPR: medication possession ratio; SD: standard deviation)

Discussion: This study had analyzed 10–years data on OAC use for stroke prevention in NVAF in a PHC database in Catalonia, Spain. They found an increasing number of NVAF diagnoses over time, which obviously increased the number of people treated with OAC. Their study also showed a progressive increase in the number of DOAC initiations and a decrease in VKA-DOAC account for >50% of the OAC initiations in NVAF.

There were more men in this study, as they are more frequently affected by AF.[49] Calderon et al. 2022,[50] reported more men with the disease but women with higher CHA_2DS_2-VASc, as in our study. Loikas et al. 2017,[51] also found that from 2011 to 2015 the number of women receiving OAC increased, except in older than 80 years, who were anticoagulated less frequently than in 2011.

We found that women were more frequently underdosed than men with all DOAC, even though they have a higher risk of stroke and the use of lower doses than recommended can presumably result in an increased rate of events.[52] They postulated that underdosing could have been due to insufficient knowledge or lack of confidence in the appropriate dose, or due to fear of the prescribers of causing harm, such as bleeding, as women present higher frequency and severity of such adverse drug reactions than men. Also, prescribers might be more concerned for bleeding risk than for stroke risk, as overdosing was less frequent.

Limitations and strengths: This study has some limitations inherent to database studies, such as missing variables, potential confounders or the lack of register of sex and gender variables.

Rather, this study has some strengths as the large number of persons included, the representativeness of the general population, complete records, long follow-up periods, and real-world data.

COMMENT

Atrial fibrillation (AF) is the most common form of chronic arrhythmia, affecting 2–3% of the population in Europe and USA.[53] It is associated with several cardiovascular complications, and it increases the risk of stroke. Men are more often affected by AF, although women have a higher risk of being affected with stroke.[48] To prevent stroke in non-valvular atrial fibrillation (NVAF), oral anticoagulants (OAC) are usually prescribed; vitamin K antagonists (VKA) have been used for years and recently, direct oral anticoagulants (DOAC) were introduced.

Considering the lack of information on gender differences in NVAF, and as sex and gender affect to all aspects of health and disease, it becomes necessary to carry out studies with gender perspective, paving way to reduce health inequalities.

This study found a high frequency of underdosing in women in compared to men. Adherence was generally high, only with higher levels in women for rivaroxaban. Persistence during the first year of treatment was also high in general, being significantly more in women than men in the case of dabigatran and edoxaban. Dose inadequacy, lack of adherence and persistence can result in less effective and safe treatments.

In the Indian perspective, we also find underdosing more common in women than men. Though this study showed more persistence to treatment with women, in our country, we encounter that more women do not persist with treatment due to socioeconomic issues.

As disease and outcomes are equal in both men and women, it is high time that we undertake such study in India to analyze the ground reality and to make amendments to improve the health care of women who are the backbone of our country.

ARTICLE 12

Maternal and Fetal Outcomes in Pregnant Patients with Mechanical and Bioprosthetic Heart Valves

Ng AP, Verma A, Sanaiha Y, Williamson CG, Afshar Y, Benharash P. Maternal and fetal outcomes in pregnant patients with mechanical and bioprosthetic heart valves.
J Am Heart Assoc. 2023;12(10):e028653.

Abstract

The purpose of this study was to determine the relationship between prosthetic valve type and maternal and fetal outcomes in pregnant patients. Author identified all adult patients hospitalized for delivery with prior heart valve implants using the 2008 to 2019 National Inpatient Sample. The primary outcome; significant adverse cardiovascular events; and secondary outcomes such as maternal and fetal problems, duration of stay, and expenses were all studied using multivariable regressions. Mechanical heart valves (MHVs) were found in 4,152 of the 39,871,862 birth hospitalizations, while biologic heart valves (BHVs) were found in 874.

Age, comorbidities, and cesarean birth rates were comparable across MHV and BHV patients. The presence of a prosthetic valve was linked with a >22-fold increase in the likelihood of significant adverse cardiovascular events [MHV: adjusted odds ratio, 22.1 (95% CI 17.3–28.2); BHV: adjusted odds ratio, 22.5 (95% CI 13.9–36.5)], as well as an increase in hospitalization time and expenses. However, there was no significant difference in the likelihood of any maternal outcome, including severe adverse cardiovascular events, hypertensive illness of pregnancy, and ante/postpartum hemorrhage, between individuals with MHVs and BHVs. Similarly, prenatal problems were more common in individuals who had valve prostheses, including a four-fold increase in the risks of stillbirth, but were comparable between MHVs and BHVs.

COMMENT

- When compared to those without a prosthetic valve, pregnant women with prior heart valve replacement are at a higher risk of significant adverse cardiovascular events, as well as increased length of stay and costs.
- The risks of poor maternal and fetal outcomes such as ante/postpartum hemorrhage, congenital abnormalities, and stillbirth are comparable with mechanical and bioprosthetic heart valves.

What are the Clinical Consequences?
- The presence of a valve prosthesis, regardless of form, increases the risk of unfavorable maternal and fetal events during delivery.
- Individuals who have had a previous valve replacement and become pregnant require specialists and multidisciplinary cardio-obstetrics care during labor and delivery.
- For patients of reproductive age with valvular heart disease, preconception counseling can assist guided shared decision-making and optimizes treatment options.

ARTICLE 13

Validation of Risk Stratification for Cardiac Events in Pregnant Women with Valvular Heart Disease

Pande SN, Suriya Y, Ganapathy S, Pillai AA, Satheesh S, Mondal N, et al. Validation of risk stratification for cardiac events in pregnant women with valvular heart disease.
J Am Coll Cardiol. 2023;82(14):1395-406.

Abstract

The majority of risk assessment algorithms for pregnant patients with heart disease was created in high-income countries and in populations with mostly congenital heart disease, and hence may not be applicable to people with valvular heart disease (VHD). From January 2019 through April 2022, the study included successive pregnancies complicated by VHD admitted to a tertiary center in a middle-income environment. The DEVI and CARPREG-II models were used to calculate individual risk for unfavorable composite cardiac events. The goal of this study was to validate and establish the clinical utility of two-risk stratification tools for predicting adverse cardiac events in pregnant VHD patients: DEVI (VHD-specific tool) and CARPREG-II. In 577 eligible pregnancies, 69 (12.1%) had a component of the composite result.

The majority of cases (94.7%) had rheumatic etiology, with mitral regurgitation being the most common lesion (48.2%). The DEVI models had an area under the receiver-operating characteristic curve of 0.884 (95% CI 0.844–0.923) and the CARPREG-II models had an area under the receiver-operating characteristic curve of 0.808 (95% CI 0.753–0.863). Calibration plots revealed that the DEVI score overestimates risk at higher probability, whereas the CARPREG-II score overestimates risk at both extremes while underestimating risk in the mean. Decision curve research revealed that both models were useful for projected probability thresholds ranging from 10 to 50%. The study concluded that pregnant women with VHD, DEVI, and CARPREG-II scores demonstrated high discriminative ability and clinical value across a wide range of probabilities. The DEVI score demonstrated higher agreement between expected and observed probability.

COMMENT

This prospective study focuses on risk stratification for pregnant women with valvular heart disease (VHD), particularly in middle-income countries, addressing a major issue in maternal health. Pregnant patients with cardiac disease were thoroughly assessed at the first antenatal appointment to establish baseline readings, then every 2 weeks until 32 weeks and weekly until birth. Patients deemed at risk were monitored by a multidisciplinary team of obstetricians and cardiologists until the fifth postpartum day.

Cardiac disease is a diverse set of congenital and acquired heart abnormalities that is a primary cause of pregnancy-related mortality and morbidity in both high- and low-to-middle-income countries (LMICs).

During the study period, there were 41,947 births, with 892 (2.1%) occurring in patients with heart illness. 577 (62.7%) of these pregnancies occurred in 512 people with VHD and were included in the analysis. Only 27 (5.3%) had congenital cardiac disease. Many VHD patients (145; 28.4%)

were diagnosed while pregnant. Heart failure was the most common adverse event ($n = 52$; 9.0%), with the majority (69.0%) occurring during the prenatal period. Arrhythmias necessitating treatment occurred in 25 (4.3%) of the patients. There were two occurrences of stroke and two cases of infective endocarditis.

There were 3 (1.8%) maternal deaths during the study period, 2 among those with mechanical heart valves (1 each from valve thrombosis and refractory supraventricular arrhythmia), and the third was secondary to infective endocarditis in a patient with severe mitral regurgitation. In relation to risk-stratification in pregnant patients with primarily rheumatic VHD in a middle-income country, the DEVI and CARPREG-II scores aid in correctly classifying those who develop adverse cardiac outcomes during pregnancy and childbirth (discrimination).

ARTICLE 14

Pregnancy Outcomes in Women with Heart Disease: The Madras Medical College Pregnancy and Cardiac (M-PAC) Registry from India

Paul GJ, Princy SA, Anju S, Anita S, Mary MC, Gnanavelu G. Pregnancy outcomes in women with heart disease: The Madras Medical College Pregnancy and Cardiac (M-PAC) Registry from India.
Eur Heart J. 2023;44(17):1530-40.

Abstract

This study aimed to assess the fetomaternal outcomes, determine predictors of adverse outcomes, and evaluate the applicability of the modified World Health Organization (mWHO) classification in pregnant women with heart disease (PWWHD) in Tamil Nadu, India. A total of 1,005 pregnant women (meanage: 26.04 ± 4.2) with 1,029 consecutive pregnancies were enrolled in the Madras Medical College Pregnancy and Cardiac (M-PAC) registry from July 2016 to December 2019. The majority (60.5%) were diagnosed with heart disease during pregnancy, with rheumatic heart disease being the most common (42%). Key outcomes included maternal mortality, composite maternal cardiac events (MCEs), fetal loss, and composite adverse fetal events (AFEs). Maternal mortality was 1.9%, with the highest rates observed in patients with prosthetic heart valves (8.6%). Left ventricular systolic dysfunction, prosthetic heart valves, severe mitral stenosis, pulmonary hypertension, and current pregnancy diagnosis of heart disease were identified as independent predictors of MCEs. The mWHO classification showed good predictive ability for MCEs and maternal death. Live births were observed in 91.2% of pregnancies, while 33.7% reported AFEs. In conclusion, maternal mortality is elevated in PWWHD in India, particularly in those with prosthetic heart valves, pulmonary hypertension, and left ventricular systolic dysfunction. The mWHO classification may need further adaptation and validation for risk stratification in the Indianpopulation.

Conclusion: This study underscores the high maternal mortality in PWWHD in India, with notable risks associated with specific cardiac conditions. The findings emphasize the importance of early detection and management of heart disease in pregnancy. The mWHO classification demonstrated promising predictive accuracy, but its suitability for the Indian population requires additional refinement and validation. Overall, the study provides valuable insights into the complex interplay between cardiac health and pregnancy outcomes, offering a foundation for further research and improvements in risk stratification strategies for this vulnerable population.

COMMENT

In this prospective study conducted in Tamil Nadu, India, 1,005 pregnant women with heart disease (PWWHD) were enrolled from 2016 to 2019. Of these, 60.5% were diagnosed with heart disease for the first time during pregnancy, and rheumatic heart disease was the most common type (42%). Pulmonary hypertension was present in 34.2% of cases. The primary outcomes assessed were maternal mortality and composite maternal cardiac events (MCEs), with secondary outcomes including fetal loss and adverse fetal events (AFEs). Maternal mortality was 1.9%, with the highest rates observed in patients with prosthetic heart valves (8.6%). Heart failure was the most common MCE, occurring in 15.2% of pregnancies. Independent predictors of MCE included left ventricular systolic dysfunction, prosthetic heart valves, severe mitral stenosis, pulmonary hypertension, and current pregnancy diagnosis of heart disease. The modified World Health Organization (mWHO) classification demonstrated good predictive ability for MCEs and maternal death. However, the study suggests that further adaptation and validation of this classification may be needed for the Indian population. Overall, the findings highlight a high maternal mortality rate in PWWHD in India, emphasizing the importance of tailored risk stratification and management strategies.

ARTICLE 15

2023 HRS Expert Consensus Statement on the Management of Arrhythmias During Pregnancy

Joglar JA, Kapa S, Saarel EV, Dubin AM, Gorenek B, Hameed AB, et al. 2023 HRS expert consensus statement on the management of arrhythmias during pregnancy.
Heart Rhythm. 2023;20(10):e175-264.

Abstract

This international multidisciplinary expert consensus statement aimed to act as comprehensive guidance that can be referenced to cardiac electrophysiologists, cardiologists, and other healthcare professionals on the management of cardiac arrhythmias in pregnant patients and in fetuses. This document covers general concepts related to arrhythmias, including both brady- and tachyarrhythmias in both the patient and the fetus during pregnancy.

Conclusion: This study underscores the high maternal mortality in PWWHD in India, with notable risks associated with specific cardiac conditions. The findings emphasize the importance

COMMENT

Sinus arrhythmia, supraventricular tachycardia, and premature beats are among the most prevalent benign arrhythmias seen in pregnant patients; in contrast, life-threatening arrhythmias like hemodynamically significant supraventricular tachycardia or ventricular tachycardia are much less frequent. The most frequent sustained arrhythmia that is newly identified during pregnancy is atrial fibrillation. A patient's hemodynamic tolerance and underlying substrate should be taken into consideration while making some therapeutic options for atrial fibrillation such as which rate control technique to use versus which rhythm control strategy to use. Other decisions such as anticoagulant medication protocols are unique to pregnancy. To improve outcomes for both the mother and the fetus/newborn, care for arrhythmias in pregnant patients should involve a multidisciplinary team of cardiologists and/or electrophysiologists, pediatric electrophysiologists, maternal–fetal medicine subspecialists, anesthesiologists, and neonatologists. Any concurrent maternal diagnoses or arrhythmias should be taken into account when making judgments about fetal arrhythmia care (e.g., fetal bradycardia in women with long QT syndrome). Typically, maternal systemic administration of antiarrhythmic agents is used to treat fetal arrhythmias. Occasionally, however, such as in cases of fetal hydrops, direct intramuscular or intraperitoneal injection of antiarrhythmic medications into the fetus may be required. The prompt application of the most effective therapy (cardioversion, antiarrhythmic drug infusion, or catheter ablation) to end the current arrhythmia and/or prevent recurrent arrhythmias should be emphasized in the management of hemodynamically significant maternal arrhythmias, along with appropriate fetal monitoring and steps to minimize radiation exposure when catheter ablation is pursued. At skilled facilities, procedures such as catheter ablation and implantable devices can be carried out with the greatest possible mitigation of radiation exposure to the fetus, which is best achieved by overall reduction of total maternal radiation, since covering the maternal abdomen with a lead apron alone is typically of no benefit. Due to the overall risk of aortocaval compression, these procedures are generally not recommended. For the sake of the safety of the fetus, antiarrhythmic medication use during pregnancy and the postpartum period should largely follow practices used in non-pregnant patients, with a few exceptions: choosing medications with the longest track records of safe use during pregnancy and lactation; using the lowest effective dose; and periodically re-evaluating the need for the same dose/type of antiarrhythmic, including during the postpartum period. To evaluate potential fetal hazards and to optimize treatment, genetic screening and counseling should be given to parents who have an inherited arrhythmia syndrome that is suspected or known, ideally by genetic counselors or physicians who are trained or specialize in genetics.

ARTICLE 16

2023 ESH Guidelines for the Management of Arterial Hypertension The Task Force for the Management of Arterial Hypertension of the European Society of Hypertension Endorsed by the International Society of Hypertension (ISH) and the European Renal Association (ERA)

Mancia G, Kreutz R, Brunström M, Burnier M, Grassi G, Januszewicz A, et al. 2023 ESH Guidelines for the management of arterial hypertension The Task Force for the management of arterial hypertension of the European Society of Hypertension: Endorsed by the International Society of Hypertension (ISH) and the European Renal Association (ERA). *J Hypertens. 2023;41(12):1874-2071.*

Abstract

The 2023 ESH guidelines aim to summarize the best available evidence for all aspects of hypertension management including defining criteria, pathophysiology and various aspects of management. The guidelines were developed by a Task Force of 59 experts representing the areas of internal medicine, cardiology, nephrology, endocrinology, general medicine, geriatrics, pharmacology, and epidemiology. The guidelines pay specific attention to gender based differences in various parameters of arterial hypertension.

COMMENT

The European Society of Hypertension (ESH) recently published guidelines for the management of arterial hypertension in the year 2013 which have focused on various gender-related aspects of hypertension. As per the guidelines, there are many gender-related differences that have an impact on the pathophysiology, epidemiology, and clinical management of hypertension.

The worldwide age-standardized prevalence of hypertension was 32% in women and 34% in men in 2019. Hypertension prevalence increases with age in both sexes, but it tends to be lower in premenopausal women than in men of the same age, with a marked rise in women after menopause. After the age of 65 years, the prevalence of hypertension in females exceeds that of male individuals. These can be explained by the contribution of estrogens in lowering blood pressure (BP) through various mechanisms including endothelial vasodilatation via upregulation of the nitric oxide pathway and inhibition of the activity of sympathetic nervous system (SNS) and renin–angiotensin system (RAS).

As per the IDACO (International Database on Ambulatory BP in Relation to Cardiovascular Outcomes) study, the absolute cardiovascular risk was lower in women than in men, while the increase in risk associated with 24-hour and night-time BP was steeper in women than in men. Thus, women may have a higher proportion of potentially preventable events by management of hypertension.

Also, according to a meta-analysis including 27,542 individuals (54% females), the increased risk for cardiovascular (CV) events, including myocardial infarction, heart failure (HF), and stroke, was found to be associated with systolic BP (SBP) elevations at lower SBP ranges in females than in male patients, suggesting that the definition of optimal SBP might differ between men and women. As per the INTERHEART study, the increased risk of myocardial infarction associated with hypertension was greater in older females than in male patients.

It was also found that left ventricular hypertrophy (LVH) is more prevalent and less modifiable by antihypertensive treatment in women than in men. A stronger association was found between an elevated SBP and incident atrial fibrillation (AF) in female than in male patients in a Norwegian study, but this finding has not been consistently confirmed by other studies.

There is also evidence that the impact of hypertension on kidney function and disease progression may have a sex-dependent component. The prevalence of albuminuria was lower in postmenopausal female individuals than in male individuals. Recent studies also suggest that stroke risk starts to increase at a lower BP in female patients. Hypertension also seems to be a stronger risk factor for dementia and cognitive decline in female individuals.

The management of hypertension whether it be non-pharmacological or pharmacological interventions is influenced by the gender of the patients. Non-pharmacological interventions such as lifestyle modifications form the cornerstone in the management of hypertension, and sex differences in their effects have been noted. According to the findings of the DASH trial, dietary sodium restriction induced pronounced BP reductions only in female individuals. Regarding physical activity, a meta-analysis of 93 trials found that exercise induced a greater BP reduction in male than in female participants.

Regarding drug therapy, there are no established differences in pharmacokinetics of antihypertensive drugs between women and men including differences in body weight and body composition among both sexes. However, women have a 50% greater risk of adverse reactions compared to men from antihypertensive drugs, e.g., angiotensin-converting enzyme (ACE) inhibitors-induced cough and calcium channel blocker (CCB)-induced ankle edema. There is no consistent data on sex differences in the efficacy of antihypertensive drugs. Therefore, drug selection and dosing should not be based on the sex.

ARTICLE 17

Sex-based Differences in Risk Factors for Incident Myocardial Infarction and Stroke in the UK Biobank

Remfry E, Ardissino M, McCracken C, Szabo L, Neubauer S, Harvey NC, et al. Sex-based differences in risk factors for incident myocardial infarction and stroke in the UK Biobank.
Eur Heart J Qual Care Clin Outcomes. 2023:qcad029.

Objective: This prospective study aimed to characterize and understand the differences in risk factors between men and women with respect to incident cardiovascular events in the UK Biobank cohort.

Materials and methods: From the UK Biobank Cohort (which recruited more than 500,000 patients aged 40–69 years from 2006 to 2010), people with risk factors known to be causative in stroke and myocardial infarction (MI) were included. The factors included: Age, ethnicity, body mass index (BMI), Townsend deprivation index, systolic and diastolic blood pressure, waist and hip circumference, waist-to-hip ratio (WHR), dyslipidemia, apolipoprotein A (ApoA), apolipoprotein B (ApoB), glycated hemoglobin (HbA1c), smoking, diabetes, and hypertension. Arterial compliance vis-a-vis arterial stiffness index (ASI) and aortic distensibility (AD) were also characterized. The primary outcomes were incident stroke and MI for each sex. Multivariable Cox proportional hazard regression models were utilized to obtain hazard ratios (HR) and 95% confidence intervals (CI). HR between men and women were compared. Incidence rates of MI and stroke per 1,000 person years by sex were calculated using Poisson regression.

Results: A total of 363,605 patients (53.8% females) were followed up for a mean of 12.66 (11.93–13.38) years. The median age was 58 years in both males and females. A total of 8,470 cases of MI (29% in women) and 7,705 cases of stroke (40.1% in women) were recorded. The unadjusted crude incidence rate of MI and stroke per 1,000 person years was 3.04 (95% CI 2.99–3.11) and 2.30 (95% CI 2.24–2.37) for men, and 1.06 (95% CI 1.02–1.10) and 1.30 (95% CI 1.26–1.35) for women, respectively. It was notable that nonconventional risk factors including ApoA and LDL-C were more strongly associated with incident cardiovascular outcomes in males while conventional risk factors such as older age, current smoking, socioeconomic deprivation, and hypertension had a higher HR for females. Arterial compliance showed a higher-baseline risk in males, and a steeper age-associated increase in risk for females. Anthropometric measurements (BMI, WHR) did not have a significant difference in HR between the sexes.

Conclusion: Both MI and stroke were more common in men. Smoking, lower socioeconomic status, hypertension, and increasing age were more strongly associated with cardiovascular events in females. Dyslipidemia and ApoA had a more potent association in males.

COMMENT

What was Known Prior to this Study?

Cardiovascular disease (CVD) is the most common cause of death in India and worldwide, leading to an age-standardized death rate of 272 per 100,000 population in India.[54] There is a persistent misconception that CVD is a men's disease. Acute coronary syndrome (ACS) is the most common cause of death in women, and CVD causes more deaths in women than breast cancer and other cancers combined.[54,55] including its accelerated buildup, the early age of disease onset in the population, and the high case fatality rate. In India, the epidemiological transition from predominantly infectious disease conditions to noncommunicable diseases has occurred over a rather brief period of time. Premature mortality in terms of years of life lost because of CVD in India increased by 59%, from 23.2 million (1990 Atypical presentations of ACS are known to occur more commonly in women and may lead to a delay in diagnosis and treatment. Thus, identifying women-specific risk factors is essential in controlling CVD.

Hypertension is known to be a major risk factor for CVD in women.[56] Almost 1 in 5 women in the reproductive age in the United States of America have hypertension.[56] Smoking, diabetes, and high LDL-C (low-density lipoprotein cholesterol) have also been shown to increase risk of CVD in women.[57] Women-specific risk factors such as early menarche, late menopause, polycystic ovarian syndromes, and complicated pregnancies have also been shown to increase CVD risk.[57] However, this data is not absolute. The INTERHEART and INTERSTROKE studies showed that smoking causes less population attributable risk, while dyslipidemia, diabetes, hypertension, and waist–hip ratio (WHR) were more significantly associated with CVD in women.[58] Nonconventional risk factors have not been studied comprehensively, especially in terms of gender differences. There was, therefore, a need to properly assess the sex-specific risk factors for CVD, which this study aimed to fulfill.

What this Study Adds?

This study included over 3.6 lakh people, 53.8% of whom were females. It was a prospective study with a mean follow-up of 12.66 years. The study reiterated the fact that CVD is more common in males than females, with 71% of myocardial infarction (MI) and 59.9% of stroke occurring in the former. LDL-C and ApoA had a higher hazard ratio in men. HDL-C (high-density lipoprotein cholesterol) was inversely associated with MI risk in men but had a paradoxical direct association with stroke risk. This was likely because of the increased apolipoprotein A (ApoA), and was neutralized when ApoA was accounted for. Age had a higher association with incident events in females. This was fortified by the arterial compliance measures, which showed both an increased basic risk in men, and a rapid increase in risk in women with age. Smoking, particularly current smoking, conferred a higher risk of CVD in women. Hypertension was associated with a higher risk of MI, but not stroke, in females. A lower socioeconomic status also led to a higher risk of cardiovascular events in females. Anthropometric measurements were not significantly different across the sexes, in contradiction to some previous studies.

Major strengths of the study: The main strength of the study was its large study population, and a gratuitous follow-up period. The study included both conventional as well as newer risk factors such as LDL-C and ApoA and examined their sex-specific significance. The use of arterial compliance measures also fortified the age-related cardiovascular event associations. Standardized disease codes also helped in proper follow-up. Incident cardiovascular events also occurred in a quantity sufficient for statistical analysis.

Limitations of the study: Almost 95% of the study population was White. As such the applicability of the results to other ethnicities is questionable. The socioeconomic status (as derived from the Townsend deprivation index) was better than the average status of England, leading to potential bias and underrepresentation of females of lower socioeconomic status which are a known vulnerable subset. Smoking status was self-reported, which could be inaccurate. Lipid parameters were unavailable in close to 5% of the population, which could affect the final outcomes. Women-specific risk factors such as pregnancy-induced hypertension (PIH), gestational diabetes mellitus (GDM), and polycystic ovarian syndrome (PCOS) were not assessed.

Implications of the findings for clinicians: To some extent, CVD is a preventable disease. Identifying the risk factors and correcting them before they translate into CVD is important in community-health building. Studies such as INTERHEART have already established important risk factors for the development of CVD.[58] This study shows the importance of smoking, hypertension, and increasing age as causative agents of CVD in women. In India, as per the National Family Healthy Surveys, the use of smokeless tobacco is high in females, and thus, it needs to be ascertained and addressed during the index patient visit.[58]

Knowledge gaps and scope for future research: Pregnancy with its associated complications (PIH, GDM) and the long-term clinical outcomes has not been studied adequately. Similarly, other risk factors exclusive to women including early menarche, late menopause, and PCOS also need to be comprehensively assessed for their association with CVD. Further, comparison of risk factors in pre- and postmenopausal women who develop CVD also warrants investigation.

The clinical profile of women who do develop MI also needs to be addressed. While atypical presentations are common, characterization of these presentations, and their association with any particular risk factor should be tested. Similarly, sex-specific angiographic profile and post angioplasty long-term clinical outcomes, especially in ACS patients are yet to be established. It may be fruitful that a large-scale study addressing these issues, or a further post-hoc analysis of this study itself, can answer these pending questions.

REFERENCES

1. Scantlebury DC, Borlaug BA. Why are women more likely than men to develop heart failure with preserved ejection fraction? Curr Opin Cardiol. 2011;26:562-8.
2. Gori M, Lam CSP, Gupta DK, Santos AB, Cheng S, Shah AM, et al.; PARAMOUNT Investigators. Sex-specific cardiovascular structure and function in heart failure with preserved ejection fraction. Eur J Heart Fail. 2014;16:535-42.
3. Beale AL, Nanayakkara S, Segan L, Mariani JA, Maeder MT, van Empel V, et al. Sex differences in heart failure with preserved ejection fraction pathophysiology: a detailed invasive hemodynamic and echocardiographic analysis. JACC Heart Fail. 2019;7:239-49.
4. McMurray JJV, Jackson AM, Lam CSP, Redfield MM, Anand IS, et al. Effects of sacubitril-valsartan versus valsartan in women compared with men with heart failure and preserved ejection fraction. Circulation. 2020;141:338-51.
5. Collet JP, Thiele H, Barbato E, Barthélémy O, Bauersachs J, Bhatt DL, et al. ESC Guidelines for the management of acute coronary syndromes in patients presenting without persistent ST-segment elevation. Eur Heart J. 2021;42:1289-367.
6. Ibanez B, James S, Agewall S, Antunes MJ, Bucciarelli-Ducci C, Bueno H, et al. 2017 ESC Guidelines for the management of acute myocardial infarction in patients presenting with ST-segment elevation: the Task Force for the management of acute myocardial infarction in patients presenting with ST-segment elevation of the European Society of Cardiology (ESC). Eur Heart J. 2018;39(2):119-77.
7. Schreuder MM, Badal R, Boersma E, Kavousi M, Roos-Hesselink J, Versmissen J, et al. Efficacy and safety of high potent P2Y(12) inhibitors Prasugrel and Ticagrelor in patients with coronary heart disease treated with dual antiplatelet therapy: a sex-specific systematic review and meta-analysis. J Am Heart Assoc. 2020;9(4):e014457.
8. Ndrepepa G, Schulz S, Neumann FJ, Byrne RA, Hoppmann P, Cassese S, et al. Bleeding after percutaneous coronary intervention in women and men matched for age, body mass index, and type of antithrombotic therapy. Am Heart J. 2013;166(3):534-40.
9. Pandie S, Mehta SR, Cantor WJ, Cheema AN, Gao P, Madan M, et al. Radial versus femoral access for coronary angiography/intervention in women with acute coronary syndromes: insights from the RIVAL Trial (Radial vs. femorAL access for coronary intervention). JACC Cardiovasc Interv. 2015;8(4):505-12.

10. Alexander KP, Chen AY, Newby LK, Schwartz JB, Redberg RF, Hochman JS, et al. Sex differences in major bleeding with glycoprotein IIb/IIIa inhibitors: results from the CRUSADE (Can Rapid risk stratification of Unstable angina patients Suppress ADverse outcomes with Early implementation of the ACC/AHA guidelines) initiative. Circulation. 2006;114(13):1380-7.

11. Osnabrugge RL, Mylotte D, Head SJ, Van Mieghem NM, Nkomo VT, LeReun CM, et al. Aortic stenosis in the elderly: Disease prevalence and number of candidates for transcatheter aortic valve replacement: A meta-analysis and modeling study. J Am Coll Cardiol 2013;62:1002-12.

12. Dobson LE, Fairbairn TA, Plein S, Greenwood JP. Sex differences in aortic stenosis and outcome following surgical and transcatheter aortic valve replacement. J. Womens Health. 2015;24:986-95.

13. Hartzell M, Malhotra R, Yared K, Rosenfield HR, Walker JD, Wood MJ. Effect of gender on treatment and outcomes in severe aortic stenosis. Am J Cardiol. 2011;107(11):1681-6.

14. Chaker Z, Badhwar V, Alqahtani F, Aljohani S, Zack CJ, Holmes DR, et al. Sex differences in the utilization and outcomes of surgical aortic valve replacement for severe aortic stenosis. J Am Heart Assoc. 2017;6:e006370.

15. Kulik A, Lam BK, Rubens FD, Hendry PJ, Masters RG, et al. Gender differences in the long-term outcomes after valve replacement surgery. Heart. 2009;95:318-26.

16. Koo BK, Kang J, Park KW, Rhee TM, Yang HM, Won KB, et al. Aspirin versus clopidogrel for chronic maintenance monotherapy after percutaneous coronary intervention (HOST-EXAM): an investigator-initiated, prospective, randomised, open-label, multicentre trial. Lancet. 2021;397:2487-96.

17. Yu J, Mehran R, Grinfeld L, Xu K, Nikolsky E, Brodie BR, et al. Sex-based differences in bleeding and long term adverse events after percutaneous coronary intervention for acute myocardial infarction: three year results from the HORIZONS-AMI trial. Catheter Cardiovasc Interv. 2015;85:359-68.

18. Conrad N, Judge A, Tran J, Mohseni H, Hedgecott D, Crespillo AP, et al. Temporal trends and patterns in heart failure incidence: a population-based study of 4 million individuals. Lancet. 2018;391:572-80.

19. Jones NR, Roalfe AK, Adoki I, Hobbs FR, Taylor CJ. Survival of patients with chronic heart failure in the community: a systematic review and meta-analysis. Eur J Heart Fail. 2019;21:1306-25.

20. Alla F, Zannad F, Filippatos G. Epidemiology of acute heart failure syndromes. Heart Fail Rev. 2007;12:91-5.

21. Anker SD, Agewall S, Borggrefe M, Calvert M, Caro JJ, Cowie MR, et al. The importance of patient-reported outcomes: a call for their comprehensive integration in cardiovascular clinical trials. Eur Heart J Oxford Univ Press. 2014;35:2001-9.

22. Walsh MN, Jessup M, Lindenfeld J. Women with heart failure: unheard, untreated, and unstudied. J Am Coll Cardiol. 2019;73:41-3.

23. Lam CSP, Arnott C, Beale AL, Chandramouli C, Hilfiker-Kleiner D, Kaye DM, et al. Sex differences in heart failure. Eur Heart J Oxford Univ Press. 2019;40:3859-68.

24. Magnussen C, Niiranen TJ, Ojeda FM, Gianfagna F, Blankenberg S, Vartiainen E, et al. Sex-specific epidemiology of heart failure risk and mortality in Europe: results from the BiomarCaRE Consortium. JACC: Heart Fail. 2019;7:204-13

25. Pandey A, Omar W, Ayers C, LaMonte M, Klein L, Allen NB, et al. Sex and race differences in lifetime risk of heart failure with preserved ejection fraction and heart failure with reduced ejection fraction. Circulation. 2018;137:1814-23.

26. Conrad N, Judge A, Tran J, Mohseni H, Hedgecott D, Crespillo AP, et al. Temporal trends and patterns in heart failure incidence: a population-based study of 4 million individuals. The Lancet. 2018;391:572-80.

27. Tsao CW, Aday AW, Almarzooq ZI, Alonso A, Beaton AZ, Bittencourt MS, et al. Heart disease and stroke statistics—2022 update: a report from the American Heart Association. Circulation. 2022;145:e153-639

28. Cheng K, Wu N. Retrospective investigation of hospitalized patients with heart failure in some parts of China in 1980, 1990 and 2000. Chin J Cardiol. 2002;8:5-9.

29. Yin Q, Zhao Y, Li J, Xue Q, Wu X, Gao L, et al. The coexistence of multiple cardiovascular diseases is an independent predictor of the 30-day mortality of hospitalized patients with congestive heart failure: a study in Beijing. Clin Cardiol. 2011;34: 442-6.

30. Ma L-Y, Chen WW, Gao RL, Liu LS, Zhu ML, Wang YJ, et al. China cardiovascular diseases report 2018: an updated summary. J Geriatric Cardiol. 2020;17:1.

31. Toggweiler S, Gurvitch R, Leipsic J, Wood DA, Willson AB, Binder RK, et al. Percutaneous aortic valve replacement: Vascular outcomes with a fully percutaneous procedure. J Am Coll Cardiol. 2012;59:113-8.

32. Pibarot P, Hahn RT, Weissman NJ, Arsenault M, Beaudoin J, Bernier M, Dahou A, et al. Association of paravalvular regurgitation with 1-year outcomes after transcatheter aortic valve replacement with the SAPIEN 3 valve. JAMA Cardiol. 2017:2:1208-16.

33. De Torres-Alba F, Kaleschke G, Diller GP, Vormbrock J, Orwat S, Radke R, et al. Changes in the Pacemaker Rate After Transition from Edwards SAPIEN XT to SAPIEN 3 Transcatheter Aortic Valve Implantation: The Critical Role of Valve Implantation Height. JACC Cardiovasc Interv. 2016;9(8):805-13.
34. Alushi B, Beckhoff F, Leistner D, Franz M, Reinthaler M, Stähli B.E et al. Pulmonary hypertension in patients with severe aortic stenosis: prognostic impact after transcatheter aortic valve replacement: pulmonary hypertension in patients undergoing TAVR JACC Cardiovasc Imaging. 2019;12:591-601.
35. Denegri A, Romano M, Petronio AS, Angelillis M, Giannini C, Fiorina C, et al. Gender differences after transcatheter aortic valve replacement (TAVR): Insights from the Italian Clinical service project. J Cardiovasc Dev Dis. 2021;8(9):114.
36. Ko D, Rahman F, Schnabel RB, Yin X, Benjamin EJ, Christophersen IE. Atrial fibrillation in women: epidemiology, pathophysiology, presentation, and prognosis. Nat Rev Cardiol. 2016;13(6):321-32.
37. Friberg L, Skeppholm M, Terént A. Benefit of anticoagulation unlikely in patients with atrial fibrillation and a CHA_2DS_2-VASc Score of 1. J Am Coll Cardiol. 2015;65:225-32.
38. Dagres N, Nieuwlaat R, Vardas PE, Andresen D, Lévy S, Cobbe S, et al. Gender-Related Differences in Presentation, Treatment, and Outcome of Patients with Atrial Fibrillation in Europe: A Report from the Euro Heart Survey on Atrial Fibrillation. J Am Coll Cardiol. 2007;49:572-7.
39. Gallù M, Marrone G, Legramante JM, De Lorenzo A, Di Daniele N, Noce A. Female sex as a thromboembolic risk factor in the era of nonvitamin K antagonist oral anticoagulants. Cardiovasc Ther. 2020;2020:1743927.
40. Dewan P, Jackson A, Lam CSP, Pfeffer MA, Zannad F, Pitt B, Solomon SD, McMurray JJV. Interactions between left ventricular ejection fraction, sex and effect of neurohumoral modulators in heart failure. Eur J Heart Fail. 2020;22:898-901.
41. Butler J, Packer M, Filippatos G, Ferreira JP, Zeller C, Schnee J, et al. Effect of empagliflozin in patients with heart failure across the spectrum of left ventricular ejection fraction. Eur Heart J. 2022;43:416-26.
42. Smedberg C, Steuer J, Leander K, Hultgren R. Sex differences and temporal trends in aortic dissection: A population-based study of incidence, treatment strategies, and outcome in Swedish patients during 15 years. Eur Heart J. 2020;41:2430-8.
43. Bossone E, Eagle KA. Epidemiology and management of aortic disease: aortic aneurysms and acute aortic syndromes. Nat Rev Cardiol. 2021;18:331-48.
44. Rylski B, Georgieva N, Beyersdorf F, Busch C, Boening A, Haunschild J, et al. German Registry for Acute Aortic Dissection Type A Working Group of the German Society of Thoracic, Cardiac, and Vascular Surgery. gender-related differences in patients with acute aortic dissection type A. J. Thorac Cardiovasc Surg. 2021;162:528-35.e1.
45. Liu Y-J, Wang X-Z, Wang Y, He R-X, Yang L, Jing Q-M. Correlation between sex and prognosis of acute aortic dissection in the Chinese population. Chin Med J. 2018;131:1430-5.
46. Chemtob RA, Hjortdal V, Ahlsson A, Gunn J, Mennander A, Zindovic I, et al. Effects of Sex on Early Outcome Following Repair of Acute Type A Aortic Dissection: Results from The Nordic Consortium for Acute Type A Aortic Dissection (NORCAAD). Aorta. 2019;7:7-14.
47. Recalde M, Rodríguez C, Burn E, Far M, García D, Carrere-Molina J et al. Data resource profile: The information system for research in primary care (SIDIAP). Int J Epidemiol. 2022;51(6):e324-36.
48. Lip GYH, Tse HF, Lane DA. Atrial fibrillation. Lancet. 2012;379(9816):648-61.
49. Hindricks G, Potpara T, Dagres N, Arbelo E, Bax JJ, Blomström-Lundqvist C, et al. 2020 ESC Guidelines for the diagnosis and management of atrial fibrillation developed in collaboration with the European Association for Cardio-Thoracic Surgery (EACTS) The Task Force for the diagnosis and management of atrial fibrillation of the European Society of Cardiology (ESC) Developed with the special contribution of the European Heart Rhythm Association (EHRA) of the ESC. Eur Heart J. 2021 Feb 1;42(5):373-498.
50. Calderon JM, Martinez F, Fernandez A, Sauri I, Diaz J, Uso R, et al. Real-world data of anticoagulant treatment in non-valvular atrial fibrillation. Front Cardiovasc Med. Sci Rep. 2022;12(1):6123.
51. Loikas D, Forslund T, Wettermark B, Schenck-Gustafsson K, Hjemdahl P, von Euler M. Sex and gender differences in thromboprophylactic treatment of patients with atrial fibrillation after the introduction of non-vitamin K oral anticoagulants. Am J Cardiol. 2017;120(8):1302-8.
52. Raccah BH, Perlman A, Zwas DR, Hochberg-Klein S, Masarwa R, Muszkat M, et al. Gender differences in efficacy and safety of direct oral anticoagulants in atrial fibrillation: Systematic review and Network meta-analysis. Ann Pharmacother. 2018;52(11):1135-42.

53. Kirchhof P. The future of atrial fibrillation management: Integrated care and stratified therapy. Lancet. 2017;390:1873-87.
54. Prabhakaran D, Jeemon P, Roy A. Cardiovascular Diseases in India: Current Epidemiology and Future Directions. Circulation. 2016;133(16):1605-20.
55. Vaccarino V, Parsons L, Every NR, Barron HV, Krumholz HM. Sex-based differences in early mortality after myocardial infarction. National Registry of Myocardial Infarction 2 Participants. N Engl J Med. 1999;341(4):217–25.
56. Ford ND, Robbins CL, Hayes DK, Ko JY, Loustalot F. Prevalence, Treatment, and Control of Hypertension Among US Women of Reproductive Age by Race/Hispanic Origin. Am J Hypertens. 2022;35(8):723-30.
57. Centers for Disease Control and Prevention. (2023). Women and heart disease. [online] Available from https://www.cdc.gov/heartdisease/women.htm. [Last accessed November, 2023].
58. Gupta R. Prevention & control of CVD in women & children in India. Indian J Med Res. 2013;138(3):281-4.

Index

A

Abortion, recurrent 59
Acetylcholine provocation testing 180
Acetylsalicylic acid 45
Activated partial thromboplastin time 87
Acute aortic dissection 199, 200
  diagnosis of 199, 200
  management of 199, 200
  presentation of 200
Acute coronary syndrome 59, 149, 168, 174, 180, 186, 190, 214
  clinical presentation of 168
Acute myocardial infarction 149, 150, 152, 159
  causes of 152
  study 154
Adiposity 142
Adverse pregnancy outcomes 6, 12
Aerobic exercise 109
Alanine aminotransferase 77
Albuminuria 26
  prevalence of 213
Aldosterone 26
Alpha-blockers 109
American College of Cardiology 50, 198
American College of Obstetricians and Gynecologists 50
  guidelines 22
American Diabetes Association guideline 115
American Heart Association 10, 69, 198
Aminophylline 161
Amlodipine 39
Androgens 144
Angina 180
Angiogram 169, 180
Angiographic frame count 109
Angiographic myocardial blush 109
Angioselective calcium channel blocker 39
Angiotensin-converting enzyme activity 26
  inhibitors 21, 29, 38, 53, 109, 160, 161, 213
Angiotensin-receptor blocker 21, 29, 198
  therapy 53
Angiotensin-receptor-neprilysin inhibitors 163, 198
Anomalous pulmonary venous return 110
Anthropometric parameters 74
Anti-anginal therapy 161
Antiarrhythmic medications 211
Antiatherosclerotic
  therapy 161
  treatment strategies 109
Antihyperglycemic agents 161
Antihypertensive 21
  drugs 23, 213
    dosage of 25
    usage of 37
  treatment 23, 27, 40, 41
Anti-ischemic treatment strategies 109
Antioxidant 43
  capacity 75
Antiplatelet
  agents 42
  monotherapy 190
Aortic dissection, acute 199, 200
Aortic distensibility 214
Aortic stenosis 188
Apolipoprotein 214, 215
Arrhythmias 180
  life-threatening 211
  management of 210
  maternal 211
  recurrent 211
Arterial function 53
Arterial hypertension 25, 37, 132
  management of 212
Arterial stiffness 26, 53-55, 143
  index 214
Artificial intelligence 114, 116-118, 120
  application of 119
  computed tomography coronary angiogram 119
  echocardiography 118
  electrocardiography 118
  magnetic resonance imaging 119
  stethoscope 118
Asanas 45
Aspartate aminotransferase 77
Aspirin 29, 45, 96, 161, 186, 190
  low-dose 23, 51, 52
  prophylaxis, use of 52
Atherosclerosis 127, 151
  biological determinant of 151
Atherosclerotic cardiovascular disease 19, 138, 151
  increased risk of 18
  occurrence of 141
Atherosclerotic coronary artery disease, progression of 181
Atrial fibrillation 128, 129, 196, 202, 206, 213
  higher risk of 27
  risk factors for 130
  therapeutic options for 211
Atrioventricular septal defect 110
Autoimmune disorders 26

B

Barker's hypothesis states 99
Baroreflex sensitivity 45
Beta-blockers 21, 27, 38, 109, 161
Bleeding
  risk 186, 187
  major 196
Blood
  flow tracers 109
  glucometers 117
  glucose 22
    fasting 77
    self-monitoring 117

lipids, temporal sequence of 81
pressure 23, 26, 27, 36, 38, 39, 41, 49, 55-57, 58, 74, 99, 132, 158
  control 37, 200
  diastolic 11, 23, 36, 39, 55, 59
  higher 38
  levels 39
  new-onset 7
  reduction 108
  regulation 25
  salt sensitivity of 33, 34
  systolic 1, 23, 30, 36, 57, 59, 184
  transitions 26
sugar, fasting 11
urea nitrogen 77
vessels 7
Body
  fat distribution 142
  mass index 1, 77, 80, 111, 113, 124, 133, 173, 194
  higher 10, 197
  weight 184
Bradyarrhythmias 210
Bradycardia, fetal 211
Breast
  arterial calcification 174, 175
  cancer 214
    evidence of 174

C

Calcium 39
  channel blockers 21, 29, 38, 109, 161, 213
  effect of 38
  intake, potential impact of 39
  oral 39
  supplements 38
    widespread use of 38
Calorie restriction 72, 73
Candesartan 54
Cardiac arrhythmias 103
  management of 210
Cardiac death, sudden 180
Cardiac disease 208
  congenital 208
Cardiac events 154
Cardiac health and pregnancy outcomes 210
Cardiac malformations, congenital 110

Cardiogenic shock 152
  incidence of 152, 153
Cardiometabolic biomarkers 1, 124, 125
Cardiometabolic profile 2
Cardiometabolic risk 131
  factors 11, 12
  levels 45
  lower 2
  maternal 1
Cardiomyopathy 23
  fetal 110
  hypertrophic 159
Cardiovascular ailments 57
Cardiovascular assessment 3, 5
Cardiovascular complications 120
  risk of 89
Cardiovascular death 197
  lesser 198
  outcomes 154
Cardiovascular disease 8, 13, 18, 25, 28, 30, 67-69, 86, 98, 98, 106, 113, 115, 117, 123, 127, 133, 135, 137, 142, 143, 146, 214
  assessment of 146
  causes of 67
  deaths 138
  development of 6
  elevated risk of 33
  episodes 95
  global burden of 30
  growing realm of 6
  higher relative risk for 102
  intervention 118
  occurrence of 69
  prediction of 123
  prevention of 14, 124, 180
  risk 12, 14, 22, 30, 68, 134, 143
  severity of 84
Cardiovascular events 140
  adverse 207
  higher risk of 215
  increased risk for 213
  primary prevention of 70
Cardiovascular health 126
Cardiovascular malformations, phenotypes of 110
Cardiovascular medicine 108
  practice of 120
Cardiovascular mortality, high risk of 124
Cardiovascular outcomes 100, 103, 104

Cardiovascular risk 59, 95, 103
  assessment of 123
  factors 3, 102, 105, 113, 151
    distribution of 25
    increased prevalence of 190
    meta-analysis of 9
    prevalence of 105
  lower 26
  prediction 124
  scores 124
Cardiovascular system 145
Cardioversion 211
Carotid intima-media thickness 143
Cerebrovascular diseases 13, 98, 99
Cerebrovascular events 13
  components of 150
Chest pain 108, 177
  anginal 160
  evaluation of 180
  severe 160
  stable 177
Chi-square test 202
Chronic coronary syndrome 170, 171
Chronic obstructive pulmonary disease 200
Cilostazol 161
Classical cardiovascular risk factors, increased risk of 4
Clopidogrel 190
Cluster analysis 116
Clustered cardiometabolic risk score 1
Cognitive behavioral therapy 109
Congenital heart defects 109
  risk of 111
Connective tissue growth factor 33
Conotruncal defects 110
Continuous cardiometabolic risk score assessment 2
Continuous glucose monitoring 117
Contraceptives 28
Coronary anatomy 173
Coronary angiography 180
  rates of 149
Coronary artery
  bypass graft 15
    surgery 14
  calcification 174
    progression of 180

calcium 181
  progression of 180
  scores 143
disease 150, 165, 168, 171, 174, 177, 178
  development of 173
  early-onset development of 176
  incidence of 172
  marker of 175
  premature 158
  presentation 170
  risk of 127
  treatment of 119
normal 108
plaque 170
size of 170
spasm 179, 180
  features of 179
  incidence of 180
stenosis, treatment of 190
Coronary Artery Risk Development in Young Adults Study 145
Coronary atherosclerosis 161
  early 176
  prevalence of 177
Coronary blood flow techniques 109
Coronary computed tomography angiography 177, 178
Coronary endothelial function 108
Coronary heart disease, higher risk of 100
Coronary microvascular disease 156
  dysfunction 108
    evidence of 161
  function, sex-specific predictors of 107
  tone 109
Coronary sinus thermodilution 109
Coronary spasm, incidence of 179
Coronary syndrome, acute 59, 149, 168, 174, 180, 186, 190, 214
Coronary Vasomotion Disorders International Study Group 161
Coronavirus disease 2019 73

Cough 27, 213
C-reactive protein 132

D

Dabigatran 203, 204
Dapagliflozin 197, 198
  effect of 198
  similar benefit of 198
Death
  cardiovascular 197
  vascular 103
Deep learning 116, 117
Deep venous thrombosis 201, 202
Diabetes Control and Complications Trial 102
Diabetes 22, 110, 173, 174, 190, 215
  incidence of 26
  maternal 110
  mellitus 26, 89, 95, 96, 98-100, 101, 103, 104, 107, 111, 113, 132, 133, 134, 143
  gestational 13, 88, 90, 91, 98-100, 215
  impact of 69
  management 98
  pregestational 109, 110, 112
  prevalence of 100, 101
  types of 102
Dietary patterns 86
Dihydropyridine calcium channel blockers 27
Diltiazem 21
Direct oral anticoagulants 187, 204-206
Doppler echocardiography 109
Drug-eluting stent 190
Dual antiplatelet therapy 186, 189
Duke activity status index, self-reported 131
Dysglycemia 132
Dyslipidemia 26, 27, 67, 73, 76, 78, 82, 83, 85, 86, 89, 105, 125, 143, 214, 215
  atherogenic 132
  higher risk of 26
  increased risk of 86
  proatherogenic 132
  risk of 83
  worsening 132

E

Echocardiogram, fetal 111
Eclampsia 46
Ejection fraction, spectrum of 198
Electrocardiographic left ventricular hypertrophy 159
Electronic medical data 69
Embryopathy, diabetic 110
Empagliflozin 184, 185, 198
  benefits of 185
Endocarditis, infective 209
Endothelial dysfunction 99, 103, 143, 151, 161
Endothelial function 170
Endothelial inflammation 10
Endothelial vascular cell adhesion molecule-1 expression 10
Endothelial vasodilatation 212
Epicardial coronary spasm 180
Epicardial fat 143
  deposition 185
  thickness 143
Epicardial vasospastic angina 156
Estrogen 151, 163
  effects of 163
  hormone levels 55
  levels of 151
European Renal Association 212
European Society of Cardiology Chronic Coronary Syndromes 156
European Society of Hypertension 212
Extracorporeal membrane oxygenation 153
Ezetimibe 132

F

Fabry's disease 159
Fasudil 161
Fat
  distribution, female pattern of 142
  regional deposition of 142
Fatty liver disease
  metabolic associated 134
  non-alcoholic 132, 134, 174
Female reproductive system, physiological effects of 145
Fetal
  arrhythmia care 211

cardiac
	abnormalities, subtypes of 110, 111
	development 110
	loss 209, 210
Fetomaternal neonatal outcomes 45, 46
Foramen ovale, persistent 110
Framingham Heart Study 59, 145
Framingham Risk Score 124

G

Gastroesophageal reflux disease 162
Genotype 73
Glucagon-like peptide-1 receptor agonist 96
Glucose 73, 74
	concentration 174
	fasting 1
	homeostasis, dysregulated 132
	intolerance 143
		first-onset 98
	lowering agents
		initiation of 95
		usage of 97
Glycation
	advanced 125
	nonenzymatic 103
Growth monitoring 111
Guideline-directed medical therapy 155

H

Health
	consequences 142
	maternal 208
Healthcare systems 2
Heart 7, 110
	anomalies, congenital 110
	defects, congenital 109
	development, fetal 112
	disease 18, 114, 209
		congenital 110
		current pregnancy diagnosis of 209, 210
		hypertensive 193
		ischemic 7, 29, 57, 104, 130, 194
	valvular 207, 208
	failure 27, 108, 138, 184, 185, 191-193, 197, 198, 209, 213

chronic 184
congestive 201
pharmacotherapies 198
prevalence of 192, 193
questionnaire 191
rate 45, 110, 158
sounds, fetal 111
valves
	biologic 207
	mechanical 207
Hemoglobin 184
	glycated 214
	levels, higher maternal glycated 110
Hemolysis, elevated liver enzymes, low platelets syndrome 49
Hemorrhage
	antepartum 207
	postpartum 207
Heterotaxia 110
High Dutch Lipid Clinic Network Score 68
High low-density lipoprotein cholesterol 86
High total cholesterol, higher risk of 86
High-density lipoprotein 11, 74, 88, 92
	antioxidant ability of 74
	cholesterol 1, 81, 82, 87, 91, 99, 215
		assessment of 91
		higher levels of 92
		levels 89, 90
Higher triglyceride-glucose index 174
High-intensity lipid-lowering therapy 68
High-resolution intracoronary imaging, use of 152
High-to-high low-density lipoprotein cholesterol 90
Hip circumference 214
Hormone replacement therapy 127, 162
Human coronary arteries 169
Hydralazine 21, 29
Hydrops, fetal 211
Hydroxymethylglutaryl coenzyme A 109
Hyperandrogenism 125
Hypercholesterolemia 133
	familial 67, 68, 84

Hyperglycemia
	degree of 110
	fetal 110
	maternal 110
	pregestational 110
Hyperinsulinemia, chronic fetal 110
Hyperketonemia 110
Hypertension 7, 8, 20, 25, 27, 28, 32, 36-39, 45, 48, 50, 53, 55, 57, 58, 99, 102, 143, 169, 173, 174, 190, 194, 215
	antepartum 23
	arterial 25, 37, 132
	chronic 20, 21, 46-48, 50, 51, 59, 133
	control of 56, 105
	diastolic 26
	effective management of 39
	essential arterial 25
	gestational 7, 22, 44, 45, 47, 58, 59
	higher prevalence of 197
	increased risk of 26, 29
	isolated systolic 26
	long-term risk of 35
	management 20, 25, 78, 212
		aspects of 212
	mild 41
	mild-to-moderate 40, 41
	new-onset 45
	optimal treatment study 27
	postpartum 3, 23
	pregnancy-induced 7, 45, 215
	pre-pregnancy 16
	prevalence of 4, 76
	pulmonary 209, 210
	severe 41
	sex-specific impact of 31
	treatment 52
	waist circumference 29
Hypertensive disorders 3, 4, 7, 8, 22, 26, 41-43, 45-47, 49, 50, 59
	occurrence of 50
	prevalence of 4, 43, 59
	risk of 44
Hypertensive profile 132
Hypertrophy, ventricular 110
Hypothesis 33
Hypothyroidism 75, 76

I

Immune expression 151
Impella 153

Infectious disease 214
Inflammation
  adipocyte-associated 185
  marker of 45
  systemic 131
Inflammatory cells 151
Inflammatory disease, higher incidence of 26
Inflammatory pathways, activation of 103
Insulin
  homeostasis 73
  resistance 45, 72, 73, 81, 82, 89, 125, 173, 174
    surrogate marker of 173
  sensitive tissues, hypertrophy of 110
Insulinemia 110
International Classification of Diseases 149
International Society of Hypertension 212
Interstitial sodium microdomains, role of 35
Intra-aortic balloon pump 153
Intracoronary acetylcholine provocation test 179
Intracranial bleeding, lower risk of 196
Intramyocardial fat deposition 185
Intrauterine growth retardation 45, 59
Intrauterine hyperglycemia, chronic 110
Intravascular ultrasound 152, 170
  studies 161
Invasive coronary angiography 174, 177
Ischemia, myocardial 108
Ischemic heart disease 7, 29, 57, 104, 130, 194
  causes of 150
  pathogenesis of 108
Ivabradine 161

K

Kansas City Cardiomyopathy Questionnaire Scores 197
Kaplan–Meier curves 202
Ketogenic diet, low-calorie 73
Kidney disease, chronic 22, 191, 195

Korean National Health Insurance Service database 150

L

Labetalol 21, 23, 29
Lacunae 146
L-arginine supplementation 109
Latin American Society of Hypertension 29
Left ventricular
  assist device 153
  ejection fraction 160, 185
  hypertrophy 26, 213
  mass index 33
  outflow tract obstruction 110
  systolic dysfunction 209, 210
Levothyroxine treatment, significance of 75
Lipid
  fasting 22
  levels 76, 80
    goals 67
  lowering therapy 67
    utilization 67
  profiles 68, 70, 72, 75, 78, 90
    adverse 76
    role of 82
Lipoprotein
  Cholesterol
    high low-density 86
    high-density 1, 81, 82, 87, 91, 99, 215
    high-to-high low-density 90
    low high-density 86
    low-density 1, 68, 74, 77, 81, 87, 99, 215
    non-high-density 77, 87
  high-density 11, 74, 88, 92
  low-density 88, 102
  metabolism 89
Lisinopril, effects of 54
Liver function, abnormal 201
Local self-governing bodies, guidance of 57
Low high-density lipoprotein cholesterol 86
Low-carbohydrate diets 73
Low-density lipoprotein 88, 102
  cholesterol 1, 68, 74, 77, 81, 87, 99, 215
  high levels of 106

M

Machine learning 116, 117
Macrosomia 110
Magnesium sulfate 29
Magnetic resonance
  imaging 109
  spectroscopy 109
Major adverse cardiac events 174
  components of 150
Major adverse cardiovascular event 130, 159, 160, 177
  higher risk of 156
Major coronary artery 108
Maternal-fetal medicine 211
Menarche, early 215
Menopausal hormone therapy 136
Menopause 26, 123, 134
  late 215
  transition 92, 126
Menstrual cycle 134
  regularity 133
Metabolic abnormalities 82
Metabolic disorders 134
  chronic 110
Metabolic dysregulation 23
Metabolic syndrome 99, 105, 108, 123, 129, 130, 132, 134, 135, 143, 173, 194
  components 143
  cumulative burden of 128
  gender-specific 132
  high risk of 107
  management of 132
  prevalence of 11, 125, 131
  scoring systems of 140
Metabolic tracers 109
Metformin 112, 161
Methyldopa 21, 23
Microvascular angina 160
  pharmacologic management of 160
Microvascular dysfunction 108, 109, 155
Microvascular vasospastic angina 156
Mineralocorticoid receptor antagonists 38, 198
Mitral regurgitation 208
  severe 209
Mitral stenosis, severe 209, 210
Modified World Health Organization 209

Monocyte chemoattractant
  protein-1 125
Mortality
  causes of 27
  maternal 209, 210
  pregnancy-related 208
Muscle mass 74
Myocardial bridge 179
  incidence of 179
Myocardial fibrosis 32
Myocardial infarction 59, 138,
    154, 157, 213-215
  acute 149, 150, 152, 159
  early 159
  incidence of 158
  nonfatal 150, 162, 171, 190
  risk of 100
  syndromes of 159
Myocardial ischemia 108
  assessment of 109
Myocardial perfusion
  imaging, sex-specific
    associations of 170
  reserve 108
  scintigraphy 171
  techniques 109
Myocardial scintigraphy 109

N

National Institute for Health and
  Care Excellence 52
Natriuretic peptide levels 184
Neural tube defects 111
Neurohormonal modulators
  198
Neurohumoral pathways 102
New York Heart Association
  classification 192
Nifedipine 21, 23, 29
Nitrates 109, 161
Nitric oxide 44, 45
Noncommunicable diseases 214
Nonobstructive coronary artery
  disease 168, 179, 180
Non-ST-elevation myocardial
  infarction 163
Non-valvular atrial fibrillation
  201, 202, 206
Nonvitamin K oral anticoagulants
  196, 197
N-terminal prohormone, levels
  of 10
Nutrition 70

Nutritional information 146
Nutritional quality serves, index
  of 70, 71

O

Obesity 2, 17, 26, 73, 108, 132,
    143, 174
Obstructive coronary artery
  disease 19, 155, 156, 159, 160,
    173, 174
  absence of 108
  clinical outcomes of 172
  evidence of 155
  pattern of 172
Obstructive sleep apnea 26
Omega-3 fatty acids 161
Optimizing anticoagulant therapy
  197
Oral anticoagulants 201-203, 206
  use of 201
Oral contraceptive
  dose of 146
  pills, estrogen-progesterone-
    based 29
Osteoporosis 79
  development of 80
  risk of 80
Ovarian physiological function 55
Overweight 2
Oxidative stress 45, 103, 174
Oxygen consumption 161

P

Pain, chest 108, 177
Percutaneous coronary
  intervention 154, 162, 172,
    186, 189, 190
  angioplasty 15
  primary 153, 165
Peripartum screening 3
  approach 4
Peripheral artery disease 85, 195
Peripheral pulse pressure 54
Phosphodiesterase inhibitors
  161
Placental abruption 41
Placental disorders 59
Placental growth factor 46
Placental maternal vascular
  malperfusion, evidence
  of 36
Placental syndrome 35, 36

Plaque
  formation 151
  morphological characteristics
    151
  progression 169
Plasminogen activator inhibitor-1
  106
Polycystic ovarian
  disease 26
  syndrome 82, 124, 125, 143,
    215
Positron emission tomography
  109
Postpartum hypertension 3, 23
  prevalence of 23
Pranayamas 45
Prazosin 21
Pre-diabetes mellitus 114
Preeclampsia 4, 7, 10, 21, 41, 45,
    46, 48, 52, 176, 177
  early-onset 10
  postpartum 23
  pregnancy 9
  prevention of 43
  treatment for 29
Pregestational diabetes mellitus
  109, 110, 112
  effect of 110
Pregnancy 1, 21, 44, 83, 98, 209,
    216
  complicated 215
  first trimester of 76, 82
  hemodynamic stress of 12
  hypertensive disorders of 3,
    4, 7, 8, 26, 41, 43, 45, 47,
    49, 59
  loss of 19
    recurrent 19
  management 28
  outcomes 44, 45, 209
Premenopausal disease 114
Preterm birth 41, 52
Progesterone 163
Proprotein convertase subtilisin/
  kexin type 9 132
Prosthetic heart valves 207, 209,
  210
Proteinuria 7
Proton-pump inhibitors 162
Pulmonary embolism 201, 202
Pulmonary valve stenosis 110
Pulse
  pressure, ratio of 26
  wave reflections 54

Index

Q
QT syndrome 211

R
Radial artery, small caliber of 187
Random blood sugar 11
Ranolazine 109, 161
Reductase inhibitors 109
Refractory supraventricular arrhythmia 209
Renal dysfunction 26
Renal function, abnormal 201
Renal impairment 41
Renin-angiotensin aldosterone system 26
   signaling pathway inhibitors 157
Reproductive disorders 146
Rheumatic heart disease 194, 209
Rho-kinase inhibitors 161
Right ventricular outflow tract obstruction 110
Rivaroxaban 204

S
Sacubitril 32, 33, 185
   benefits of 185
   treatment 33
Seizures 23
Serum creatinine 77
Serum lipid 87
   levels 85, 86
   profile 79
Serum lipoprotein profile 88
Severe adverse cardiovascular events 207
Sex chromosomes 25
Sex hormones 25, 102
Sexual maturity 34
Shock, cardiogenic 152
Short-term maternal cardiovascular disease risk factors, development of 6
Sildenafil 161
Single antiplatelet therapy 190
Sinus arrhythmia 211
Sleep apnea 26, 132
Small-for-gestational-age 36, 41
   births 52
SMARTTOOL techniques 119
Sodium-glucose cotransporter-2 inhibitors 10, 95, 96, 161, 163, 197, 198

Spectrophotometers 80
Spontaneous coronary artery dissection 14, 15, 152, 162
   incidence of 152
Stable angina, chronic 169
Statins 161
   benefits of 132
   usage of 96
ST-elevation myocardial infarction 154
Stent thrombosis, incidence of 186
Stillbirth, risk of 207
Stress electrocardiography test 109
Stroke 22, 23, 29, 57, 100, 103, 138, 200, 201, 206, 213
   ischemic 103, 159
   nonfatal 150, 177
   occurrence of 209
   volume index 26
ST-segment elevation
   acute coronary syndrome 169
   myocardial infarction 165
Supraventricular tachycardia 211
Surgical aortic valve replacement 188
Sympathetic nervous system, activity of 212

T
Tachyarrhythmias 210
Tachycardia, ventricular 211
Target vessel revascularization 150, 165
Thoracic endovascular repair 200
Thromboembolic events, risk factors for 196
Thromboembolic risk 196
Thromboembolism, risk of 196
Thrombolysis in myocardial infarction thrombus grade 154
Thrombophiliac disorders 106
Thrombus aspiration 154
Thyroid dysfunction 76
Ticagrelor 187
Total cholesterol 77, 81, 90
Transcatheter aortic valve replacement 194, 195
Transcatheter heart valves
   early-generation 195
   newer generation of 194, 195

Transforming growth factor-beta 33
Transmyocardial metabolic studies 109
Tricyclic antidepressants, low-dose 161
Triglyceride 74, 81, 90
   glucose index 173
   high 86
   levels 90
Tumor necrosis factor-alpha 99

U
Uric acid 132, 184

V
Valsartan 32, 33, 185
   treatment 33
Valve
   defect 110
   prostheses 207
   replacement 207
Vascular disease 104, 201
Vascular dysfunction 35
Vascular endothelial
   dysfunction 45
   marker of 46
Vascular endothelial growth factor 46
Vascular function 54
Vascular smooth muscle cell proliferation 151
Vascular stiffness 27
Vasodilators, direct-acting 29
Vasopressors 153
Vasospasm 155
Venous thromboembolic disease 22
Venous thromboembolism 13
Ventricular pressure overload 188
Ventricular segmentation 119
Ventricular septal defect 110
Verapamil 29
Vessel calcification 175
Visceral fat 143
Vitamin
   D 112
      supplementation 38, 39, 161
   K antagonists 196, 202, 206

W

Waist circumference 113, 214
Waist-hip ratio 214, 215
Weight
　gain, gestational 1
　loss 108

Women's Ischemia Syndrome
　　Evaluation Prospective 131
Women's Reproductive
　　Milestones and
　　Cardiovascular Disease Risk
　　144
Women's Self-Help Groups 56

Y

Yoga
　effects of 44
　practice 46
　regimen 45